STROKE
SOURCEBOOK
FIFTH EDITION

Health Reference Series

STROKE
SOURCEBOOK
FIFTH EDITION

Basic Consumer Health Information about Brain and Stroke, Ischemic Stroke, Hemorrhagic Stroke, Recurrent Stroke, and Its Causes with Information about Stroke Risk Factors and Prevention, Diagnostic Tests, Poststroke Complications, Rehabilitative Treatments, Such as Stroke Medications, Surgeries, and Therapies

Along with Life after Stroke, Tips for Caregivers, Managing Financial and Legal Issues, Advance Care Planning, and End-of-life Care after Stroke, a Glossary of Related Medical Terms, and a Directory of Resources for Further Help and Information

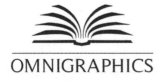

OMNIGRAPHICS
615 Griswold St., Ste. 520, Detroit, MI 48226

Bibliographic Note

Because this page cannot legibly accommodate all the copyright notices,
the Bibliographic Note portion of the Preface constitutes an extension
of the copyright notice.

* * *

OMNIGRAPHICS
Kevin Hayes, *Managing Editor*

* * *

Copyright © 2020 Omnigraphics

ISBN 978-0-7808-1802-6
E-ISBN 978-0-7808-1803-3

Library of Congress Cataloging-in-Publication Data

Library of Congress Cataloging-in-Publication Data

Title: Stroke sourcebook: basic consumer health information about ischemic stroke, hemorrhagic stroke, transient ischemic attack, and other forms of brain attack, with information about stroke risk factors and prevention, diagnostic tests, post-stroke complications, and acute and rehabilitative treatments, such as stroke medications, surgeries, and therapies ; along with tips on regaining independence, restoring cognitive function, and dealing with depression after stroke, a glossary of related medical terms, and a directory of resources for further help and information.

Description: Fifth edition. | Detroit, MI: Omnigraphics, Inc., 2020. | Series: Health reference series | Includes index. | Summary: "Provides primary health information on stroke, types, symptoms, disparities, risk factors, prevention, treatment, along with complications and rehabilitation, with tips on coping methods, financial and legal issues, and advance care planning and end of life care. Includes a glossary of terms and directory of organizations for additional help and information"-- Provided by publisher.

Identifiers: LCCN 2020010444 (print) | LCCN 2020010445 (ebook) | ISBN 9780780818026 (library binding) | ISBN 9780780818033 (ebook)

Subjects: LCSH: Cerebrovascular disease--Popular works.

Classification: LCC RC388.5.S8566 2020 (print) | LCC RC388.5 (ebook) | DDC 616.8/1--dc23

LC record available at https://lccn.loc.gov/2020010444
LC ebook record available at https://lccn.loc.gov/2020010445

Table of Contents

OCT 2 1 2020

Preface

ABOUT THIS BOOK

According to the statistics provided by the Centers for Disease Control and Prevention (CDC), stroke kills nearly 150,000 of the 860,000 Americans who die of cardiovascular diseases each year—that is 1 in every 19 deaths from all causes. The southeastern United States has the highest death rates from stroke. Stroke is the fifth leading cause of death in the United States and the leading cause of serious long-term disability. This is disturbing because about 80 percent of strokes are preventable. Every year, about 800,000 people in the United States have a stroke—and about 1 in 4 of those strokes are recurrent strokes.

Stroke Sourcebook, Fifth Edition provides detailed information about stroke, its causes and types such as ischemic, hemorrhagic, and cerebral aneurysm. The risk factors, lifestyle changes, health conditions to control and prevent stroke are also discussed. It also explains the diagnosis and treatment of stroke which includes neurological tests and procedures, medications, surgical procedures and its emerging treatments along with poststroke complications, rehabilitation, life after stroke, and clinical trials and research on stroke along with a glossary of related terms, and a directory of organizations that provide information to stroke patients and their caregivers.

HOW TO USE THIS BOOK

This book is divided into parts and chapters. Parts focus on broad areas of interest. Chapters are devoted to single topics within a part.

Part 1: Introduction to Stroke and Its Types provides information about stroke symptoms, its nonmodifiable risk factors, stroke statistics, racial and ethnic stroke disparities, types of stroke including ischemic stroke, hemorrhagic stroke, cerebral aneurysm along with the impact of stroke in different geographic regions and preventing stroke deaths.

Part 2: Stroke Risk Factors and Prevention discusses the stroke risk profile, modifiable risk factors for stroke such as atrial fibrillation, cardiovascular disease, diabetes, and hypertension including conditions that increase stroke risk and stroke prevention such as managing high blood pressure, high cholesterol, the role of physical activity in stroke prevention, dietary pattern, and nutritional status.

Part 3: Diagnosis and Treatment of Stroke offers information about the first 24 hours of a stroke and its diagnoses including the neurological diagnostic tests and procedures used to identify a stroke along with the medications used to treat stroke, treatments that can improve recovering from a stroke, other surgical interventions for stroke prevention, and advances in stroke care and research.

Part 4: Poststroke Complications and Rehabilitation discusses the numerous physical complications, cognitive impairment that stroke often causes, and mental-health issues. It also provides information about outpatient rehabilitation, rehabilitation facilities, stroke care, and management. The part concludes with facts about therapies used to help patients manage their physical complications and cognitive problems.

Part 5: Life after Stroke identifies common concerns of stroke patients and their families for physical needs, a healthier life, becoming more independent, and includes tips for caregivers. It also covers points on respite care, long-term care housing, and stroke support groups. The part also examines financial and legal issues and how to manage advance care planning and end-of-life care.

Part 6: Clinical Trials and Research on Stroke discusses the clinical trials and research on stroke such as combination therapy, hibernating ground squirrels for new stroke treatment, and immune cells that may heal bleeding brains after stroke.

Part 7: Additional Help and Information provides a glossary of important terms related to stroke and a directory of organizations that offer information to stroke patients and their families and caregivers.

BIBLIOGRAPHIC NOTE

This volume contains documents and excerpts from publications issued by the following U.S. government agencies: Administration for Community Living (ACL); Agency for Healthcare Research and Quality (AHRQ);

Centers for Disease Control and Prevention (CDC); Centers for Medicare & Medicaid Services (CMS); *Eunice Kennedy Shriver* National Institute of Child Health and Human Development (NICHD); Genetic and Rare Diseases Information Center (GARD); National Heart, Lung, and Blood Institute (NHLBI); National Highway Traffic Safety Administration (NHTSA); National Institute of Diabetes and Digestive and Kidney Diseases (NIDDK); National Institute of Mental Health (NIMH); National Institute of Neurological Disorders and Stroke (NINDS); National Institute on Aging (NIA); National Institutes of Health (NIH); National Institute on Deafness and Other Communication Disorders (NIDCD); *NIH News in Health*; Office of Minority Health (OMH); Office on Women's Health (OWH); Rehabilitation Research & Development Service (RR&D); U.S. Department of Agriculture (USDA); U.S. Department of Health and Human Services (HHS); U.S. Department of Veterans Affairs (VA); and U.S. Food and Drug Administration (FDA).

It may also contain original material produced by Omnigraphics and reviewed by medical consultants.

ABOUT THE *HEALTH REFERENCE SERIES*

The *Health Reference Series* is designed to provide basic medical information for patients, families, caregivers, and the general public. Each volume provides comprehensive coverage on a particular topic. This is especially important for people who may be dealing with a newly diagnosed disease or a chronic disorder in themselves or in a family member. People looking for preventive guidance, information about disease warning signs, medical statistics, and risk factors for health problems will also find answers to their questions in the *Health Reference Series*. The *Series*, however, is not intended to serve as a tool for diagnosing illness, in prescribing treatments, or as a substitute for the physician–patient relationship. All people concerned about medical symptoms or the possibility of disease are encouraged to seek professional care from an appropriate healthcare provider.

A NOTE ABOUT SPELLING AND STYLE

Health Reference Series editors use *Stedman's Medical Dictionary* as an authority for questions related to the spelling of medical terms and *The Chicago Manual of Style* for questions related to grammatical structures, punctuation, and other editorial concerns. Consistent adherence is not always possible, however, because the individual volumes within the *Series* include many documents from a wide variety of different producers, and the editor's primary goal is to present material from each source as accurately as is possible. This sometimes means that information in different chapters or sections may follow other guidelines and alternate spelling authorities. For example, occasionally a copyright holder may require that eponymous terms be shown in possessive forms (Crohn's disease vs. Crohn disease) or that British spelling norms be retained (leukaemia vs. leukemia).

MEDICAL REVIEW

Omnigraphics contracts with a team of qualified, senior medical professionals who serve as medical consultants for the *Health Reference Series*. As necessary, medical consultants review reprinted and originally written material for currency and accuracy. Citations including the phrase "Reviewed (month, year)" indicate material reviewed by this team. Medical consultation services are provided to the *Health Reference Series* editors by:

Dr. Vijayalakshmi, MBBS, DGO, MD
Dr. Senthil Selvan, MBBS, DCH, MD
Dr. K. Sivanandham, MBBS, DCH, MS (Research), PhD

OUR ADVISORY BOARD

We would like to thank the following board members for providing initial guidance on the development of this series:

- Dr. Lynda Baker, Associate Professor of Library and Information Science, Wayne State University, Detroit, MI
- Nancy Bulgarelli, William Beaumont Hospital Library, Royal Oak, MI
- Karen Imarisio, Bloomfield Township Public Library, Bloomfield Township, MI
- Karen Morgan, Mardigian Library, University of Michigan-Dearborn, Dearborn, MI
- Rosemary Orlando, St. Clair Shores Public Library, St. Clair Shores, MI

HEALTH REFERENCE SERIES UPDATE POLICY

The inaugural book in the *Health Reference Series* was the first edition of *Cancer Sourcebook* published in 1989. Since then, the *Series* has been enthusiastically received by librarians and in the medical community. In order to maintain the standard of providing high-quality health information for the layperson the editorial staff at Omnigraphics felt it was necessary to implement a policy of updating volumes when warranted.

Medical researchers have been making tremendous strides, and it is the purpose of the *Health Reference Series* to stay current with the most recent advances. Each decision to update a volume is made on an individual basis. Some of the considerations include how much new information is available and the feedback we receive from people who use the books. If there is a topic you would like to see added to the update list, or an area of medical concern you feel has not been adequately addressed, please write to:

Managing Editor
Health Reference Series
Omnigraphics
615 Griswold St., Ste. 520
Detroit, MI 48226

Part 1 | Introduction to Stroke and Its Types

Chapter 1 | Brain and the Stroke

The brain is like a committee of experts. All the parts of the brain work together, but each part has its own special properties. The brain can be divided into three basic units: the forebrain, the midbrain, and the hindbrain.

The hindbrain includes the upper part of the spinal cord, the brain stem, and a wrinkled ball of tissue called the "cerebellum." The hindbrain controls the body's vital functions such as respiration and heart rate. The cerebellum coordinates movement and is involved in learned rote movements. When you play the piano or hit a tennis ball you are activating the cerebellum. The uppermost part of the brainstem is the midbrain, which controls some reflex actions and is part of the circuit involved in the control of eye movements and other voluntary movements. The forebrain is the largest and most highly developed part of the human brain: it consists primarily of the cerebrum and the structures hidden beneath it.

When people see pictures of the brain it is usually the cerebrum that they notice. The cerebrum sits at the topmost part of the brain and is the source of intellectual activities. It holds your memories, allows you to plan, enables you to imagine and think. It allows you to recognize friends, read books, and play games.

If you are like most Americans, you plan your future. When you take a job, you examine its benefit plan. When you buy a home,

This chapter contains text excerpted from the following sources: Text in this chapter begins with excerpts from "Brain Basics: Know Your Brain," National Institute of Neurological Disorders and Stroke (NINDS), February 13, 2020; Text beginning with the heading "What Is a Stroke?" is excerpted from "Brain Basics: Preventing Stroke," National Institute of Neurological Disorders and Stroke (NINDS), January 19, 2020.

3

you consider its location and condition so that your investment is safe. Nowadays, more and more Americans are protecting their most important asset—their brain.

Stroke ranks as the fourth leading killer in the United States. A stroke can be devastating to individuals and their families, robbing them of their independence. It is the most common cause of adult disability. Each year approximately 795,000 Americans have a stroke, with about 160,000 dying from stroke-related causes.

WHAT IS A STROKE?

A stroke, or "brain attack," occurs when blood circulation to the brain fails. Brain cells can die from decreased blood flow and the resulting lack of oxygen. There are two broad categories of stroke: those caused by a blockage of blood flow and those caused by bleeding into the brain. A blockage of a blood vessel in the brain or neck, called an "ischemic stroke," is the most frequent cause of stroke and is responsible for about 80 percent of strokes. These blockages stem from three conditions: the formation of a clot within a blood vessel of the brain or neck, called "thrombosis;" the movement of a clot from another part of the body, such as the heart to the brain, called "embolism;" or a severe narrowing of an artery in or leading to the brain, called "stenosis." Bleeding into the brain or the spaces surrounding the brain causes the second type of stroke, called "hemorrhagic stroke."

Two key steps you take will lower your risk of death or disability from stroke: control stroke's risk factors and know stroke's warning signs. Scientific research conducted by the National Institute of Neurological Disorders and Stroke (NINDS) has identified warning signs and a large number of risk factors.

WHAT ARE WARNING SIGNS OF A STROKE?

Warning signs are clues your body sends that your brain is not receiving enough oxygen. If you observe one or more of these signs of a stroke or "brain attack," do not wait, call a doctor.
- Sudden numbness or weakness of face, arm, or leg, especially on one side of the body

- Sudden confusion, or trouble talking or understanding speech
- Sudden trouble seeing in one or both eyes
- Sudden trouble walking, dizziness, or loss of balance or coordination
- Sudden severe headache with no known cause

Other danger signs that may occur include double vision, drowsiness, and nausea or vomiting. Sometimes the warning signs may last only a few moments and then disappear. These brief episodes, known as "transient ischemic attacks" or "TIAs," are sometimes called "ministrokes." Although brief, they identify an underlying serious condition that is not going away without medical help. Unfortunately, since they clear up, many people ignore them. Do not. Paying attention to them can save your life.

WHAT ARE RISK FACTORS FOR A STROKE?

A risk factor is a condition or behavior that occurs more frequently in those who have, or are at greater risk of getting, a disease than in those who do not. Having a risk factor for stroke does not mean you will have a stroke. On the other hand, not having a risk factor does not mean you will avoid a stroke. But, your risk of stroke grows as the number and severity of risk factors increases.

Some factors for stroke cannot be modified by medical treatment or lifestyle changes.

- **Age.** Stroke occurs in all age groups. Studies show the risk of stroke doubles for each decade between the ages of 55 and 85. But, strokes also can occur in childhood or adolescence. Although stroke is often considered a disease of aging, the risk of stroke in childhood is actually highest during the perinatal period, which encompasses the last few months of fetal life and the first few weeks after birth.
- **Gender.** Men have a higher risk for stroke in young and middle age, but, rates even out at older ages, and more women die from stroke. Men generally do not live as long as women, so men are usually younger when they

5

have their strokes and, therefore, have a higher rate of survival.

- **Race.** People from certain ethnic groups have a higher risk of stroke. For African Americans, stroke is more common and more deadly—even in young and middle-aged adults—than for any ethnic or other racial group in the United States. Studies show that the age-adjusted incidence of stroke is about twice as high in African Americans and Hispanic Americans as in Caucasians, and while stroke incidence has declined for whites since the 1990s, there has not been a decline for Hispanics or black Americans. An important risk factor for African Americans is sickle cell disease, which can cause a narrowing of arteries and disrupt blood flow. The incidence of the various stroke subtype also varies considerably in different ethnic groups.
- **Family history of stroke.** Stroke seems to run in some families. Several factors may contribute to familial stroke. Members of a family might have a genetic tendency for stroke risk factors, such as an inherited predisposition for high blood pressure (hypertension) or diabetes. The influence of a common lifestyle among family members also could contribute to familial stroke.

WHAT ARE THE TREATABLE RISK FACTORS?

Some of the most important treatable risk factors for stroke are:

- **High blood pressure, or hypertension.** Hypertension is by far the most potent risk factor for stroke. Hypertension causes a twofold to fourfold increase in the risk of stroke before 80 years of age. If your blood pressure is high, you and your doctor need to work out an individual strategy to bring it down to the normal range. Some ways that work:
  - Maintain proper weight.
  - Avoid drugs known to raise blood pressure.
  - Eat right. Cut down on salt and eat fruits and vegetables to increase potassium in your diet.

- Exercise more.
- Your doctor may prescribe medicines that help lower blood pressure. Controlling blood pressure will also help you avoid heart disease, diabetes, and kidney failure.
- **Cigarette smoking.** Cigarette smoking causes about a twofold increase in the risk of ischemic stroke and up to a fourfold increase in the risk of hemorrhagic stroke. It has been linked to the buildup of fatty substances (atherosclerosis) in the carotid artery, the main neck artery supplying blood to the brain. Blockage of this artery is the leading cause of stroke in Americans. Also, nicotine raises blood pressure; carbon monoxide from smoking reduces the amount of oxygen your blood can carry to the brain; and cigarette smoke makes your blood thicker and more likely to clot. Smoking also promotes aneurysm formation. Your doctor can recommend programs and medications that may help you quit smoking. By quitting, at any age, you also reduce your risk of lung disease, heart disease, and a number of cancers including lung cancer.
- **Heart disease.** Common heart disorders such as coronary artery disease, valve defects, irregular heartbeat (atrial fibrillation), and enlargement of one of the heart's chambers can result in blood clots that may break loose and block vessels in or leading to the brain. Atrial fibrillation—which is more prevalent in older people—is responsible for one in four strokes after 80 years of age, and is associated with higher mortality and disability. The most common blood vessel disease is atherosclerosis. Hypertension promotes atherosclerosis and causes mechanical damage to the walls of blood vessels. Your doctor will treat your heart disease and may also prescribe medication, such as aspirin, to help prevent the formation of clots. Your doctor may recommend surgery to clean out a clogged neck artery if you match a particular risk profile. If you are over 50 years of age, the National Institute of

7

Neurological Disorders and Stroke (NINDS) scientists believe you and your doctor should make a decision about aspirin therapy. A doctor can evaluate your risk factors and help you decide if you will benefit from aspirin or other blood-thinning therapy.

- **Warning signs or history of transient ischemic attacks (TIA) or stroke.** If you experience a TIA, get help at once. If you have previously had a TIA or stroke, your risk of having a stroke is many times greater than someone who has never had one. If you have had a stroke in the past, it is important to reduce your risk of a second stroke. Your brain helps you recover from a stroke by asking the unaffected brain regions to do double duty. That means a second stroke can be twice as bad.

- **Diabetes.** In terms of stroke and cardiovascular disease, having diabetes is the equivalent of aging 15 years. You may think this disorder affects only the body's ability to use sugar, or glucose. But, it also causes destructive changes in the blood vessels throughout the body, including the brain. Also, if blood glucose levels are high at the time of a stroke, then brain damage is usually more severe and extensive than when blood glucose is well-controlled. Hypertension is common among diabetics and accounts for much of their increased stroke risk. Treating diabetes can delay the onset of complications that increase the risk of stroke.

- **Cholesterol imbalance.** Low-density lipoprotein (LDL) cholesterol carries cholesterol (a fatty substance) through the blood and delivers it to cells. Excess LDL can cause cholesterol to build up in blood vessels, leading to atherosclerosis. Atherosclerosis is the major cause of blood vessel narrowing, leading to both heart attack and stroke.

- **Physical inactivity and obesity.** Obesity and inactivity are associated with hypertension, diabetes, and heart disease. Waist circumference to hip circumference ratio equal to or above the mid-value for the population increases the risk of ischemic stroke threefold.

8

Chapter 2 | Stroke Symptoms and What You Should Do If Someone Has Them

During a stroke, every minute counts! Fast treatment can lessen the brain damage that stroke can cause.

By knowing the signs and symptoms of stroke, you can take quick action and perhaps save a life—maybe even your own.

SIGNS OF STROKE IN MEN AND WOMEN
- Sudden numbness or weakness in the face, arm, or leg, especially on one side of the body
- Sudden confusion, trouble speaking, or difficulty understanding speech
- Sudden trouble seeing in one or both eyes
- Sudden trouble walking, dizziness, loss of balance, or lack of coordination
- Sudden severe headache with no known cause

ACTING F.A.S.T. IS THE KEY FOR STROKE
Acting F.A.S.T. can help stroke patients get the treatments they desperately need. The stroke treatments that work best are available

This chapter includes text excerpted from "Stroke Signs and Symptoms," Centers for Disease Control and Prevention (CDC), January 31, 2020.

9

only if the stroke is recognized and diagnosed within three hours of the first symptoms. Stroke patients may not be eligible for these if they do not arrive at the hospital in time.

If you think someone may be having a stroke, act F.A.S.T. and do the following simple test:

- **F—Face.** Ask the person to smile. Does one side of the face droop?
- **A—Arms.** Ask the person to raise both arms. Does one arm drift downward?
- **S—Speech.** Ask the person to repeat a simple phrase. Is the speech slurred or strange?
- **T—Time.** If you see any of these signs, call the doctor right away.

Note the time when any symptoms first appear. This information helps healthcare providers determine the best treatment for each person. Do not drive to the hospital or let someone else drive you. Call an ambulance so that medical personnel can begin life-saving treatment on the way to the emergency room.

TREATING A TRANSIENT ISCHEMIC ATTACK

If your symptoms go away after a few minutes, you may have had a transient ischemic attack (TIA). Although brief, a TIA is a sign of a serious condition that will not go away without medical help.

Unfortunately, because TIAs clear up, many people ignore them. But paying attention to a TIA can save your life. Tell your healthcare team about your symptoms right away.

Chapter 3 | Nonmodifiable Risk Factors for Stroke

It is a myth that stroke occurs only in elderly adults. In actuality, stroke strikes all age groups, from fetuses still in the womb to centenarians. It is true, however, that older people have a higher risk for stroke than the general population and that the risk for stroke increases with age. For every decade after 55 years of age, the risk of stroke doubles, and two-thirds of all strokes occur in people over 65 years of age. People over 65 years of age also have a sevenfold greater risk of dying from stroke than the general population. And the incidence of stroke is increasing proportionately with the increase in the elderly population. When the baby boomers move into the over 65 age group, stroke and other diseases will take on even greater significance in the healthcare field.

Gender also plays a role in risk for stroke. Men have a higher risk for stroke, but more women die from stroke. The stroke risk for men is 1.25 times higher than that for women. But, men do not live as long as women, so men are usually younger when they have their strokes and, therefore, have a higher rate of survival than women. In other words, even though women have fewer strokes than men, women are generally older when they have their strokes and are more likely to die from them.

Stroke seems to run in some families. Several factors might contribute to familial stroke risk. Members of a family might have

This chapter contains text excerpted from the following sources: Text in this chapter begins with excerpts from "Stroke: Hope through Research," Know Stroke, National Institute of Neurological Disorders and Stroke (NINDS), February 1, 2001, Reviewed May 2020; Text beginning with the heading "Risk Variation" is excerpted from "Stroke: Challenges, Progress, and Promise," Know Stroke, National Institute of Neurological Disorders and Stroke (NINDS), February 2009, Reviewed May 2020; Text beginning with the heading "Family History and Other Characteristics" is excerpted from "Family History and Other Characteristics That Increase Risk for Stroke," Centers for Disease Control and Prevention (CDC), January 31, 2020.

a genetic tendency for stroke risk factors, such as an inherited predisposition for hypertension or diabetes. The influence of a common lifestyle among family members could also contribute to familial stroke.

The risk for stroke varies among different ethnic and racial groups. The incidence of stroke among African Americans is almost double that of white Americans, and twice as many African Americans who have a stroke die from the event compared to white Americans. African Americans between the ages of 45 and 55 have four to five times the stroke death rate of whites. After age 55 the stroke mortality rate for whites increases and is equal to that of African Americans.

Compared to white Americans, African Americans have a higher incidence of stroke risk factors, including high blood pressure and cigarette smoking. African Americans also have a higher incidence and prevalence of some genetic diseases, such as diabetes and sickle cell anemia, that predispose them to stroke.

Hispanics and Native Americans have stroke incidence and mortality rates more similar to those of white Americans. In Asian Americans, stroke incidence and mortality rates are also similar to those in white Americans, even though Asians in Japan, China, and other countries of the Far East have significantly higher stroke incidence and mortality rates than white Americans. This suggests that environment and lifestyle factors play a large role in stroke risk.

RISK VARIATION

The risk of stroke varies by age, sex, race, and even where people live. Although these risk factors are considered unmodifiable, they help inform stroke prevention strategies at the individual and population levels.

STROKE AND AGE

The effects of age on the cardiovascular system, combined with the insidious nature of other types of risk over the lifespan, make it a key risk factor for stroke. A major source of information about stroke risk is the Framingham Heart Study, which began tracking the cardiovascular health of some 5,000 individuals from the Framingham, Massachusetts area in 1948 and has since expanded to include their children. The study, which receives primary support from the National Institutes of Health's (NIH) National Heart, Lung, and Blood Institute (NHLBI) and support for its stroke component from the National Institute of Neurological Disorders and Stroke (NINDS), has shown that the risk of stroke doubles for each decade between the ages of 55 and 85.

Stroke in young adults is relatively infrequent, but it does happen. The Northern Manhattan Study, supported by the NINDS, found that, among people living in that area in the mid-1990s, the annual incidence of stroke was about two per 10,000 among people 20 to 44 years of age, and about 56 per 10,000 among people 45 years of age and older. The researches in the United States have found that hemorrhagic and ischemic strokes tend to occur in roughly equal proportion in young people. The increased risk of stroke that occurs with age, therefore, appears to be mostly an increased risk of ischemic stroke.

STROKE ACROSS RACES AND REGIONS

People from certain ethnic groups have a higher risk of stroke. Many studies show that the age-adjusted incidence of stroke is about twice as high in African Americans and Hispanic Americans as in Caucasians. Moreover, several studies have found that, on average, African and Hispanic Americans tend to experience stroke at younger ages than Caucasians. The stroke mortality rate is higher in African Americans than in Caucasians or Hispanics. The incidence of the various stroke subtypes also varies considerably in different ethnic groups.

Stroke is a global health problem. In some Eastern European countries and in the Far East, stroke rates are much higher than in the United States. Within the United States, stroke mortality is unusually high in people living in a cluster of Southeastern states-Alabama, Arkansas, Georgia, Louisiana, Mississippi, North Carolina, South Carolina, and Tennessee—known as the "Stroke Belt." A study funded by NIH's National Institute on Aging suggests that the "belt" is worn from childhood. That is, people who lived in the Stroke Belt during grade school but later moved away had the elevated stroke risk characteristic of the area, while people who moved to the Stroke Belt as adults did not have an elevated stroke risk.

Although clearly influenced by differences in the prevalence of known stroke risk factors, the basis for these ethnic and geographic trends is not fully understood. For example, higher rates of hypertension and diabetes explain some, but not all, of the increased stroke risk among African Americans and residents of the Stroke Belt. Socioeconomic disadvantages in income and education level also appear to play a role. However, within a given geographic area, the most disadvantaged groups do not necessarily have the highest stroke risk. Finally, the relatively high percentage of African Americans living in Stroke Belt states does not explain the Stroke Belt's existence, since Caucasians living there also have an increased risk of stroke.

With an eye toward improving stroke prevention in high-risk communities, the NINDS is supporting two studies to confront these issues: the Reasons for Geographic and Racial Differences in Stroke (REGARDS) study and the Northern Manhattan Study (NOMAS). Launched in 2003, REGARDS has enrolled more than 30,000 participants (including 12,000 African Americans), with half of the participants coming from the Stroke Belt and half from the 40 other mainland states. REGARDS investigators have found that, in individuals with hypertension, awareness, and treatment of it is more common in African Americans, but that effective treatment; lowering blood pressure to the normal range is more common in Caucasians. They have also found evidence that strokes are more likely to occur without diagnosis in African Americans than in Caucasians, and in Stroke Belt residents than in nonresidents. Thus, a lack of awareness about stroke and a failure to intervene at the first signs of disease may explain the high stroke mortality of certain groups.

Launched in 1990, the NOMAS study has been tracking stroke incidence, risk factors, and outcomes in Northern Manhattan, where about 60 percent of residents now identify themselves as Hispanic and 15 percent identify as African American. NOMAS investigators have found that AF has an especially high impact on stroke risk in Caucasians, while a trend for hypertension and diabetes has a higher impact in Hispanics and African Americans. Physical inactivity appears to be a strong risk factor in all three ethnic groups.

FAMILY HISTORY AND OTHER CHARACTERISTICS

Family members share genes, behaviors, lifestyles, and environments that can influence their health and their risk for disease. Stroke risk can be higher in some families than in others, and your chances of having a stroke can go up or down depending on your age, sex, and race or ethnicity.

GENETICS AND FAMILY HISTORY

When members of a family pass traits from one generation to another through genes, that process is known as "heredity."

Genetic factors likely play some role in high blood pressure, stroke, and other related conditions. Several genetic disorders can cause a stroke, including sickle cell disease. People with a family history of stroke are also likely to share common environments and other potential factors that increase their risk.

The chances for stroke can increase even more when heredity combines with unhealthy lifestyle choices, such as smoking cigarettes and eating an unhealthy diet.

Family health history is a record of the diseases and health conditions that happen in your family. Family health history is a useful tool for understanding health risks and preventing health problems. To help people collect and organize their family history information, the Centers for Disease Control and Prevention's (CDC) Office of Public Health Genomics worked with the U.S. Surgeon General and other federal agencies to develop a web-based tool called "My Family Health Portrait."

Chapter 4 | Stroke in Children

Despite growing appreciation by neurologists that cerebrovascular disorders occur more often in children than once suspected, the study of stroke in children and adolescents has remained largely descriptive. Child neurologists often encounter children with a cerebrovascular lesion, yet large scale clinical research is difficult because these disorders are less common than in adults and arise from diverse causes. Three fundamental problems hinder both clinical research and the routine clinical care of children with cerebrovascular disease:

1. The infrequency of cerebrovascular disorders in children makes it difficult to organize multicenter controlled clinical trials of the sort done in adults in recent years. The relative rarity of stroke in children also contributes to the still remaining reluctance of some clinicians to consider the diagnosis in individual children.
2. The causes of cerebrovascular disease in children are legion, and no one risk factor predominates. Thus, not only is stroke less common in children, but the diversity of risk factors creates a heterogeneous patient population which hinders clinical research.
3. Despite improved diagnostic techniques which make rapid, noninvasive diagnosis of cerebrovascular disease possible, many physicians still know very little about cerebrovascular disorders in children. This lack

This chapter includes text excerpted from "Recognition and Treatment of Stroke in Children," National Institute of Neurological Disorders and Stroke (NINDS), September 10, 2008. Reviewed May 2020.

17

of awareness contributes to delayed diagnosis and in the near future will make it more difficult to use thrombolytic agents or other treatments which require early diagnosis and treatment.

FREQUENCY OF PEDIATRIC STROKE

Although cerebrovascular disorders or stroke occur less often in children than in adults, recognition of stroke in children has probably increased because of the widespread application of noninvasive diagnostic studies such as magnetic resonance imaging (MRI), magnetic resonance angiography (MRA), computed tomography (CT) and, in the neonate, cranial ultrasound studies. These studies allow confirmation of a diagnosis that would not have been suspected or at least not recognized as a vascular lesion. Also, the number of patients with cerebrovascular lesions from certain risk factors may have increased as more effective treatments for some causes of stroke have allowed patients to survive long enough to develop vascular complications. Patients with sickle cell disease or with leukemia, for example, now have a longer life expectancy, and during this time they may have a stroke.

Most of the pediatric cerebrovascular literature consists of single case reports or small groups of children with a common etiology. These reports offer some insight into the relative frequency of various causes of stroke and draw attention to individual risk factors, but their usefulness is otherwise limited. Larger series of children selected for a common anatomic lesion or a single cause offer additional insight into the unique features of cerebrovascular lesions in children, but patients collected from large medical centers may not be representative of all children with stroke. None of these studies can accurately judge the incidence of cerebrovascular disease in children.

Schoenberg and colleagues studied cerebrovascular disease in children of Rochester, Minnesota from 1965 through 1974. Excluding strokes related to intracranial infection, trauma or birth, they found three hemorrhagic strokes and one ischemic stroke in an average at risk population of 15,834, for an estimated average annual incidence rate of 1.89/100,000/year and 0.63/100,000/year for hemorrhagic and ischemic strokes respectively. Their overall average annual incidence rate for children through 14 years of age was 2.52/100,000/year. In this population, hemorrhagic strokes occurred more often than ischemic strokes, while in the Mayo Clinic referral population, ischemic strokes were more common. The risk of childhood cerebrovascular disease in this study is about half the risk for neoplasms of the central nervous system of children, but neonates and children with traumatic lesions are excluded. Despite the impression that cerebrovascular disorders are recognized more often in children than in previous years, Broderick and colleagues found an incidence of 2.7 cases/1 00,000/year, similar to the figure reported by Schoenberg and colleagues. In the Canadian Pediatric Ischemic Stroke Registry incidence of arterial and venous occlusion is estimated to be 1.2/100,000 children/year.

The frequency of several individual risk factors for stroke in children is known, but in most instances, the occurrence of secondary cerebrovascular disease is so variable that it is difficult to assess the relative contribution of each risk factor to the problem of cerebrovascular disease as a whole. In one report which included both children and young adults, children were less likely than young adult stroke patients to have identifiable risk factors and more often fall victim to infectious or inflammatory disorders. The implication is that children may have additional, as yet unknown, risk factors.

ETIOLOGY OF STROKE IN CHILDREN

Congenital heart disease and sickle cell disease, for example, are common causes of stroke in children, while atherosclerosis is rare in children. No cause can be detected in about a fifth of the children with ischemic infarction, yet many of these children seem to do well. The recognized causes of cerebrovascular disorders in children are numerous and the probability of identifying the cause depends on the thoroughness of the evaluation. The source of an intracranial hemorrhage is even more likely to be found.

The most common cause of stroke in children is probably congenital or acquired heart disease. In the Canadian Pediatric Ischemic Stroke Registry, heart disease was found in 40 of 228 (19%) of the children with arterial thrombosis. Many of these children are already known to have heart disease prior to their stroke, but in other instances a less obvious cardiac lesion is discovered only after a stroke. Complex cardiac anomalies involving both the valves and chambers are collectively the biggest problem, but virtually any cardiac lesion can sometimes lead to a stroke. Of particular concern are cyanotic lesions with polycythemia, which increase the risk of both thrombosis and embolism.

Both the frequency and the cause of pediatric stroke may depend somewhat on both the geographic location and the specific hospital setting. The Canadian Pediatric Ischemic Stroke Registry, for example, lists only five children (2%) with cerebral infarction due to sickle cell anemia. A large metropolitan hospital in the United States might care for this many patients in a year, but early estimates that cerebral infarction occurred in 17 percent of people with sickle cell disease proved far higher than the four to five percent figure derived from more representative samples in Jamaica and in Africa.

PREHOSPITAL EMERGENCY CARE

Lack of general awareness of cerebrovascular disorders in children probably delays medical attention for children with cerebrovascular disorders. It is not unusual, for example, for children with a cerebral infarction to be brought to a physician several days after the onset of symptoms. In contrast, family members are usually well aware of the significance of an acute neurological impairment in older individuals, and these patients are typically seen by a physician earlier than children with a similar lesion.

Venous Occlusion was discovered a bit more quickly than arterial occlusion, at least in younger children, perhaps because of the common occurrence of epileptic seizures in children with venous thrombosis. This seems to be fairly typical of the pattern seen in the United States as well. The typical adult with a new onset neurological deficit from cerebrovascular disease undoubtedly sees a physician much sooner. It is likely that this delay in the diagnosis of children reflects a lack of awareness by both physicians and families that cerebrovascular disease occurs in children. To the extent that treatment might be improved by earlier evaluation and treatment, prompt recognition and treatment could improve management.

Chapter 5 | **Women and Stroke**

Stroke kills about twice as many women as breast cancer each year. In fact, stroke is the third leading cause of death for women. Stroke also kills more women than men each year. A stroke can leave you permanently disabled. But many strokes are preventable and treatable. Every woman can take steps to prevent stroke by knowing her risk factors and making healthy changes.

A stroke is sometimes called a "brain attack." Stroke happens when blood flow to a part of the brain stops or is blocked by a blood clot or plaque, and brain cells begin to die.

STROKE RISK FACTORS UNIQUE TO WOMEN
Age and Menopause
As a woman ages, her risk of stroke goes up each year by 10 percent.
- When you are younger, your arteries have smooth linings and flexible walls that allow blood to flow freely. As you age, the linings get stiff and the walls thicken, which can make it harder for blood to flow. This is mainly caused by plaque buildup in your arteries, a process called "atherosclerosis." Atherosclerosis begins in childhood. The older you are, the more likely your arteries will be narrowed or blocked enough to cause problems.

This chapter includes text excerpted from "Stroke and Women," Office on Women's Health (OWH), U.S. Department of Health and Human Services (HHS), June 7, 2019.

- Your chance of surviving a stroke also goes down as you get older. This is usually because you are more likely to have other health problems when you are older such as high blood pressure, high cholesterol, or diabetes. These health conditions make it harder for your body to recover from stroke.
- Menopause raises your risk of stroke because your ovaries stop making estrogen. Estrogen is a hormone that may help keep blood vessels relaxed and open and help the body maintain a healthy balance of good and bad cholesterol. Without estrogen, cholesterol may start building up on artery walls. This can lead to stroke and other types of heart disease.

MENOPAUSAL HORMONE THERAPY

Many women take menopausal hormone therapy to help relieve menopause symptoms, such as hot flashes. Results from a large study called the "Women's Health Initiative" showed that women taking menopausal hormone therapy with estrogen plus progesterone had a higher risk of stroke, serious blood clots, heart attacks, and other serious health problems. The risks were found to be much higher for women 60 years of age and older.

If you decide to use menopausal hormone therapy, talk to your doctor. The U.S. Food and Drug Administration (FDA) advises women who want to try menopausal hormone therapy to use the lowest dose that works for the shortest time needed.

Personal and Family Health History

Having already had a stroke is the biggest risk factor for having another stroke.

Your family history also puts you at risk of a stroke. Your risk of stroke is higher if one of your parents, especially your mother, had a stroke.

If stroke runs in your family, it may be because your family carries genes that raise your risk. An example would be a gene that makes your blood more likely to clot. Talk to your doctor about your family health history.

Race and Ethnicity

Women who are black and non-Hispanic are more likely to have a stroke and die from stroke than white women. The reason for this is not totally clear. It is partly because many of the other risk factors for stroke are more common in black women than white women, including diabetes, obesity, high blood pressure, and high cholesterol. Black women are also less likely to get to the hospital in time for treatment with tPA, a clot-busting drug that must be given within three to four and half hours of the onset of symptoms. Black women are also less likely to be treated with tPA if they do get to the hospital in time.

Some of these risk factors are also more common among women who are American Indian/Alaska Native and Hispanic. No matter your racial or ethnic group, you can take the same steps as any other woman to control your risk factors for stroke.

Pregnancy

During and soon after pregnancy, your risk of stroke is higher. Although pregnancy-related stroke is not common, the number of women who have a stroke during or soon after pregnancy is going up. This is likely because more women have other risk factors for stroke, including heart disease, overweight and obesity, and high blood pressure, during pregnancy.

The increased risk of stroke during pregnancy comes from several changes that happen to your body during pregnancy, such as increased blood clotting. Your body also makes more blood during pregnancy. After birth, these changes reverse rapidly, and this can trigger a stroke.

Some women are more at risk of pregnancy-related stroke. You may be more at risk if you already have risk factors for stroke, such as high blood pressure, and you:
- Are African American
- Are older than 35 years of age
- Have lupus
- Have migraine headaches

The best way to lower the risk of stroke during pregnancy is to control your stroke risk factors before you get pregnant.

Pregnancy History

Some health problems can happen during pregnancy and raise your risk of stroke later in life:

- **Preeclampsia.** Preeclampsia is a health problem that can happen during pregnancy. It is unexpected high blood pressure and problems with your kidneys called ("protein in the urine"). If you have ever had preeclampsia, you are at a higher risk of stroke even decades later. Having preeclampsia before 32 weeks of pregnancy is especially risky. This may be because women who get preeclampsia have other problems with their blood vessels that can also lead to stroke. Another reason could be that preeclampsia causes long-term changes in the blood vessels. If you have had preeclampsia, you are more likely to develop high blood pressure later in life, the number one stroke risk factor.
- **Gestational high blood pressure** (sometimes called **"gestational hypertension"**). High blood pressure during pregnancy can happen in some women who do not normally have high blood pressure. Gestational high blood pressure goes away after birth, but raises your risk of stroke later in life, after pregnancy is over. Gestational high blood pressure can also lead to preeclampsia.
- **Gestational diabetes.** Having gestational diabetes (diabetes during pregnancy) puts you at higher risk of having type 2 diabetes later in life, after pregnancy is over. Diabetes is a major risk factor for stroke.

Migraine Headaches

Having a migraine with aura (seeing bright flashing lights or spots that are not real) raises your risk of stroke, especially if you are younger than 55 years of age or if you smoke. Women on hormonal birth control pills who have migraine with aura are also at risk of stroke. Researchers are studying whether migraine raises stroke risk for women on other forms of hormonal birth control, like the patch or ring.

However, the overall risk of stroke for otherwise healthy women who get migraine is still low. The type of stroke that happens most often in women with migraine is also less serious. If you have migraine, talk to your doctor about your stroke risk.

Chapter 6 | Men and Stroke

Stroke is the fifth leading cause of death in men, killing almost the same number of men each year as prostate cancer and Alzheimer disease combined. Stroke is also a leading cause of long-term disability and is more common in younger men under 44 years of age than in younger women.

These facts are alarming, but there is good news: about four in five strokes are preventable. That is why it is important to know your risk for stroke and take action to reduce the risk.

WHAT PUTS MEN AT RISK FOR STROKE

Hypertension, also called "high blood pressure," is a main risk factor for stroke. About one in three men have stage 2 hypertension (having a blood pressure greater than or equal to 140/90 mmHg), and more than half do not have it under control.

Other risk factors for stroke include:

- **Smoking.** Smoking damages blood vessels, which can cause a stroke. About one in six men smoke. Men are also more likely to be smokers than women.
- **Overweight and obesity.** Having overweight or obesity increases stroke risk. About three in four men in the United States have overweight or obesity.
- **Diabetes.** Diabetes increases stroke risk because it can harm blood vessels in the brain. About one in eight men have diabetes.
- **Too much alcohol.** Drinking too much alcohol can raise blood pressure levels and increase the risk for stroke. It also increases levels of triglycerides, a form of

This chapter includes text excerpted from "Men and Stroke," Centers for Disease Control and Prevention (CDC), July 25, 2019.

fat in your blood that can harden your arteries. Men are more likely than women to drink too much alcohol.

- **Not enough physical activity.** Not getting enough physical activity can lead to other health conditions that can raise the risk for stroke. Only one in four men gets enough physical activity, including muscle strengthening exercises, according to the 2018 Physical Activity Guidelines for Americans. In 2017, fewer than one in three men met the guidelines (for aerobics and muscle strengthening).

WHY ARE AFRICAN-AMERICAN MEN AT HIGHER RISK FOR STROKE?

Almost half of African Americans have a risk factor that can lead to a stroke.

- Two in five African-American men have stage 2 hypertension—a main risk factor for stroke. High blood pressure is more severe in African-American men than in white men. More than three in five African-American men with stage 2 hypertension do not have it under control.
- About one in eight African-American men have been diagnosed with diabetes, and many more have the disease but do not know it.
- Sickle cell disease, a common genetic disorder in African Americans, can lead to a stroke. About one in 365 black or African-American babies are born with sickle cell disease.
- About one in five African-American men smoke.
- About seven in 10 African-American men are overweight or obese.
- Eating too much salt, or sodium, can raise your blood pressure, putting you at higher risk of stroke. Researchers think there may be a gene that makes African Americans more sensitive to the effects of salt, which in turn increases the risk of developing high blood pressure.

WHY ARE HISPANIC MEN AT RISK FOR STROKE?

- One in four Hispanic men has stage 2 hypertension—a major risk factor for stroke. More than half of Hispanic men with high blood pressure do not have it under control.
- About one in eight Hispanic men have been diagnosed with diabetes, and many more have the disease, but do not know it. Diabetes is also more common in people of Mexican and Puerto Rican ancestry than in people of Cuban or Central/South American ancestry.
- About one in seven Hispanic men smoke.
- About four in five Hispanic men are overweight or obese.

HOW CAN MEN PREVENT STROKE?

Most strokes can be prevented by keeping medical conditions under control and making healthy lifestyle changes.

Know your ABCS of heart and brain health:

- **Aspirin.** Aspirin may help reduce your risk for stroke, but you should check with your doctor before taking aspirin, because it can make some types of stroke worse. Before taking aspirin, talk with your doctor about whether it is right for you.
- **Blood pressure.** Control your blood pressure with healthy lifestyle changes. If a blood pressure medicine is prescribed, take it as directed.
- **Cholesterol.** Manage your blood cholesterol with healthy lifestyle changes. If a cholesterol medicine is prescribed, take it as directed.
- **Smoking.** Do not smoke. If you smoke, learn how to quit.

Make lifestyle changes:

- **Eat healthy.** Choose healthy foods, including foods with less salt, or sodium, to lower your blood pressure and foods that are rich in fiber and whole grains to manage your cholesterol.
- **Get regular physical activity.** Regular physical activity helps you reach and maintain a healthy weight and

keeps your heart and blood vessels healthier. Adults 18 years of age and older should get at least 150 minutes (or 2 hours and 30 minutes) of physical activity each week and do muscle-strengthening activities on two or more days each week.

Work with your healthcare team:
- Talk with your doctor about your chances of having a stroke, including your age and whether anyone in your family has had a stroke.
- Get other health conditions under control, such as diabetes or heart disease.

Chapter 7 | Statistics of Stroke in Older Adults

The elderly population is rapidly growing all around the world, and stroke incidences are starting to increase twofold in octogenarians. The number of people older than 85 years of age, who currently constitute two percent of the total population in the United States, will double by 2060. The aging population is high, particularly in Western Europe and North America. By 2050, it is predicted that 35 percent of the European population will be over 65 years of age.

Globally, those who are more than 60 years of age will number 2 billion by 2050 and 56.9 million will be more than 90 years of age. Hence, the number of strokes is expected to escalate over the course of the next century.

STROKE EPIDEMIOLOGY

There were about 16.9 million first-ever strokes, 5.9 million stroke-related deaths, and about 4 million stroke survivors in 2010. The amount of stroke survivors is expected to be 7.8 million by 2030. The Get With The Guidelines (GWTG) stroke database showed that 168,000 stroke patients (33.5%) admitted to hospital were over the 80 years of age, in 2010.

STROKE IN OLDER ADULTS

- A study shows that stroke patients who are more than 85 years of age, constitute 17 percent of all stroke patients.

"Statistics of Stroke in Older Adults," © 2020 Omnigraphics. Reviewed May 2020.

- Between the 60- to 79-year-old age group, 6.5 percent of males and 5.4 percent of females have had a stroke between 2013 and 2016.
- Among people over 80 years of age, the following have had a stroke: 11.5 percent of males; 13.4 percent of females.
- In 2014, among people who were above 85 years of age, females constituted 66 percent of all stroke patients.
- Very elderly patients have more prolonged hospitalizations, have higher risk-adjusted mortality, have a more significant disability, receive less evidenced-based care, and are less likely to be discharged to their original place of residence.
- The prevalence of stroke survivors is anticipated to increase, especially among elderly females, due to the surge in the aging population.
- A study shows that between 2010 and 2050, the number of strokes is expected to increase, with the majority being the elderly (aged ≥75 years) and minority groups.

ELDERLY STROKE SURVIVORS OUTCOME

The better the prestroke cognitive function at the time of stroke, the better functional outcome for an elderly patient. Stroke recovery requires neuroplasticity (ability of brain to adapt) to occur; however, animal studies have suggested that with increasing age, there is a reduction in neurogenesis (formation of new neurons).

The potential for a good outcome following stroke treatments such as thrombolysis (removing blood clots), endovascular intervention (replacing a diseased aorta), or a hemicraniectomy (brain surgery) is more significant in older people than in younger patients. However, despite the positive outcomes, all studies report that with increasing age, and comorbidities, there is a higher risk of poor functional outcome and mortality, following a stroke.

STROKE COMPLICATIONS IN OLDER PEOPLE

Stroke is a chronic condition and is associated with many frequently unmet needs, including isolation, depression, poor quality of life, fatigue, and apathy. Complications following stroke are common and include visual disturbance, dysphagia, chest infection, venous thromboembolism (blood clots in veins), confusion, and bowel and bladder disturbance. These complications are prevalent in weak old people and may be challenging to manage. Patients with delirium also tended to stay longer in hospital compared to those who did not and were more likely to be discharged to a nursing home or other institutions.

References

1. "2019 Heart Disease and Stroke Statistical Update Fact Sheet," American Heart Association (AHA), January 31, 2019.
2. "Stroke Facts," Centers for Disease Control and Prevention (CDC), January 31, 2020.
3. "Stroke in Frail Older People," Multidisciplinary Digital Publishing Institute (MDPI), December 4, 2012.

Chapter 8 | Racial and Ethnic Stroke Disparities

STROKE IN AFRICAN AMERICANS

- African Americans are 50 percent more likely to have a stroke (cerebrovascular disease), as compared to their white adult counterparts.
- Black men are 60 percent more likely to die from a stroke as compared to non-Hispanic whites.
- African-American women are twice as likely to have a stroke as compared to non-Hispanic white women.

Diagnosed Cases of Stroke

Table 8.1. Age-Adjusted Percentages of Stroke among Persons 18 Years of Age and Over, 2018

	Non-Hispanic Black	Non-Hispanic White	Non-Hispanic Black/Non-Hispanic White Ratio
Men	3.2	3.1	1
Women	4.6	2.3	2
Total	4	2.7	1.5

(Source: Centers for Disease Control and Prevention (CDC), 2020. Summary Health Statistics: National Health Interview Survey (NHIS): 2018)

This chapter contains text excerpted from the following sources: Text under the heading "Stroke In African Americans" is excerpted from "Stroke and African Americans," Office of Minority Health (OMH), U.S. Department of Health and Human Services (HHS), February 3, 2020; Text under the heading "Stroke In American Indians/Alaska Natives" is excerpted from "Stroke and American Indians/Alaska Natives," Office of Minority Health (OMH), U.S. Department of Health and Human Services (HHS), February 3, 2020; Text under the heading "Stroke and Asian Americans" is excerpted from "Stroke in Asian Americans," Office of Minority Health (OMH), U.S. Department of Health and Human Services (HHS), February 3, 2020; Text under the heading "Stroke and Hispanic Americans" is excerpted from "Stroke and Hispanic Americans," Office of Minority Health (OMH), U.S. Department of Health and Human Services (HHS), February 3, 2020; Text under the heading "Stroke In Native Hawaiians/Pacific Islanders" is excerpted from "Stroke and Native Hawaiians/Pacific Islanders," Office of Minority Health (OMH), U.S. Department of Health and Human Services (HHS), February 3, 2020.

Death Rate

Table 8.2. Age-Adjusted Stroke Death Rates per 100,000 (2017)

	Non-Hispanic Black	Non-Hispanic White	Non-Hispanic Black/Non-Hispanic White Ratio
Men	57.9	36	1.6
Women	48.3	26	1.3
Total	52.7	36.4	1.4

(Source: Centers for Disease Control and Prevention (CDC), 2019. National Vital Statistics Report (NVSR))

STROKE IN AMERICAN INDIANS/ALASKA NATIVES

In general, American Indians/Alaska Natives and non-Hispanic whites have similar rates of strokes (cerebrovascular disease) and stroke-related deaths.

Diagnosed Cases of Stroke

Table 8.3. Age-Adjusted Percentages of Stroke among Persons 18 Years of Age and Over, 2018

American Indian/ Alaska Native	Non-Hispanic White	American Indian/Alaska Native/ Non-Hispanic White Ratio
3	2.7	1.1

(Source: Centers for Disease Control and Prevention (CDC), 2020. Summary Health Statistics: National Health Interview Survey (NHIS): 2018)

Death Rate

Table 8.4. Age-Adjusted Stroke Death Rates per 100,000 (2017)

	Non-Hispanic American Indian/Alaska Native	Non-Hispanic White	Non-Hispanic American Indian/ Alaska Native/Non-Hispanic White Ratio
Men	33.3	36	0.9
Women	34.4	36	1
Total	34.1	36.4	0.9

(Source: Centers for Disease Control and Prevention (CDC), 2019. National Vital Statistics Report (NVSR))

STROKE IN ASIAN AMERICANS

- Overall, Asian-American adults are about 20 percent less likely than white adults to die from a stroke (cerebrovascular disease).
- In general, Asian-American adults have lower rates of being overweight or obese, lower rates of hypertension, and they are less likely to be current cigarette smokers— all risk factors for having a stroke (cerebrovascular disease).

Diagnosed Cases of Stroke

Table 8.5. Age-Adjusted Percentages of Stroke among Persons 18 Years of Age and Over, 2018

Asian	Non-Hispanic White	Asian/Non-Hispanic White Ratio
2.7	2.7	1

(Source: Centers for Disease Control and Prevention (CDC), 2020. Summary Health Statistics: National Health Interview Survey (NHIS): 2018)

Death Rate

Table 8.6. Age-Adjusted Stroke Death Rates per 100,000 (2017)

	Non-Hispanic Asian	Non-Hispanic White	Non-Hispanic Asian/Pacific Islander/ Non- Hispanic White Ratio
Men	32.1	36	0.8
Women	28.7	36	0.8
Total	30.3	36.4	0.8

(Source: Centers for Disease Control and Prevention (CDC), 2019. National Vital Statistics Report (NVSR))

STROKE IN HISPANIC AMERICANS

Hispanics and non-Hispanic whites have similar rates of strokes (cerebrovascular disease) and stroke-related deaths.

Diagnosed Cases of Stroke

Table 8.7. Age-Adjusted Percentages of Stroke among Persons 18 Years of Age and Over, 2018

	Hispanic	Non-Hispanic White	Hispanic/Non-Hispanic White Ratio
Men	2.8	3.1	0.9
Women	2.3	2.3	1
Total	2.5	2.7	0.9

(Source: Centers for Disease Control and Prevention (CDC), 2020. Summary Health Statistics: National Health Interview Survey (NHIS): 2018)

Death Rate

Table 8.8. Age-Adjusted Stroke Death Rates per 100,000 (2017)

	Hispanic	Non-Hispanic White	Hispanic/Non-Hispanic White Ratio
Men	34	36	0.9
Women	29.6	36	0.8
Total	31.8	36.4	0.9

(Source: Centers for Disease Control and Prevention (CDC), 2019. National Vital Statistics Report (NVSR))

STROKE IN NATIVE HAWAIIANS/PACIFIC ISLANDERS

- Native Hawaiians/Pacific Islanders were almost four times more likely than non-Hispanic white adults to have a stroke in 2014.
- In general, Native Hawaiian/Pacific Islander adults have developed several of the high-risk factors which can lead to heart attacks and stroke, such as higher rates of obesity, hypertension, and cigarette smoking.
- Cerebrovascular disease can be more prevalent in some U.S. island territories. For example, the death rate from stroke is 20 percent higher in the Northern Marianas, as compared to the non-Hispanic white population nationally.

Racial and Ethnic Stroke Disparities

Diagnosed Cases of Stroke

Table 8.9. Age-Adjusted Percentages of Stroke among Persons 18 Years of Age and Over, 2014

Native Hawaiian/Pacific Islander	Non-Hispanic White	Native Hawaiian/Pacific Islander/ Non-Hispanic White Ratio
8.6*	2.2	3.9

(Source: Centers for Disease Control and Prevention (CDC), 2020. Summary Health Statistics: National Health Interview Survey (NHIS): 2014)
*Estimates are considered unreliable. Data shown have a relative standard error of greater than 30 percent.

Death Rate
National data is not available at this time.

United States Territories

Table 8.10. Age-Adjusted Stroke Death Rates per 100,000 (2018)

	Territory	Non-Hispanic White (U.S. National)	Territory/Non-Hispanic White Ratio
Guam	31.1	36.4	0.9
American Samoa	—	36.4	—
Northern Marianas	44	36.4	1.2

(Source: Centers for Disease Control and Prevention (CDC), 2019. National Vital Statistics Report (NVSR))

Chapter 9 | Geography and Stroke: The Stroke Belt

About 795,000 strokes occur in the United States each year, causing more than 130,000 fatalities and making it the fifth leading cause of death in the country. Although in most cases it is difficult to predict or prevent a stroke, there are a number of risk factors that are known to contribute to the likelihood of having one, including high blood pressure, age, obesity, and smoking. But in the 1950s medical researchers began to document another factor: geography.

WHAT IS THE STROKE BELT?

It has been found that people living in a region generally comprising the southeastern part of the United States have about an 18 percent higher risk of experiencing a stroke than people with similar traits (age, sex, race, etc.) living in other areas. Since the initial findings in the 1950s, additional research has been conducted by a number of organizations, and most, including studies by the Centers for Disease Control and Prevention (CDC) and the National Institutes of Health (NIH), have confirmed that geography does, indeed, appear to be a factor in the risk of stroke. The exact statistics and individual states involved have varied with time and sources, but the following states have been included in what has become known as the "Stroke Belt:"

- Alabama
- Arkansas
- Georgia
- Indiana

"Geography and Stroke: The Stroke Belt," © 2017 Omnigraphics. Reviewed May 2020.

- Kentucky
- Louisiana
- Mississippi
- North Carolina
- South Carolina
- Tennessee
- Virginia

Some researchers have reported that individuals from Georgia, North Carolina, and South Carolina have an even higher stroke risk than those in the other Stroke Belt states, with the death rates for some age groups in those states being as much as twice as high as the rest of the country. And further study by the NIH has also demonstrated that those who lived in the Stroke Belt from childhood carry the elevated stroke risk with them even if they move out of the area, while people who move to the Stroke Belt as adults do not have an elevated risk.

WHAT IS THE EXPLANATION FOR THE STROKE BELT?

Even though the existence of the Stroke Belt has been confirmed by a number of independent studies, the reason for its existence is not fully understood. Many theories have been proposed, but so far none has been definitively proven, although it is fairly certain that the reasons are regional, rather than state-specific. Researchers have examined ethnicity, access to healthcare, and even climate as possible contributing factors but have been unable to make a positive determination.

The National Institute of Health (NIH) has concluded that the Stroke Belt is most likely the result of a combination of genetic and lifestyle factors, including smoking, a sedentary lifestyle, and a diet rich in saturated fats, all of which contribute to conditions like high blood pressure and high cholesterol, which can mean a higher risk of stroke. The so-called "Southern Diet" has been identified by several studies as one plausible explanation for the geographic trend. A study by the American Stroke Association found that this type of diet, characterized by "a high intake of foods such as fried chicken, fried fish, fried potatoes, bacon, ham, liver and gizzards, and sugary drinks, such as sweet tea," resulted in a significantly higher risk of stroke. Those who ate these foods about six times per week had a 41 percent higher stroke risk compared to those who ate them just once a month. But it is worth pointing out that this nationwide study also concluded that people who maintain this type of diet are at higher risk for stroke no matter where they live, although the southern cultural tradition may account for its prevalence in that region.

PREVENTION OF STROKE

No matter where you live, some risk factors for stroke cannot be changed, including age, gender, genetic makeup, and ethnicity. But there are a number of lifestyle changes you can make to help lessen your risk for stroke. These include:

- **Maintain a healthy diet.** Generally, this includes eating a variety of vegetables, fruits, whole grains, lean protein, and the "good fats," such as certain oils, nuts, fatty fish, and cheese, while staying away from foods that contain saturated fats, trans fats, added sugars, and excess sodium.
- **Get enough physical activity.** The CDC recommends 150 minutes of moderate activity—such as brisk walking, water aerobics, or bicycling—plus at least two or more days of muscle-strengthening activities, per week. The alternative is 75 minutes of more vigorous activity—like jogging, running, or swimming laps—plus two or more days of muscle-strengthening activities per week.
- **Stop smoking.** If you smoke, quitting can cut your risk of stroke in half. Smoking can thicken blood, increase clot formation, and cause the buildup of plaque in the arteries, all of which can be contributing factors to stroke.
- **Drink alcohol in moderation.** A number of studies have shown that alcohol can increase blood pressure and, therefore, escalate the risk of stroke. Experts recommend no more than two drinks per day for men

and one drink per day for women. One drink equates to approximately 1½ ounces of liquor, 5 ounces of wine, or 12 ounces of beer.

References

1. "Geography: The Stroke Belt," Hearthealthywomen.org, n.d.
2. Lambert, Katie. "Loosening the Stroke Belt," Bestofatlanta. com, n.d.
3. "Prevalence of Stroke: United States, 2006–2010," Centers for Disease Control and Prevention (CDC), May 25, 2012.
4. "Southern Diet Could Raise Your Risk of Stroke," American Heart Association (AHA), February 7, 2013.
5. "Stroke," Centers for Disease Control and Prevention (CDC), December 28, 2016.
6. "Stroke: Challenges, Progress, and Promise," National Institutes of Health (NIH), February 2009.
7. "The Stroke Belt," Saebo.com, September 16, 2015.

Chapter 10 | Statistics on Stroke in the United States

STROKE STATISTICS
- Stroke kills about 140,000 Americans each year—that is 1 in every 20 deaths.
- Someone in the United States has a stroke every 40 seconds. Every 4 minutes, someone dies of a stroke.
- Every year, more than 795,000 people in the United States have a stroke. About 6,10,000 of these are first or new strokes.
- About 185,000 strokes—nearly 1 in 4—are in people who have had a previous stroke.
- About 87 percent of all strokes are ischemic strokes, in which blood flow to the brain is blocked.
- Stroke costs the United States an estimated $34 billion each year. This total includes the cost of healthcare services, medicines to treat stroke, and missed days of work.
- Stroke is a leading cause of serious long-term disability. Stroke reduces mobility in more than half of stroke survivors 65 years of age and over.

STROKE STATISTICS BY RACE AND ETHNICITY
- Stroke is the fifth leading cause of death in Americans, but the risk of having a stroke varies with race and ethnicity.

This chapter includes text excerpted from "Stroke Facts," Centers for Disease Control and Prevention (CDC), September 6, 2017.

- Risk of having a first stroke is nearly twice as high for blacks as for whites, and blacks have the highest rate of death due to stroke.
- Though stroke death rates have declined for decades among all race/ethnicities, Hispanics have seen an increase in death rates since 2013.

STROKE RISK VARIES BY AGE

- Stroke risk increases with age, but strokes can—and do—occur at any age.
- In 2009, 34 percent of people hospitalized for stroke were less than 65 years old.

EARLY ACTION IS IMPORTANT FOR STROKE

Know the warning signs and symptoms of stroke so that you can act fast if you or someone you know might be having a stroke. The chances of survival are greater when emergency treatment begins quickly.

- In one survey, most respondents—93 percent—recognized sudden numbness on one side as a symptom of stroke. Only 38 percent were aware of all major symptoms.
- Patients who arrive at the emergency room within 3 hours of their first symptoms often have less disability 3 months after a stroke than those who received delayed care.

AMERICANS AT RISK FOR STROKE

High blood pressure, high cholesterol, smoking, obesity, and diabetes are leading causes of stroke. One in three U.S. adults have at least one of these conditions or habits.

Chapter 11 | Types of Stroke

Chapter Contents

Section 11.1 | Ischemic Stroke

This section contains text excerpted from the following sources: Text in this section begins with excerpts from "Types of Stroke," Centers for Disease Control and Prevention (CDC), January 31, 2020; Text under the heading "About Ischemic Stroke" is excerpted from "Stroke: Hope through Research," Know Stroke, National Institute of Neurological Disorders and Stroke (NINDS), February 1, 2001, Reviewed May 2020; Text beginning with the heading "Types of Ischemic Stroke" is excerpted from "Stroke," National Heart, Lung, and Blood Institute (NHLBI), February 11, 2020.

Most strokes (87%) are ischemic strokes. An ischemic stroke happens when blood flow through the artery that supplies oxygen-rich blood to the brain becomes blocked.

Blood clots often cause the blockages that lead to ischemic strokes.

ABOUT ISCHEMIC STROKE

An ischemic stroke occurs when an artery supplying the brain with blood becomes blocked, suddenly decreasing or stopping blood flow and ultimately causing a brain infarction. This type of stroke accounts for approximately 80 percent of all strokes. Blood clots are the most common cause of artery blockage and brain infarction. The process of clotting is necessary and beneficial throughout the body because it stops bleeding and allows repair of damaged areas of arteries or veins. However, when blood clots develop in the wrong place within an artery they can cause devastating injury by interfering with the normal flow of blood. Problems with clotting become more frequent as people age.

Blood clots can cause ischemia and infarction in two ways. A clot that forms in a part of the body other than the brain can travel through blood vessels and become wedged in a brain artery. This free-roaming clot is called an "embolus" and often forms in the heart. A stroke caused by an embolus is called an "embolic stroke." The second kind of ischemic stroke, called a "thrombotic stroke," is caused by thrombosis—the formation of a blood clot in one of the cerebral arteries that stays attached to the artery wall until it grows large enough to block blood flow.

Ischemic strokes can also be caused by stenosis, or a narrowing of the artery due to the buildup of plaque (a mixture of fatty substances, including cholesterol and other lipids) and blood clots along the artery wall. Stenosis can occur in large arteries and small arteries and is, therefore, called "large vessel disease" or "small vessel disease," respectively. When a stroke occurs due to small vessel disease, a very small infarction results, sometimes called a "lacunar infarction," from the French word "lacune" meaning "gap" or "cavity."

The most common blood vessel disease that causes stenosis is atherosclerosis. In atherosclerosis, deposits of plaque build up along the inner walls of large and medium-sized arteries, causing thickening, hardening, and loss of elasticity of artery walls and decreased blood flow.

TYPES OF ISCHEMIC STROKE

The two types of ischemic stroke are thrombotic and embolic.
1. In a **thrombotic stroke**, a blood clot (thrombus) forms in an artery that supplies blood to the brain.
2. In an **embolic stroke**, a blood clot or other substance (such as plaque, a fatty material) travels through the bloodstream to an artery in the brain. (A blood clot or piece of plaque that travels through the bloodstream is called an "embolus.")

With both types of ischemic stroke, the blood clot or plaque blocks the flow of oxygen-rich blood to a portion of the brain.

TREATING AN ISCHEMIC STROKE

Treatment for an ischemic stroke or transient ischemic attack (TIA) may include medicines and medical procedures.

Medicines

The main treatment for an ischemic stroke is a medicine called "tissue plasminogen activator" (tPA). It breaks up the blood clots that block blood flow to your brain. A doctor will inject tPA into a vein in your arm. This type of medicine must be given within 3 hours after your symptoms start. In some cases, it is given up to 4.5 hours. The sooner the treatment begins, the better your chances of recovery.

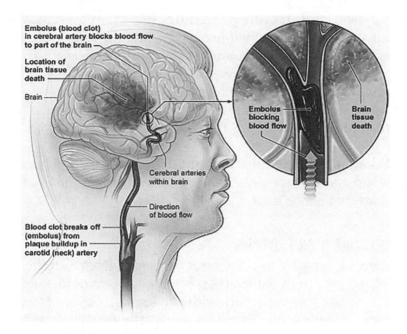

Figure 11.1. Ischemic Stroke

The image shows how an ischemic stroke can occur in the brain. If a blood clot breaks away from plaque buildup in a carotid (neck) artery, it can travel to and lodge in an artery in the brain. The clot can block blood flow to part of the brain, causing brain tissue death.

If you cannot have tPA, your doctor may give an anticoagulant or blood-thinning medicine, such as aspirin or clopidrogrel. This helps stop blood clots from forming or getting larger. The main side effect of these medicines is bleeding.

Medical Procedures

You may need a procedure to open up blocked arteries and restore blood flow to the brain. This can be done several ways.

A thrombectomy removes the clot from the blood vessel. A surgeon will put a long, flexible tube called a "catheter" into your groin (upper thigh) and thread it to the blocked artery in your neck or brain. They will then use angioplasty and stenting or a device called a "stent retriever" to open up the blocked artery.

- **Angioplasty and stenting procedures** use a thin tube to deliver a balloon or small mesh tube into the artery. Inflating the balloon or expanding the mesh tube clears space for blood to flow more easily to the brain.
- **The stent retriever** is a wire mesh inside the catheter that traps the clot. The stent retriever and the blood clot are then pulled out through the tube.

If carotid artery disease caused your stroke, your doctor may suggest carotid endarterectomy, a surgery to remove plaque from the carotid artery in your neck.

TREATING STROKE RISK FACTORS

It can take weeks, months, or even years to recover from a stroke. Some people recover fully, while others have long-term or lifelong disabilities. A stroke team will work with you to manage your care. Your team may include specialists in neurology (brain, spinal cord, and nerves), rehabilitation, or mental health. You will also want to take steps to prevent another stroke and be aware of possible long-term complications. Call 911 if you have any signs of another stroke.

Healthy Lifestyle Changes

Heart-healthy lifestyle changes can help you recover from a stroke and may help prevent another one.

- Choose heart-healthy foods
- Aim for a healthy weight
- Manage stress
- Get regular physical activity
- Quit smoking
- Get enough good-quality sleep

Section 11.2 | **Hemorrhagic Stroke**

This section contains text excerpted from the following sources: Text in this section begins with excerpts from "Types of Stroke," Centers for Disease Control and Prevention (CDC), January 31, 2020; Text under the heading "About Hemorrhagic Stroke" is excerpted from "Stroke: Hope through Research," Know Stroke, National Institute of Neurological Disorders and Stroke (NINDS), February 1, 2001, Reviewed May 2020; Text beginning with the heading "Types of Hemorrhagic Stroke" is excerpted from "Stroke," National Heart, Lung, and Blood Institute (NHLBI), February 11, 2020.

A hemorrhagic stroke happens when an artery in the brain leaks blood or ruptures (breaks open). The leaked blood puts too much pressure on brain cells, which damages them.

High blood pressure and aneurysms—balloon-like bulges in an artery that can stretch and burst—are examples of conditions that can cause a hemorrhagic stroke.

ABOUT HEMORRHAGIC STROKE

In a healthy, functioning brain, neurons do not come into direct contact with blood. The vital oxygen and nutrients the neurons need from the blood come to the neurons across the thin walls of the cerebral capillaries. The glia (nervous system cells that support and protect neurons) form a blood-brain barrier, an elaborate meshwork that surrounds blood vessels and capillaries and regulates which elements of the blood can pass through to the neurons.

When an artery in the brain bursts, blood spews out into the surrounding tissue and upsets not only the blood supply but the delicate chemical balance neurons require to function. This is called a "hemorrhagic stroke." Such strokes account for approximately 20 percent of all strokes.

Hemorrhage can occur in several ways. One common cause is a bleeding aneurysm, a weak or thin spot on an artery wall. Over time, these weak spots stretch or balloon out under high arterial pressure. The thin walls of these ballooning aneurysms can rupture and spill blood into the space surrounding brain cells.

Hemorrhage also occurs when arterial walls break open. Plaque-encrusted artery walls eventually lose their elasticity and become brittle and thin, prone to cracking. Hypertension, or high blood

53

pressure, increases the risk that a brittle artery wall will give way and release blood into the surrounding brain tissue.

A person with an arteriovenous malformation (AVM) also has an increased risk of hemorrhagic stroke. AVMs are a tangle of defective blood vessels and capillaries within the brain that have thin walls and can, therefore, rupture.

Bleeding from ruptured brain arteries can either go into the substance of the brain or into the various spaces surrounding the brain. Intracerebral hemorrhage occurs when a vessel within the brain leaks blood into the brain itself. Subarachnoid hemorrhage is bleeding under the meninges, or outer membranes, of the brain into the thin fluid-filled space that surrounds the brain.

The subarachnoid space separates the arachnoid membrane from the underlying pia mater membrane. It contains a clear fluid (cerebrospinal fluid or CSF) as well as the small blood vessels that supply to the outer surface of the brain. In a subarachnoid hemorrhage, one of the small arteries within the subarachnoid space bursts, flooding the area with blood and contaminating the cerebrospinal fluid. Since the CSF flows throughout the cranium, within the spaces of the brain, subarachnoid hemorrhage can lead to extensive damage throughout the brain. In fact, subarachnoid hemorrhage is the most deadly of all strokes.

TYPES OF HEMORRHAGIC STROKE

The two types of hemorrhagic stroke are intracerebral and subarachnoid.

1. In an **intracerebral hemorrhage**, a blood vessel inside the brain leaks blood or ruptures.
2. In a **subarachnoid hemorrhage**, a blood vessel on the surface of the brain leaks blood or ruptures. When this happens, bleeding occurs between the inner and middle layers of the membranes that cover the brain.

In both types of hemorrhagic stroke, the leaked blood causes swelling of the brain and increased pressure in the skull. The swelling and pressure damage cells and tissues in the brain.

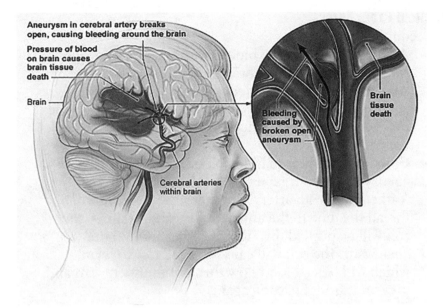

Figure 11.2. Hemorrhagic Stroke

The image shows how a hemorrhagic stroke can occur in the brain. An aneurysm in a cerebral artery breaks open, which causes bleeding in the brain. The pressure of the blood causes brain tissue death.

TREATING AN HEMORRHAGIC STROKE

Hemorrhagic stroke can happen suddenly and grow worse quickly. Just as with an ischemic stroke, getting treatment as quickly as possible is essential for a full recovery. The type of treatment you receive depends on what part of your brain is bleeding and how severe it is.

Medicines

You may be given blood pressure medicine to lower the pressure and strain on blood vessels in the brain. You will also be taken off any anticoagulant or blood-thinning medicines that may have led to bleeding. Depending on the type of medicine you were taking, you may be given vitamin K to help stop bleeding.

Medical Procedures

Procedures may include:

- **Aneurysm clipping** to block off the aneurysm from the blood vessels in the brain. This surgery helps stop bleeding from an aneurysm. It can also help prevent the aneurysm from bursting again. During the procedure, a surgeon places a tiny clamp at the base of the aneurysm.
- **Coil embolization** to block blood flow to or seal an aneurysm. The surgeon will insert a tube called a "catheter" into an artery in the groin. She or he will thread the tube to the aneurysm in your brain. A tiny coil will be pushed through the tube and into the aneurysm. The coil will cause a blood clot to form, which will block blood flow through the aneurysm and prevent it from bursting again.
- **Blood transfusion**
- **Draining excess fluid** that collects in the brain. Fluid can build up after a stroke, pushing the brain against the skull and causing damage. Draining the fluid can relieve that pressure.
- **Surgery or radiation** to remove or shrink an arteriovenous malformation (AVM). An AVM is a tangle of arteries and veins that can break open in the brain.
- **Surgery to remove pooled blood.** Typically, the stroke team will use surgery only if you show signs of getting worse.
- **Surgery to temporarily remove part of the skull,** if you have a lot of swelling. This allows room for the brain to swell without putting pressure on the brain.

Section 11.3 | Intracerebral and Subarachnoid Hemorrhagic Stroke

"Intracerebral and Subarachnoid Hemorrhagic Stroke," © 2017 Omnigraphics. Reviewed May 2020.

There are two types of strokes, ischemic and hemorrhagic. The ischemic type results from a blockage in a blood vessel to the brain, while a hemorrhagic stroke occurs when a blood vessel either bursts or leaks, allowing blood to accumulate and compress the brain. Although hemorrhagic strokes are far less common, accounting for just 13 percent of all strokes, they are responsible for about 40 percent of stroke fatalities. They can be caused by a wide variety of conditions, including high blood pressure, atherosclerosis (hardened arteries), overtreatment with anticoagulants, and heavy alcohol or drug use, or they may be the result of a congenital condition (one present at birth). Hemorrhagic strokes are divided into two types, intracerebral and subarachnoid.

INTRACEREBRAL HEMORRHAGIC STROKE

Intracerebral hemorrhagic strokes occur when a blood vessel inside the brain bursts and allows blood to leak into the surrounding brain tissue, creating pressure, which damages brain cells and causes them to malfunction. This type of hemorrhagic stroke accounts for about 10 percent of all strokes but is responsible for a much higher percentage of fatalities. Intracerebral hemorrhagic strokes are most often caused by high blood pressure but may also result from trauma, malformed blood vessels, the overuse of anticoagulants, and other conditions.

Symptoms

Symptoms of intracerebral hemorrhagic stroke can include:
- Sudden, severe headache, or a mild but long-lasting headache
- Headache resulting from head trauma
- Weakness or partial paralysis
- Numbness
- Vision impairment

- Confusion
- Drowsiness
- Persistent vomiting
- Seizure
- Loss of consciousness

Diagnosis

Common tests used to diagnose intracerebral hemorrhagic stroke include:

- **Computed tomography (CT).** This test uses specialized x-rays to confirm that a hemorrhagic stroke has taken place and show details of its location and impact.
- **Magnetic resonance imaging (MRI).** An MRI uses a strong magnetic field to provide a detailed view of the brain and also confirm the diagnosis and provide additional details.
- **CT angiography.** This x-ray test can help determine whether the hemorrhage is spreading.
- **Blood sugar level.** This checks for low blood sugar, a condition whose symptoms can sometimes mimic those of a stroke.

Treatment

Intracerebral hemorrhagic stroke is a serious medical emergency. Almost half of patients with a large hemorrhage die within a few days, and those who survive may not recover all brain function. Treatment includes:

- **Surgery.** Usually, a small hole is drilled into the skull to relieve pressure. In some cases, more invasive surgery is required to remove blood and effect repairs, although this is very risky, since it can cause further damage.
- **Medication.** Typical medications used to treat intracerebral hemorrhagic stroke include anticoagulants to prevent clotting, steroids to reduce swelling, and anticonvulsants if the patient had

seizures. In some cases medication may be used to lower blood pressure, but only if it is very high, since parts of the brain have already been deprived of blood flow.
- **Follow-up therapy.** Physical, occupational, and speech therapies are often required after intracerebral hemorrhagic stroke to help patients recover or improve cognitive function and physical abilities.

SUBARACHNOID HEMORRHAGIC STROKE

Subarachnoid hemorrhagic strokes occur when a burst vessel in the brain causes blood to fill the space between the brain and the thin tissues that surround it, creating pressure that builds up and damages the brain. This condition makes up about 15 percent of all strokes, accounting for almost one-quarter of stroke fatalities. Women and middle-aged people are those most likely to be affected. Subarachnoid hemorrhagic strokes are most often the result of a burst aneurysm, a bulge in a blood vessel, but other causes can include malformed blood vessels, head injury, bleeding disorders, and the overuse of anticoagulants.

Symptoms

Aneurysms often cause no symptoms until they actually rupture, unless they happen to be pressing on a nerve or begin leaking. Subsequent symptoms can include:
- Sudden severe headache
- Pain in the face or eyes
- Vision problems
- Vomiting
- Loss of consciousness

Diagnosis

The diagnosis of subarachnoid hemorrhagic strokes is essentially the same as that for intracerebral hemorrhagic strokes, including CT and MRI scans and CT angiography. In some instances, a lumbar puncture (spinal tap) may also be performed, but this could be risky if the pressure in the skull is too great.

Treatment

Subarachnoid hemorrhagic strokes are also a serious medical emergency. About 35 percent of patients who arrive at a hospital die shortly thereafter. Among survivors, about half experience long-term neurological problems. And repeat hemorrhages can be a risk. Treatment may include:

- **Surgery.** A plastic tube called a "shunt" might be inserted into the skull to drain fluid and relieve pressure. To repair an aneurysm, a tiny coil may be threaded through an artery and into the affected blood vessel to effect a repair. In some instances, a metal clip might be placed around the aneurysm to prevent rupturing.
- **Medication.** Some of the medications used to treat subarachnoid hemorrhagic strokes include pain relievers, calcium blockers to prevent vasospasms—arterial spasms that can lead to ischemic strokes—and medication to adjust blood pressure to optimal levels.
- **Follow-up therapy.** Physical, occupational, and speech therapies are often required after subarachnoid hemorrhagic stroke to help patients recover or improve cognitive function and physical abilities

References

1. Carey, Elea. "Intracranial Hemorrhages," Healthline.com, November 23, 2015.
2. Giraldo, Elias A., MD, MS. "Intracerebral Hemorrhage," Merckmanuals.com, n.d.
3. Giraldo, Elias A., MD, MS. "Subarachnoid Hemorrhage," Merckmanuals.com, n.d.
4. "Hemorrhagic Stroke," National Stroke Association, n.d.
5. "Hemorrhagic Strokes (Bleeds)," American Stroke Association, November 9, 2016.

6. "Stroke," Mayo Clinic, February 21, 2017.
7. "What Is a Hemorrhagic Stroke?" Joe Niekro Foundation, n.d.

Section 11.4 | Cerebral Aneurysm

This section includes text excerpted from "Cerebral Aneurysms Fact Sheet," National Institute of Neurological Disorders and Stroke (NINDS), March 13, 2020.

WHAT IS A CEREBRAL ANEURYSM?

A cerebral aneurysm (also known as a "brain aneurysm") is a weak or thin spot on an artery in the brain that balloons or bulges out and fills with blood. The bulging aneurysm can put pressure on the nerves or brain tissue. It may also burst or rupture, spilling blood into the surrounding tissue (called a "hemorrhage"). A ruptured aneurysm can cause serious health problems such as hemorrhagic stroke, brain damage, coma, and even death.

Some cerebral aneurysms, particularly those that are very small, do not bleed or cause other problems. These types of aneurysms are usually detected during imaging tests for other medical conditions. Cerebral aneurysms can occur anywhere in the brain, but the most form in the major arteries along the base of the skull.

Brain aneurysms can occur in anyone and at any age. They are most common in adults between the ages of 30 and 60 and are more common in women than in men. People with certain inherited disorders are also at higher risk.

All cerebral aneurysms have the potential to rupture and cause bleeding within the brain or surrounding area. Approximately 30,000 Americans per year suffer a brain aneurysm rupture. Much less is known about how many people have cerebral aneurysms, since they do not always cause symptoms. There are no proven statistics but a consensus of scientific papers indicate that between three and five percent of Americans may have an aneurysm in their lifetime.

WHAT ARE THE SYMPTOMS?
Unruptured Aneurysm

Most cerebral aneurysms do not show symptoms until they either become very large or rupture. Small unchanging aneurysms generally will not produce symptoms.

A larger aneurysm that is steadily growing may press on tissues and nerves causing:

- Pain above and behind the eye
- Numbness
- Weakness
- Paralysis on one side of the face
- A dilated pupil in the eye
- Vision changes or double vision

Ruptured Aneurysm

When an aneurysm ruptures (bursts), one always experiences a sudden and extremely severe headache (e.g., the worst headache of one's life) and may also develop:

- Double vision
- Nausea
- Vomiting
- Stiff neck
- Sensitivity to light
- Seizures
- Loss of consciousness (this may happen briefly or may be prolonged)
- Cardiac arrest

Leaking Aneurysm

Sometimes an aneurysm may leak a small amount of blood into the brain (called a "sentinel bleed"). Sentinel or warning headaches may result from an aneurysm that suffers a tiny leak, days or weeks prior to a significant rupture. However, only a minority of individuals have a sentinel headache prior to rupture.

If you experience a sudden, severe headache, especially when it is combined with any other symptoms, you should seek immediate medical attention.

HOW ARE ANEURYSMS CLASSIFIED?
Types
There are three types of cerebral aneurysms:
- **Saccular aneurysm.** A saccular aneurysm is a rounded sac containing blood, that is attached to a main artery or one of its branches. Also known as a "berry aneurysm" (because it resembles a berry hanging from a vine), this is the most common form of cerebral aneurysm. It is typically found on arteries at the base of the brain. Saccular aneurysms occur most often in adults.
- **Fusiform aneurysm.** A fusiform aneurysm balloons or bulges out on all sides of the artery.
- **Mycotic aneurysm.** A mycotic aneurysm occurs as the result of an infection that can sometimes affect the arteries in the brain. The infection weakens the artery wall, causing a bulging aneurysm to form.

Size
- Aneurysms are also classified by size: small, large, and giant.
- Small aneurysms are less than 11 millimeters in diameter (about the size of a large pencil eraser).
- Large aneurysms are 11 to 25 millimeters (about the width of a dime).
- Giant aneurysms are greater than 25 millimeters in diameter (more than the width of a quarter).

WHAT CAUSES A CEREBRAL ANEURYSM
Cerebral aneurysms form when the walls of the arteries in the brain become thin and weaken. Aneurysms typically form at branch points in arteries because these sections are the weakest. Occasionally, cerebral aneurysms may be present from birth, usually resulting from an abnormality in an artery wall.

Risk Factors for Developing an Aneurysm
Sometimes cerebral aneurysms are the result of inherited risk factors, including:

63

- Genetic connective tissue disorders that weaken artery walls
- Polycystic kidney disease (in which numerous cysts form in the kidneys)
- Arteriovenous malformations (snarled tangles of arteries and veins in the brain that disrupt blood flow. Some AVMs develop sporadically, or on their own.)
- History of aneurysm in a first-degree family member (child, sibling, or parent)

Other risk factors develop over time and include:
- Untreated high blood pressure
- Cigarette smoking
- Drug abuse, especially cocaine or amphetamines, which raise blood pressure to dangerous levels. Intravenous drug abuse is a cause of infectious mycotic aneurysms.
- Age over 40

Less common risk factors include:
- Head trauma
- Brain tumor
- Infection in the arterial wall (mycotic aneurysm)

Additionally, high blood pressure, cigarette smoking, diabetes, and high cholesterol puts one at risk of atherosclerosis (a blood vessel disease in which fats build up on the inside of artery walls), which can increase the risk of developing a fusiform aneurysm.

Risk Factors for an Aneurysm to Rupture

Not all aneurysms will rupture. Aneurysm characteristics such as size, location, and growth during follow-up evaluation may affect the risk that an aneurysm will rupture. In addition, medical conditions may influence aneurysm rupture.

Risk factors include:
- **Smoking.** Smoking is linked to both the development and rupture of cerebral aneurysms. Smoking may even cause multiple aneurysms to form in the brain.

- **High blood pressure.** High blood pressure damages and weakens arteries, making them more likely to form and to rupture.
- **Size.** The largest aneurysms are the ones most likely to rupture in a person who previously did not show symptoms.
- **Location.** Aneurysms located on the posterior communicating arteries (a pair of arteries in the back part of the brain) and possibly those on the anterior communicating artery (a single artery in the front of the brain) have a higher risk of rupturing than those at other locations in the brain.
- **Growth.** Aneurysms that grow, even if they are small, are at increased risk of rupture.
- **Family history.** A family history of aneurysm rupture suggests a higher risk of rupture for aneurysms detected in family members. The greatest risk occurs in individuals with multiple aneurysms who have already suffered a previous rupture or sentinel bleed.

HOW ARE CEREBRAL ANEURYSMS DIAGNOSED?

Most cerebral aneurysms go unnoticed until they rupture or are detected during medical imaging tests for another condition.

If you have experienced a severe headache or have any other symptoms related to a ruptured aneurysm your doctor will order tests to determine if blood has leaked into the space between the skull bone and brain.

Several tests are available to diagnose brain aneurysms and determine the best treatment. These include:

- **Computed tomography (CT).** This fast and painless scan is often the first test a physician will order to determine if blood has leaked into the brain. CT uses x-rays to create two-dimensional images, or "slices," of the brain and skull. Occasionally a contrast dye is injected into the bloodstream prior to scanning to assess the arteries, and look for a possible aneurysm. This process, called "CT angiography" (CTA), produces sharper, more detailed images of blood flow in the brain arteries. CTA can show the size, location, and shape of an unruptured or a ruptured aneurysm.

- **Magnetic resonance imaging (MRI).** An MRI uses computer-generated radio waves and a magnetic field to create two- and three-dimensional detailed images of the brain and can determine if there has been bleeding into the brain. Magnetic resonance angiography (MRA) produces detailed images of the brain arteries and can show the size, location, and shape of an aneurysm.

- **Cerebral angiography.** This imaging technique can find blockages in arteries in the brain or neck. It also can identify weak spots in an artery, like an aneurysm. The test is used to determine the cause of the bleeding in the brain and the exact location, size, and shape of an aneurysm. Your doctor will pass a catheter (long, flexible tube) typically from the groin arteries to inject a small amount of contrast dye into your neck and brain arteries. The contrast dye helps the x-ray create a detailed picture of the appearance of an aneurysm and a clear picture of any blockage in the arteries.

- **Cerebrospinal fluid (CSF) analysis.** This test measures the chemicals in the fluid that cushions and protects the brain and spinal cord (cerebrospinal fluid). Most often a doctor will collect the CSF by performing a spinal tap (lumbar puncture), in which a thin needle is inserted into the lower back (lumbar spine) and a small amount of fluid is removed and tested. The results will help detect any bleeding around the brain. If bleeding is detected, additional tests would be needed to identify the exact cause of the bleeding.

WHAT ARE THE COMPLICATIONS OF A RUPTURED CEREBRAL ANEURYSM?

Aneurysms may rupture and bleed into the space between the skull and the brain (subarachnoid hemorrhage) and sometimes into the brain tissue (intracerebral hemorrhage). These are forms of stroke called "hemorrhagic stroke." The bleeding into the brain can cause a wide spectrum of symptoms, from a mild headache to permanent damage to the brain, or even death.

After an aneurysm has ruptured it may cause serious complications such as:

- **Rebleeding.** Once it has ruptured, an aneurysm may rupture again before it is treated, leading to further bleeding into the brain, and causing more damage or death.
- **Change in sodium level.** Bleeding in the brain can disrupt the balance of sodium in the blood supply and cause swelling in brain cells. This can result in permanent brain damage.
- **Hydrocephalus.** Subarachnoid hemorrhage can cause hydrocephalus. Hydrocephalus is a buildup of too much cerebrospinal fluid in the brain, which causes pressure that can lead to permanent brain damage or death. Hydrocephalus occurs frequently after subarachnoid hemorrhage because the blood blocks the normal flow of cerebrospinal fluid. If left untreated, increased pressure inside the head can cause coma or death.
- **Vasospasm.** This occurs frequently after subarachnoid hemorrhage when the bleeding causes the arteries in the brain to contract and limit blood flow to vital areas of the brain. This can cause strokes from lack of adequate blood flow to parts of the brain.
- **Seizures.** Aneurysm bleeding can cause seizures (convulsions), either at the time of bleed or in the immediate aftermath. While most seizures are evident, on occasion they may only be seen by sophisticated brain testing. Untreated seizures or those that do not respond to treatment can cause brain damage.

HOW ARE CEREBRAL ANEURYSMS TREATED?

Not all cerebral aneurysms require treatment. Some very small unruptured aneurysms that are not associated with any factors suggesting a higher risk of rupture may be safely left alone and monitored with MRA or CTA to detect any growth. It is important to aggressively treat any coexisting medical problems and risk factors.

Treatments for unruptured cerebral aneurysms that have not shown symptoms have some potentially serious complications and should be carefully weighed against the predicted rupture risk.

Treatment Considerations for Unruptured Aneurysms

A doctor will consider a variety of factors when determining the best option for treating an unruptured aneurysm, including:
- Type, size, and location of the aneurysm
- Risk of rupture
- The person's age and health
- Personal and family medical history
- Risk of treatment

Individuals should also take the following steps to reduce the risk of aneurysm rupture:
- Carefully control blood pressure.
- Stop smoking.
- Avoid cocaine use or other stimulant drugs.

Treatments for Unruptured and Ruptured Cerebral Aneurysms

Surgery, endovascular treatments, or other therapies are often recommended to manage symptoms and prevent damage from unruptured and ruptured aneurysms.

Surgery

There are a few surgical options available for treating cerebral aneurysms. These procedures carry some risk such as possible damage to other blood vessels, the potential for aneurysm recurrence and rebleeding, and a risk of stroke.
- **Microvascular clipping.** This procedure involves cutting off the flow of blood to the aneurysm and requires open brain surgery. A doctor will locate the blood vessels that feed the aneurysm and place a tiny,

metal, clothespin-like clip on the aneurysm's neck to stop its blood supply. Clipping has been shown to be highly effective, depending on the location, size, and shape of the aneurysm. In general, aneurysms that are completely clipped do not recur.

Endovascular Treatment

- **Platinum coil embolization.** This procedure is a less invasive procedure than microvascular surgical clipping. A doctor will insert a hollow plastic tube (a catheter) into an artery, usually in the groin, and thread it through the body to the brain aneurysm. Using a wire, the doctor will pass detachable coils (tiny spirals of platinum wire) through the catheter and release them into the aneurysm. The coils block the aneurysm and reduce the flow of blood into the aneurysm. The procedure may need to be performed more than once during the person's lifetime because aneurysms treated with coiling can sometimes recur.
- **Flow diversion devices.** Other endovascular treatment options include placing a small stent (flexible mesh tube) similar to those placed for heart blockages, in the artery to reduce blood flow into the aneurysm. A doctor will insert a hollow plastic tube (a catheter) into an artery, usually in the groin, and thread it through the body to the artery on which the aneurysm is located. This procedure is used to treat very large aneurysms and those that cannot be treated with surgery or platinum coil embolization.

Other Treatments

Other treatments for a ruptured cerebral aneurysm aim to control symptoms and reduce complications. These treatments include:

- **Antiseizure drugs (anticonvulsants).** These drugs may be used to prevent seizures related to a ruptured aneurysm.

69

- **Calcium channel-blocking drugs.** Risk of stroke by vasospasm can be reduced with calcium channel-blocking drugs.
- **A shunt,** which funnels cerebrospinal fluid from the brain to elsewhere in the body, may be surgically inserted into the brain following rupture if the buildup of cerebrospinal fluid (hydrocephalus) is causing harmful pressure on surrounding brain tissue.

Rehabilitative Therapy

Individuals who have suffered a subarachnoid hemorrhage often need physical, speech, and occupational therapy to regain lost function and learn to cope with any permanent disability.

WHAT IS THE PROGNOSIS?

An unruptured aneurysm may go unnoticed throughout a person's lifetime and not cause symptoms.

After an aneurysm bursts, the person's prognosis largely depends on:

- Age and general health
- Preexisting neurological conditions
- Location of the aneurysm
- Extent of bleeding (and rebleeding)
- Time between rupture and medical attention
- Successful treatment of the aneurysm

About 25 percent of individuals whose cerebral aneurysm has ruptured do not survive the first 24 hours; another 25 percent die from complications within 6 months. People who experience subarachnoid hemorrhage may have permanent neurological damage. Other individuals recover with little or no disability. Diagnosing and treating a cerebral aneurysm as soon as possible will help increase the chances of making a full recovery. Recovery from treatment or rupture may take weeks to months.

Chapter 12 | Recurrent Stroke

As the name implies, a recurrent stroke is one that takes place after the original stroke has been stabilized. According to the National Stroke Association, of more than 750,000 U.S. patients who experience a stroke each year, 5 to 14 percent will have a second occurrence within one year. And 42 percent of men and 24 percent of women will have a recurrence within five years. Additionally, recurrent strokes often result in higher fatality and disability rates because parts of the brain have already been damaged by the first stroke. So awareness and monitoring for recurrence is an important part of any stroke recovery plan.

RISK FACTORS FOR RECURRENT STROKE

There are multiple risk factors that increase the chances of having a recurrent stroke. Among these are:
- Age (being over 55)
- Gender (men are more likely to experience recurrence)
- Race (African American patients are more at risk)
- Family history of strokes
- Hypertension (high blood pressure)
- Atrial fibrillation (abnormal heart rhythm)
- Diabetes
- Smoking
- Excess alcohol consumption
- Sedentary lifestyle
- Obesity
- High cholesterol

"Recurrent Stroke," © 2017 Omnigraphics. Reviewed May 2020.

MANAGING RISK FACTORS TO PREVENT RECURRENT STROKE

Although some risk factors such as age, gender, and race, are out of a patient's control, others can be managed to help reduce the chances of having a recurrent stroke. For example:

- **Hypertension.** Studies show that lowering blood pressure can reduce the risk of stroke by 30 to 40 percent. But it's also one of the most easily controlled risk factors through a variety of methods, including regular aerobic exercise, eating healthy foods, limiting salt and alcohol intake, losing weight, and medication.

- **Atrial fibrillation (AF).** An irregular heartbeat can cause blood to collect in the heart and possibly form clots, which can travel to the brain and cause a stroke. Treatment for AF can include electrical shocks or surgical procedures, but most often it is controlled through medication.

- **Diabetes.** Patients with diabetes (high glucose—or sugar—levels) are estimated to be four times as likely to have a recurrent stroke as other individuals, so it's important to keep the condition under control. Typically, this means maintaining a healthy diet, exercising, reducing blood pressure, losing weight, and taking insulin or oral hypoglycemic drugs to keep glucose levels in check.

- **Smoking.** Smokers are not only more at risk for a first stroke but are twice as likely to experience recurrent stroke than nonsmokers. Cigarette smoking causes atherosclerosis (buildup of plaque within the arteries) and other artery damage, constricting the blood vessels and reducing the flow of blood to the brain.

- **Alcohol consumption.** Very moderate alcohol use may actually help prevent ischemic stroke by increasing high-density lipoprotein ("good cholesterol") levels, but according to some studies, more than two drinks per day could increase stroke risk by 50 percent. Heavy drinking increases blood pressure, reduces blood flow to the brain, and can cause atrial fibrillation.

- **High cholesterol.** Elevated total cholesterol levels or low-density lipoprotein ("bad cholesterol") levels increase stroke risk by causing plaque to build up in the arteries and restrict blood flow to the brain. Medications called "statins" can help reduce cholesterol levels, as can lifestyle modifications, such as decreasing the intake of saturated fats, losing weight, and increasing physical activity.
- **Obesity.** There is still some debate about whether obesity directly increases the chances of having either an initial or recurrent stroke, but experts agree that obesity contributes to risk factors, such as hypertension and diabetes. Exercise and healthy eating habits are the best way to both lose weight and reduce stroke risk.
- **Sedentary lifestyle.** Studies show that patients who exercise five or more times per week are clearly less likely to have a recurrent stroke. Aerobic exercise improves cardiovascular fitness and reduces blood pressure, while strength training has the added benefit of improving balance and mobility after a stroke.

OTHER WAYS TO PREVENT RECURRENT STROKE

Although lifestyle changes and managing diseases to control risk factors are almost always suggested to help prevent recurrent stroke, doctors may recommend other methods, as well, depending on the details of the patient's original stroke, medical history, and overall physical condition. These might include:

- **Medication.** Drugs prescribed to help prevent recurrent stroke can include anticlotting medications, such as aspirin, dipyridamole, ticlopidine, and warfarin, as well as drugs to control hypertension, including diuretics, beta-blockers, angiotensin II receptor blockers (ARBs), calcium channel blockers, and renin inhibitors.
- **Surgery.** Various surgical options are available to help prevent another stroke. Depending on the cause of the initial stroke, these can include carotid endarterectomy

73

(removing a blockage in the carotid artery), extracranial or intracranial bypass (creating a new path around a damaged artery), and balloon angioplasty with stenting (expanding the artery and inserting a wire mesh tube to keep it open).

- **Physical therapy.** In patients for whom a sedentary lifestyle was a contributing factor to the original stroke and continues to put them at risk for a recurrent stroke, physical therapy might be recommended to help them make lifestyle changes. Many individuals find it easier to begin developing healthy habits by working with a trained professional, rather than trying to exercise on their own.

References

1. Dickerson, Lori M., PharmD, Peter J. Carek, MD, MS, and Robert Glen Quattlebaum, MD, MPH. "Prevention of Recurrent Ischemic Stroke," *American Family Physician*, April 1, 2007.
2. Jeffrey, Susan. "Risk for Recurrent Stroke, Death High in Hospitalized Stroke Patients" Medscape.com, February 25, 2010.
3. "New Guidelines for the Prevention of Recurrent Stroke," *Harvard Heart Letter*, July 2014.
4. "Preventing Another Stroke," National Stroke Association, n.d.
5. "Recovery after Stroke: Recurrent Stroke," National Stroke Association, 2014.

Chapter 13 | **Preventing Stroke Deaths**

After decades of decline, progress has slowed in preventing stroke deaths. Almost 800,000 people have a stroke each year, more than 140,000 die and many survivors face disability. This is disturbing because about 80 percent of strokes are preventable. High blood pressure is the single most important treatable risk factor for stroke. Preventing, diagnosing, and controlling it through lifestyle changes and medicine is critical to reducing strokes. Health systems (hospitals, doctors, rehabilitation specialists, emergency medical technicians [EMTs], pharmacists) can help address stroke risk factors and improve patient outcomes if a stroke occurs. When a stroke happens, minutes count. Health systems can treat strokes fast if patients get to the hospital in time. Reducing stroke risk factors and improving the quality of stroke care are needed to continue the decline in stroke deaths.

Health systems can:
- Use system-wide approaches to find patients with undiagnosed or unmanaged stroke risk factors
- Work with community members and emergency medical technicians (EMTs) to quickly identify strokes and get patients to the hospital fast
- Implement a coordinated system of care that effectively treats patients from the first symptom of a stroke through recovery

This chapter includes text excerpted from "Preventing Stroke Deaths," Centers for Disease Control and Prevention (CDC), September 6, 2017.

75

PROBLEM
Stroke Deaths Have Stopped Declining
STROKES ARE COMMON AND PREVENTABLE

- Stroke is the fifth leading cause of death and a leading cause of serious, long-term disability, with an estimated cost of $34 billion annually.
- One in 20 adult deaths are due to stroke. Many of these deaths are preventable.
- When stroke happens, parts of the brain become damaged and can start to die within minutes.

STROKES HAPPEN MORE IN SOME POPULATIONS AND GEOGRAPHIC AREAS

- Stroke death declines have stalled in three in every four states.
- Blacks have the highest stroke death rates among all races or ethnicities.
- Stroke death rates among Hispanics have increased by six percent each year from 2013 to 2015.
- Stroke deaths increased in southern states.

STROKES ARE HAPPENING AT YOUNGER AGES

- Risk factors such as high blood pressure, high cholesterol, obesity, and diabetes are happening at younger ages.
- Risk factors may not be recognized and treated in middle-aged adults (35–64 years of age).
- Recent studies also suggest that over the last 15 years younger adults (18–54 years of age) have had increases in stroke hospitalizations, along with increases in stroke risk factors among those hospitalized with stroke.

WHAT CAN BE DONE?
The Federal Government

- Manages the Paul Coverdell National Acute Stroke Program (Coverdell Program) that partners with

state health departments, emergency medical services (EMS), and hospitals to implement data driven quality improvement programs for stroke care.
- Leads the Million Hearts® initiative to prevent one million heart attacks and strokes by 2022.
- Provides resources to all 50 states to address chronic disease prevention, including heart disease and stroke.
- Funds stroke research in treatment, recovery, and prevention, and supports the Mind Your Risks public education campaign.

Health Systems
- Use system-wide approaches to find patients with undiagnosed or unmanaged stroke risk factors.
- Work with community members and emergency medical technicians (EMTs) to quickly identify strokes and get patients to the hospital fast.
- Implement a coordinated system of care that effectively treats patients from the first symptom of a stroke through recovery.

Doctors, Nurses, and Healthcare Professionals
- Identify and treat high blood pressure, obesity, diabetes, high cholesterol, smoking, and other risk factors for stroke.
- Help patients control their blood pressure, cholesterol, and diabetes by taking medicines as directed and making lifestyle changes that can help prevent stroke.
- Refer patients to community resources, such as smoking quitlines and obesity and diabetes prevention programs that will support their lifestyle behavior changes.
- Educate patients on the signs and symptoms of stroke.

State Health Departments
- Prioritize coordinated stroke systems of care and adopt successful strategies of the Coverdell Program.

- Use data to identify and improve gaps in stroke care to drive quality improvements.
- Train community members and emergency medical technicians (EMTs) to identify the signs of stroke and understand the importance of getting patients to the hospital quickly.
- Increase awareness of risk factors for stroke and lifestyle changes needed among high-risk populations.

Everyone
- Recognize the signs and symptoms of stroke.
- Control blood pressure and cholesterol by taking medicines as prescribed.
- Manage other medical conditions, such as obesity and diabetes.
- Avoid smoking and secondhand smoke, which increases your risk for stroke.
- Eat a healthy diet low in salt and sugar with lots of fresh fruits and vegetables, increase physical activity, and maintain a healthy weight.

Part 2 | Stroke Risk Factors and Prevention

Chapter 14 | **Your Stroke Risk Profile**

DO YOU KNOW YOUR STROKE RISK?

Some of the most important risk factors for stroke can be determined during a physical exam at your doctor's office. If you are over 55 years of age, the tables in this chapter can help you estimate your risk of stroke and show the benefit of risk factor control.

The worksheet was developed at the National Institute of Neurological Disorders and Stroke (NINDS)-supported work in the well-known Framingham Study. Working with your doctor, you can develop a strategy to lower your risk to average or even below average for your age.

Many risk factors for stroke can be managed, some very successfully. Although risk is never zero at any age, by starting early and controlling your risk factors you can lower your risk of death or disability from stroke. With good control, the risk of stroke in most age groups can be kept below that for accidental injury or death.

Americans have shown that stroke is preventable and treatable. A better understanding of the causes of stroke has helped Americans make lifestyle changes that have cut the stroke death rate nearly in half.

Scientists at the National Institute of Neurological Disorders and Stroke (NINDS) predict that, with continued attention to reducing the risks of stroke and by using currently available therapies and developing new ones, Americans should be able to prevent 80 percent of all strokes.

This chapter includes text excerpted from "Brain Basics: Preventing Stroke," National Institute of Neurological Disorders and Stroke (NINDS), April 16, 2020.

Table 14.1. Score Your Stroke Risk for the Next 10 Years: MEN

Points	0	1	2	3	4	5	6	7	8	9	10
Age	55–56	57–59	60–62	63–65	66–68	69–72	73–75	76–78	79–81	83–84	85
SBP-untrd	97–105	106–115	116–125	126–135	136–145	146–155	156–165	166–175	176–185	186–195	196–205
or SBP-trtd	97–105	106–112	113–117	118–123	124–129	130–135	136–142	143–150	151–161	162–176	177–205
Diabetes	No		Yes								
Cigarettes	No			Yes							
CVD	No				Yes						
AF	No				Yes						
LVH	No					Yes					

Table 14.2. Points with 10-Year Probability for Men

Your Points	10-Year Probability
1	3%
2	3%
3	4%
4	4%
5	5%
6	5%
7	6%
8	7%
9	8%
10	10%
11	11%
12	13%
13	15%
14	17%
15	20%
16	22%
17	26%
18	29%
19	33%
20	37%
21	42%
22	47%
23	52%
24	57%
25	63%

Table 14.2. Continued

Your Points	10-Year Probability
26	68%
27	74%
28	79%
29	84%
30	88%

Table 14.3. Age Group and Average 10-Year Probability of Stroke for Men

Compare with Your Age Group	Average 10-Year Probability of Stroke
55–59	5.90%
60–64	7.80%
65–69	11.00%
70–74	13.70%
75–79	18.00%
80–84	22.30%

To Know Your Stroke Risk for the Next 10 Years-Men

Key: **SBP** = systolic blood pressure (score one line only, untreated or treated); **Diabetes** = history of diabetes; **Cigarettes** = smokes cigarettes; **CVD** (cardiovascular disease) = history of heart disease; **AF** = history of atrial fibrillation; **LVH** = diagnosis of left ventricular hypertrophy

To Know Your Stroke Risk for the Next 10 Years-Women

Key: **SBP** = systolic blood pressure (score one line only, untreated or treated); **Diabetes** = history of diabetes; **Cigarettes** = smokes cigarettes; **CVD** (cardiovascular disease) = history of heart disease; **AF** = history of atrial fibrillation; **LVH** = diagnosis of left ventricular hypertrophy

Table 14.4. Score Your Stroke Risk for the Next 10 Years: WOMEN

Points	0	1	2	3	4	5	6	7	8	9	10
Age	55–56	57–59	60–62	63–64	65–67	68–70	71–73	74–76	77–78	79–81	82–84
SBP-untrd		95–106	107–118	119–130	131–143	144–155	156–167	168–180	181–192	193–204	205–216
or SBP-trtd		95–106	107–113	114–119	120–125	126–131	132–139	140–148	149–160	161–204	205–216
Diabetes	No			Yes							
Cigarettes	No			Yes							
CVD	No		Yes								
AF	No						Yes				
LVH	No				Yes						

Table 14.5. Points with 10-Year Probability for Women

Your Points	10-Year Probability
1	1%
2	1%
3	2%
4	2%
5	2%
6	3%
7	4%
8	4%
9	5%
10	6%
11	8%
12	9%
13	11%
14	13%
15	16%
16	19%
17	23%
18	27%
19	32%
20	37%
21	43%
22	50%
23	57%
24	64%
25	71%

Table 14.5. Continued

Your Points	10-Year Probability
26	78%
27	84%

Table 14.6. Age Group and Average 10-Year Probability of Stroke for Women

Compare with Your Age Group	Average 10-Year Probability of Stroke
55–59	3.00%
60–64	4.70%
65–69	7.20%
70–74	10.90%
75–79	15.50%
80–84	23.90%

This example helps you assess your risk of stroke. Tally your points to score your stroke risk over the next 10 years.

Martha, age 65, wanted to determine her risk for having a stroke, so she took this stroke risk profile. This is how she arrived at her 10-year probability risk for having a stroke:

Table 14.7. Score Your Stroke Risk for the Next 10 Years: WOMEN

Age 65	4 points
SBP-treated, 107–113	2 points
Diabetes—No	0 points
Cigarettes—Yes	3 points
CVD—No	0 points
AF—Yes	6 points
LVH—No	0 points
TOTAL	15 points

Interpretation. 15 points carries a 16 percent, 10-year probability of having a stroke. If Martha quits smoking she can reduce her points to 12, which carries a 9 percent, 10-year probability of having a stroke.

Her current point total does not mean Martha will have a stroke, but serves as a wake-up call to ways she can lower her risk or even prevent a stroke. A lower percent score does not mean that Martha would not have a stroke, only that she is at a lower risk of having one.

No matter what your score is, it is important to work on reducing your risk factors as Martha did in this example by quitting smoking.

Many risk factors for stroke can be managed, some very successfully. Although risk is never zero at any age, by starting early and controlling your risk factors you can lower your risk of death or disability from stroke. With good control, the risk of stroke in most age groups can be kept below that for accidental injury or death.

Americans have shown that stroke is preventable and treatable. In recent years, a better understanding of the causes of stroke has helped Americans make lifestyle changes that have cut the stroke death rate nearly in half.

Chapter 15 | Modifiable Risk Factors for Stroke

Chapter Contents

Section 15.1 | Atrial Fibrillation and Stroke Risk

This section includes text excerpted from "Atrial Fibrillation and Stroke Information Page," National Institute of Neurological Disorders and Stroke (NINDS), March 27, 2019.

WHAT IS ATRIAL FIBRILLATION?

Atrial fibrillation (AF) describes the rapid, irregular beating of the left atrium (upper chamber) of the heart. These rapid contractions of the heart are weaker than normal contractions, resulting in slow flow of blood in the atrium. The blood pools and becomes sluggish and can result in the formation of blood clots. If a clot leaves the heart and travels to the brain, it can cause a stroke by blocking the flow of blood through cerebral arteries. Some people with AF have no symptoms, but others may experience a fluttering feeling in the area of the chest above the heart, chest pain, lightheadedness or fainting, shortness of breath, and fatigue. AF is diagnosed by an electrocardiogram (ECG), a device that records the heart's electrical activity. Other tests are often performed to rule out contributing causes such as high blood pressure, an overactive thyroid gland, heart failure, faulty heart valves, lung disease, and stimulant or alcohol abuse. Some people will have no identifiable cause for their AF.

TREATMENT OF ATRIAL FIBRILLATION

Within a few hours after the onset of a stroke, treatment with drugs or devices that dissolve or break up the clot can restore blood flow to the brain and lead to a better recovery. To prevent strokes related to AF, doctors often prescribe medications to prevent the formation of clots in the heart, which can travel to the brain and cause stroke. Immediately after a stroke, doctors may temporarily administer heparin by injection, while starting an oral medication for long-term protection from clots. The most commonly used drug has been warfarin. People taking warfarin must be closely monitored to make sure their blood is thin enough to prevent clots, but not so thin as to promote bleeding. Since some foods, vitamin supplements, and medications can affect warfarin action, keeping the blood just thin enough can be tricky. A number of new blood thinners, including dabigatran, rivaroxaban, and apixaban, have been shown to be as effective as warfarin in stroke prevention. These newer medications do not require regular blood test monitoring and may have less tendency to cause bleeding due to making the blood too thin. Some individuals with AF may have a lower risk of stroke and may be treated with aspirin, either alone or with another antiplatelet agency, such as clopidogrel. Other treatments for AF include medications, such as beta-blockers or calcium channel blockers to slow the heartbeat, and anti-arrhythmic drugs or electrical cardioversion (which delivers an electrical shock to the heart) to normalize the heartbeat.

PROGNOSIS FOR ATRIAL FIBRILLATION
Atrial fibrillation which affects as many as 2.2 million Americans, increases an individual's risk of stroke by 4 to 6 times on average. The risk increases with age. In people over 80 years of age, AF is the direct cause of one in four strokes. Treating individuals with warfarin or new blood thinners reduces the rate of stroke for those who have AF by approximately one-half to two-thirds. People with AF can have multiple strokes, including silent strokes (strokes that do not show physical symptoms, but show up on a brain scan) that, over time, can cause dementia, so prevention is important.

Section 15.2 | Cardiovascular Disease and Stroke Risk

This section includes text excerpted from "Silent Heart Attacks May Help Explain Strokes of Mysterious Origin," National Institute on Aging (NIA), National Institutes of Health (NIH), July 12, 2019.

Silent heart attacks—those that occur but, are not detected—are a cause of increased risk for strokes, especially strokes of unknown origin that can baffle healthcare providers, according to the National Institute on Aging (NIA)-led study. A comparison of heart and brain imaging data from a longitudinal study of older adults in Iceland showed that while undetected heart attacks are not noticeable enough to send patients to the hospital, they can scar and damage heart tissue in ways that may raise the risk of a stroke.

These undetected heart attacks were closely associated with a type of stroke known as "embolic stroke of undetermined source" (ESUS). ESUS strokes account for one-third of all ischemic strokes, which are caused by loss of blood supply to the brain. They seem to be triggered by clots or other vascular debris in the body, possibly a byproduct of the cardiac scarring caused by undetected heart attacks. ESUS strokes make it more difficult to target the most effective prevention or treatment strategy.

Section 15.3 | **Cholesterol and Stroke Risk**

This section includes text excerpted from "LDL and HDL Cholesterol: "Bad" and "Good" Cholesterol," Centers for Disease Control and Prevention (CDC), January 31, 2020.

Cholesterol travels through the blood on proteins called "lipoproteins." Two types of lipoproteins carry cholesterol throughout the body:

- **Low-density lipoprotein (LDL)**, sometimes called "bad" cholesterol, makes up most of your body's cholesterol. High levels of LDL cholesterol raise your risk for heart disease and stroke.
- **High-density lipoprotein (HDL)**, or "good" cholesterol, absorbs cholesterol and carries it back to the liver. The liver then flushes it from the body. High levels of HDL cholesterol can lower your risk for heart disease and stroke.

When your body has too much LDL cholesterol, the LDL cholesterol can build up on the walls of your blood vessels. This buildup is called "plaque." As your blood vessels build up plaque over time, the insides of the vessels narrow. This narrowing blocks blood flow to and from your heart and other organs. When blood flow to the heart is blocked, it can cause angina (chest pain) or a heart attack.

LOWERING YOUR RISK

- If you have high LDL cholesterol levels, your healthcare team may recommend cholesterol-lowering medicine and lifestyle changes to lower your risk for heart disease and stroke.
- If you have low HDL cholesterol levels, talk to your doctor about lifestyle changes that may help raise your levels.

Section 15.4 | Diabetes and Stroke Risk

This section includes text excerpted from "Diabetes, Heart Disease, and Stroke," National Institute of Diabetes and Digestive and Kidney Diseases (NIDDK), February 2017.

Having diabetes means that you are more likely to develop heart disease and have a greater chance of a heart attack or a stroke. People with diabetes are also more likely to have certain conditions, or risk factors, that increase the chances of having heart disease or stroke, such as high blood pressure or high cholesterol. If you have diabetes, you can protect your heart and health by managing your blood glucose, also called "blood sugar," as well as your blood pressure and cholesterol. If you smoke, get help to stop.

WHAT IS THE LINK BETWEEN DIABETES, HEART DISEASE, AND STROKE?

Over time, high blood glucose from diabetes can damage your blood vessels and the nerves that control your heart and blood vessels. The longer you have diabetes, the higher the chances that you will develop heart disease.

People with diabetes tend to develop heart disease at a younger age than people without diabetes. In adults with diabetes, the most common causes of death are heart disease and stroke. Adults with diabetes are nearly twice as likely to die from heart disease or stroke as people without diabetes.

The good news is that the steps you take to manage your diabetes also help to lower your chances of having heart disease or stroke.

WHAT ELSE INCREASES THE CHANCES OF HEART DISEASE OR STROKE IF YOU HAVE DIABETES?

If you have diabetes, other factors add to your chances of developing heart disease or having a stroke.

Smoking

Smoking raises your risk of developing heart disease. If you have diabetes, it is important to stop smoking because both smoking and diabetes narrow blood vessels. Smoking also increases your chances of developing other long-term problems, such as lung disease. Smoking also can damage the blood vessels in your legs and increase the risk of lower leg infections, ulcers, and amputation.

High Blood Pressure

If you have high blood pressure, your heart must work harder to pump blood. High blood pressure can strain your heart, damage blood vessels, and increase your risk of heart attack, stroke, eye problems, and kidney problems.

Abnormal Cholesterol Levels

Cholesterol is a type of fat produced by your liver and found in your blood. You have two kinds of cholesterol in your blood: LDL and HDL.

LDL, often called "bad" cholesterol, can build up and clog your blood vessels. High levels of LDL cholesterol raise your risk of developing heart disease.

Another type of blood fat, triglycerides, also can raise your risk of heart disease when the levels are higher than recommended by your healthcare team.

Obesity and Belly Fat

Being overweight or obese can affect your ability to manage your diabetes and increase your risk for many health problems, including heart disease and high blood pressure. If you are overweight, a healthy eating plan with reduced calories often will lower your glucose levels and reduce your need for medications.

Excess belly fat around your waist, even if you are not overweight, can raise your chances of developing heart disease.

You have excess belly fat if your waist measures:
- More than 40 inches and you are a man
- More than 35 inches and you are a woman

Family History of Heart Disease

A family history of heart disease may also add to your chances of developing heart disease. If one or more of your family members had a heart attack before 50 years of age, you may have an even higher chance of developing heart disease.

You cannot change whether heart disease runs in your family, but if you have diabetes, it is even more important to take steps to protect yourself from heart disease and decrease your chances of having a stroke.

HOW CAN YOU LOWER THE CHANCES OF A HEART ATTACK OR STROKE IF YOU HAVE DIABETES?

Taking care of your diabetes is important to help you take care of your heart. You can lower your chances of having a heart attack or stroke by taking the following steps to manage your diabetes to keep your heart and blood vessels healthy.

Manage Your Diabetes ABCS

Knowing your diabetes ABCS will help you manage your blood glucose, blood pressure, and cholesterol. Stopping smoking if you have diabetes is also important to lower your chances for heart disease.
- **A is for the A1C test.** The A1C test shows your average blood glucose level over the past 3 months. This is different from the blood glucose checks that you do every day. The higher your A1C number, the higher your blood glucose levels have been during the past 3 months. High levels of blood glucose can harm your heart, blood vessels, kidneys, feet, and eyes. The A1C goal for many

people with diabetes is below 7 percent. Some people may do better with a slightly higher A1C goal. Ask your healthcare team what your goal should be.

- **B is for blood pressure.** Blood pressure is the force of your blood against the wall of your blood vessels. If your blood pressure gets too high, it makes your heart work too hard. High blood pressure can cause a heart attack or stroke and damage your kidneys and eyes. The blood pressure goal for most people with diabetes is below 140/90 mm Hg. Ask what your goal should be.
- **C is for cholesterol.** You have two kinds of cholesterol in your blood: LDL and HDL. LDL or "bad" cholesterol can build up and clog your blood vessels. Too much bad cholesterol can cause a heart attack or stroke. HDL or "good" cholesterol helps remove the "bad" cholesterol from your blood vessels. Ask your healthcare team what your cholesterol numbers should be. If you are over 40 years of age, you may need to take medicine, such as a statin to lower your cholesterol and protect your heart. Some people with very high LDL ("bad") cholesterol may need to take medicine at a younger age.
- **S is for stop smoking.** Not smoking is especially important for people with diabetes because both smoking and diabetes narrow blood vessels, so your heart has to work harder. If you quit smoking:
  - You will lower your risk for heart attack, stroke, nerve disease, kidney disease, eye disease, and amputation.
  - Your blood glucose, blood pressure, and cholesterol levels may improve.
  - Your blood circulation will improve.
  - You may have an easier time being physically active.

If you smoke or use other tobacco products, stop. Ask for help so you do not have to do it alone.

Ask your healthcare team about your goals for A1C, blood pressure, and cholesterol, and what you can do to reach these goals.

97

Learn to Manage Stress

Managing diabetes is not always easy. Feeling stressed, sad, or angry is common when you are living with diabetes. You may know what to do to stay healthy, but may have trouble sticking with your plan over time. Long-term stress can raise your blood glucose and blood pressure, but you can learn ways to lower your stress. Try deep breathing, gardening, taking a walk, doing yoga, meditating, doing a hobby, or listening to your favorite music.

Take Medicine to Protect Your Heart

Medicines may be an important part of your treatment plan. Your doctor will prescribe medicines based on your specific needs. Medicines may help you:

- Meet your A1C (blood glucose), blood pressure, and cholesterol goals.
- Reduce your risk of blood clots, heart attack, or stroke.
- Treat angina, or chest pain that is often a symptom of heart disease. (Angina can also be an early symptom of a heart attack.)

Ask your doctor whether you should take aspirin. Aspirin is not safe for everyone. Your doctor can tell you whether taking aspirin is right for you and exactly how much to take.

Statins can reduce the risk of having a heart attack or stroke in some people with diabetes. Statins are a type of medicine often used to help people meet their cholesterol goals. Talk with your doctor to find out whether taking a statin is right for you.

Talk with your doctor if you have questions about your medicines. Before you start a new medicine, ask your doctor about possible side effects and how you can avoid them. If the side effects of your medicine bother you, tell your doctor. Do not stop taking your medicines without checking with your doctor first.

Section 15.5 | Hypertension and Stroke Risk

This section includes text excerpted from "High Blood Pressure: It May Be Riskier Than You Think," Know Stroke, National Institute of Neurological Disorders and Stroke (NINDS), 2016. Reviewed May 2020.

THE CONNECTION BETWEEN HIGH BLOOD PRESSURE AND STROKE

We may face many risks in daily lives but you take steps to lower only some of them. We put on a seatbelt when you get into a car. We apply sunscreen when you are enjoying the day outside. Many people with high blood pressure know about the health risks they face, including stroke, heart attack, and kidney problems. So they take steps to follow a healthier lifestyle. But, let us face it; high blood pressure can be hard to control on a daily basis and only 50 percent of people with hypertension have their blood pressure controlled.

The research says that having high blood pressure when you are middle-aged may raise your risk for cognitive impairment and dementia, as well as stroke, later in life. Conversely, people with lower blood pressure appear to have a lower risk of cognitive impairment and dementia.

RISKS OF HIGH BLOOD PRESSURE

Over years, the wear and tear of high blood pressure causes the brain's blood vessels to become scarred, narrowed, and diseased. This can affect the bloodstream's ability to provide the nerve cells with the oxygen and nutrients they need or to remove toxic products.

This condition leads to chronic brain injury in the form of damage to the nerve fibers and their insulation that affect communications across the central nervous system (diffuse white matter disease). It also leads to multiple, small, usually "silent" strokes.

Stroke Causes Vascular Dementia

With aging, damage to the brain's blood vessels, silent strokes, and diffuse white matter disease add to the changes that occur with Alzheimer disease (AD) and result in dementia. In some cases, extensive stroke damage itself causes vascular dementia, making this one the most common forms of dementia after AD.

Preventable Risk Factor for Stroke

High blood pressure is the most important preventable risk factor for stroke. In people with vascular risk factors, aspirin and other drugs may be effective at decreasing the risk of stroke and heart attack. Treating high blood pressure and keeping it under control is good for the brain.

STROKE RATES

Over the past five decades, stroke rates in the United States have decreased by 70 percent as blood pressure control has become the standard of care. A number of studies have reported decreased dementia incidence rates in the United States and other developed countries. Although the cause of this decline is not entirely clear, many believe it is related to decreasing stroke rates. Because only 50 percent of people with hypertension have their blood pressure controlled, there is work to be done.

REDUCING THE RISKS OF STROKE

Take these steps now to "mind your risks" and reduce your chance of stroke, cognitive impairment, dementia, and heart disease later in life.

1. Talk to your healthcare provider about your risk for stroke, dementia, and heart disease.
2. Work with your provider to develop a plan to control your blood pressure and other risk factors.
3. Stick to the plan. This is the hard part, but keeping your heart and brain healthy will lead to better health in old age. A healthy heart and a healthy brain are both crucial to a healthy old age.

GOALS TO REDUCE YOUR RISK

From staying active to taking medication prescribed by your doctor, these seven simple and effective lifestyle changes can help keep your heart and brain healthy.

- Take blood pressure medicines as instructed by your healthcare provider.

Modifiable Risk Factors for Stroke

- Eat healthy and keep active.
- Exercise regularly and manage your weight.
- Quit smoking.
- Lower your cholesterol levels.
- Take blood pressure medicines as instructed by your healthcare provider.
- Manage your diabetes.
- Find out whether daily low-dose aspirin is right for you.

Chapter 16 | Other Conditions That Increase Stroke Risk

Chapter Contents

Section 16.1 | Mini-Stroke: Transient Ischemic Attack (TIA)

This section includes text excerpted from "Transient Ischemic Attack Information Page," National Institute of Neurological Disorders and Stroke (NINDS), March 27, 2019.

WHAT IS TRANSIENT ISCHEMIC ATTACK?

A transient ischemic attack (TIA) is a transient stroke that lasts only a few minutes. It occurs when the blood supply to part of the brain is briefly interrupted. TIA symptoms, which usually occur suddenly, are similar to those of stroke but do not last as long. Most symptoms of a TIA disappear within an hour, although they may persist for up to 24 hours. Symptoms can include numbness or weakness in the face, arm, or leg, especially on one side of the body; confusion or difficulty in talking or understanding speech; trouble seeing in one or both eyes; and difficulty with walking, dizziness, or loss of balance and coordination.

TREATMENT FOR TRANSIENT ISCHEMIC ATTACK

As there is no way to tell whether symptoms are from a TIA or an acute stroke, patients should assume that all stroke-like symptoms signal an emergency and should not wait to see if they go away. A prompt evaluation (within 60 minutes) is necessary to identify the cause of the TIA and determine appropriate therapy. Depending on a patient's medical history and the results of a medical examination, the doctor may recommend drug therapy or surgery to reduce the risk of stroke in people who have had a TIA. The use of antiplatelet agents, particularly aspirin, is a standard treatment for patients at risk for stroke. People with atrial fibrillation (irregular beating of the heart) may be prescribed anticoagulants.

PROGNOSIS OF TRANSIENT ISCHEMIC ATTACK

The TIAs are often warning signs that a person is at risk for a more serious and debilitating stroke. About one-third of those who have a TIA will have an acute stroke sometime in the future. Many strokes can be prevented by heeding the warning signs of TIAs and treating underlying risk factors. The most important treatable factors linked to TIAs and stroke are high blood pressure, cigarette smoking, heart disease, carotid artery disease, diabetes, and heavy use of alcohol. Medical help is available to reduce and eliminate these factors. Lifestyle changes such as eating a balanced diet, maintaining a healthy weight, exercising, and enrolling in smoking and alcohol cessation programs can also reduce these factors.

Section 16.2 | Sickle Cell Disease and Stroke Risk

This section includes text excerpted from "Sickle Cell Disease," Office on Women's Health (OWH), U.S. Department of Health and Human Services (HHS), April 26, 2019.

WHAT IS SICKLE CELL DISEASE?

Sickle cell disease (SCD) is a group of red blood cell disorders that are passed down from your parents. This means that it is a genetic disease, and you are born with it.

People with SCD have some red blood cells that are shaped like a "sickle" or crescent, instead of round. Normal, round red blood cells are flexible enough to move through blood vessels to carry oxygen to the body. Sickle-shaped red blood cells can stick to each other inside blood vessels, blocking blood flow and causing pain and problems in many different parts of the body. People with SCD also have fewer red blood cells, because sickle cells die sooner than normal red blood cells. Over time, blocked blood flow and lack of oxygen can cause serious health problems and organ damage.

WHEN SHOULD YOU GO TO THE HOSPITAL FOR YOUR SICKLE CELL DISEASE SYMPTOMS?

People with SCD should go to the hospital for:
- A pain crisis (also called a "pain episode") that cannot be treated with over-the-counter (OTC) pain medicines or your own prescription pain medicine
- A fever over 101°F
- Stroke symptoms, such as:
  - Numbness or weakness in the face, arm, or leg, especially on only one side of the body

- Confusion, or trouble speaking or understanding
- Trouble seeing in one or both eyes
- Trouble walking, dizziness, or loss of balance or coordination
- Severe headache with no known cause

RISK FACTORS LEADING TO STROKE
Hydroxyurea and the Risk of Stroke

The most commonly used medicine for SCD is a prescription medicine you take every day, called "hydroxyurea." Hydroxyurea may help prevent problems from SCD, such as pain crises, stroke, and acute chest syndrome. Hydroxyurea may also make these problems less serious when they happen. Experts recommend that children with SCD over 9 months old and all adults who have severe SCD take hydroxyurea, unless there is a medical reason they should not take it. Most people do not have any serious side effects from the medicine. Hydroxyurea may lower the number of white blood cells and platelets in your body, which is usually higher in people with SCD and may cause pain crises. Lowering the number of white blood cells and platelets may put you at higher risk of infection and bleeding. White blood cells help you fight infections. Platelets help your blood clot when you get a cut or other injury. The long-term effects of this medicine are still unknown. Pregnant women, or women trying to become pregnant, should not take hydroxyurea.

Blood Transfusions and the Risk of Stroke

You may get a red blood cell transfusion if you have sickle cell disease complications or health problems caused by SCD, such as anemia, acute chest syndrome, or stroke. Some people with SCD who had a stroke in the past may need regular blood transfusions to help prevent another stroke. Regular blood transfusions are also used to prevent crises in people who cannot take hydroxyurea. But blood transfusions can lead to dangerously high iron levels in the blood that can damage the heart and lungs. If this happens, you may need a medicine called "iron chelation therapy" to lower the iron levels in your blood.

Reproductive Health and the Risk of Stroke
MENSTRUAL CYCLE AND THE RISK OF STROKE

Many women with SCD do not have heavy periods. But, if you have heavy periods, heavy bleeding may increase your risk of iron-deficiency anemia. Doctors often prescribe birth control pills to lessen heavy menstrual bleeding. But not all birth control pills are OK for women with SCD due to a higher risk of stroke. Talk to your doctor or nurse about progesterone-only birth control. Birth control with progesterone combined with estrogen may increase your risk of stroke.

SEXUAL HEALTH AND THE RISK OF STROKE

Women who have SCD can use normal birth control methods. Some doctors do not recommend combination hormonal birth control (with a combination of two types of hormones), because it slightly increases the risk of blood clots and stroke in all women. Some women who have SCD have reported pain crises that happen more often with combination hormonal birth control. Birth control methods using only one type of hormone, like progesterone, may lower risk and may help control SCD pain crises.

PREGNANCY AND THE RISK OF STROKE

Women who have SCD and become pregnant are at greater risk of experiencing SCD complications during pregnancy. The risks are higher for those with more severe SCD. Possible sickle cell complications during pregnancy include:
- Anemia getting worse
- Higher risk of blood clots
- Higher risk of infections, such as urinary tract infections
- More frequent pain crises
- Acute chest syndrome
- Stroke

Section 16.3 | Carotid Artery Disease and Stroke Risk

This section includes text excerpted from "Carotid Artery Disease," National Heart, Lung, and Blood Institute (NHLBI), December 26, 2011. Reviewed May 2020.

WHAT IS CAROTID ARTERY DISEASE?

Carotid artery disease is a disease in which a waxy substance called "plaque" builds up inside the carotid arteries. You have two common carotid arteries, one on each side of your neck. Each of them divide into internal and external carotid arteries.

The internal carotid arteries supply oxygen-rich blood to your brain. The external carotid arteries supply oxygen-rich blood to your face, scalp, and neck.

Carotid artery disease is serious because it can cause a stroke, also called a "brain attack." A stroke occurs if blood flow to your brain is cut off.

If blood flow is cut off for more than a few minutes, the cells in your brain start to die. This impairs the parts of the body that the brain cells control. A stroke can cause lasting brain damage; long-term disability, such as vision or speech problems or paralysis (an inability to move); or death.

CAUSES OF CAROTID ARTERY DISEASE

Carotid artery disease seems to start when damage occurs to the inner layers of the carotid arteries. Major factors that contribute to damage include:

- Smoking
- High levels of certain fats and cholesterol in the blood
- High blood pressure
- High levels of sugar in the blood due to insulin resistance or diabetes
- When damage occurs, your body starts a healing process. The healing may cause plaque to build up where the arteries are damaged.

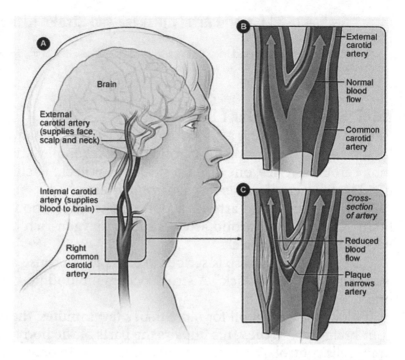

Figure 16.1. Carotid Arteries

Figure A shows the location of the right carotid artery in the head and neck. Figure B shows the inside of a normal carotid artery that has normal blood flow. Figure C shows the inside of a carotid artery that has plaque buildup and reduced blood flow.

The plaque in an artery can crack or rupture. If this happens, blood cell fragments called "platelets" will stick to the site of the injury and may clump together to form blood clots.

The buildup of plaque or blood clots can severely narrow or block the carotid arteries. This limits the flow of oxygen-rich blood to your brain, which can cause a stroke.

SCREENING AND PREVENTION OF CAROTID ARTERY DISEASE

Taking action to control your risk factors can help prevent or delay carotid artery disease and stroke. Your risk for carotid artery disease increases with the number of risk factors you have.

110

SYMPTOMS OF CAROTID ARTERY DISEASE
Transient Ischemic Attack (Mini-Stroke)

For some people, having a transient ischemic attack (TIA), or "mini-stroke," is the first sign of carotid artery disease. During a mini-stroke, you may have some or all of the symptoms of a stroke. However, the symptoms usually go away on their own within 24 hours.

Stroke and mini-stroke symptoms may include:
- A sudden, severe headache with no known cause
- Dizziness or loss of balance
- Inability to move one or more of your limbs
- Sudden trouble seeing in one or both eyes
- Sudden weakness or numbness in the face or limbs, often on just one side of the body
- Trouble speaking or understanding speech

Even if the symptoms stop quickly, call 911 for emergency help. Do not drive yourself to the hospital. It is important to get checked and to get treatment started as soon as possible.

A mini-stroke is a warning sign that you are at high risk of having a stroke. You should not ignore these symptoms. Getting medical care can help find possible causes of a mini-stroke and help you manage risk factors. These actions might prevent a future stroke.

Although a mini-stroke may warn of a stroke, it does not predict when a stroke will happen. A stroke may occur days, weeks, or even months after a mini-stroke.

DIAGNOSIS OF CAROTID ARTERY DISEASE
Medical History

Your doctor will find out whether you have any of the major risk factors for carotid artery disease. She or he also will ask whether you have had any signs or symptoms of a mini-stroke or stroke.

Diagnostic Tests
- **Carotid ultrasound** (also called "sonography") is the most common test for diagnosing carotid artery disease. It

is a painless, harmless test that uses sound waves to create pictures of the inside of your carotid arteries. This test can show whether plaque has narrowed your carotid arteries and how narrow they are. A standard carotid ultrasound shows the structure of your carotid arteries. A Doppler carotid ultrasound shows how blood moves through your carotid arteries.

- **Carotid angiography** is a special type of x-ray. This test may be used if the ultrasound results are unclear or do not give your doctor enough information. For this test, your doctor will inject a substance (called "contrast dye") into a vein, most often in your leg. The dye travels to your carotid arteries and highlights them on x-ray pictures.
- **Magnetic resonance angiography (MRA)** uses a large magnet and radio waves to take pictures of your carotid arteries. Your doctor can see these pictures on a computer screen. For this test, your doctor may give you contrast dye to highlight your carotid arteries on the pictures.
- **Computed tomography angiography,** or CT angiography, takes x-ray pictures of the body from many angles. A computer combines the pictures into two- and three-dimensional images. For this test, your doctor may give you contrast dye to highlight your carotid arteries on the pictures.

MEDICATIONS FOR CAROTID ARTERY DISEASE

Treatments for carotid artery disease may include heart-healthy lifestyle changes, medicines, and medical procedures. The goals of treatment are to stop the disease from getting worse and to prevent a stroke. Your treatment will depend on your symptoms, how severe the disease is, and your age and overall health.

If you have a stroke caused by a blood clot, you may be given a clot-dissolving, or clot-busting, medication. This type of medication must be given within four hours of symptom onset. The sooner treatment occurs, the better your chances of recovery. If you think you are having a stroke, call 911 right away for emergency care.

Medicines to prevent blood clots are the mainstay treatment for people who have carotid artery disease. They prevent platelets from clumping together and forming blood clots in your carotid arteries, which can lead to a stroke. Two common medications are:
- Aspirin
- Clopidogrel

Sometimes lifestyle changes alone are not enough to control your cholesterol levels. For example, you also may need statin medications to control or lower your cholesterol. By lowering your blood cholesterol level, you can decrease your chance of having a heart attack or stroke.

Doctors usually prescribe statins for people who have:
- Diabetes
- Heart disease or have had a stroke
- High LDL cholesterol levels

Doctors may discuss beginning statin treatment with those who have an elevated risk for developing heart disease or having a stroke.

You may need other medications to treat diseases and conditions that damage the carotid arteries. Your doctor also may prescribe medications to:
- Lower your blood pressure
- Lower your blood sugar level
- Prevent blood clots from forming, which can lead to stroke
- Prevent or reduce inflammation

Take all medicines regularly, as your doctor prescribes. Do not change the amount of your medicine or skip a dose unless your doctor tells you to. Your healthcare team will help find a treatment plan that is right for you.

LIVING WITH CAROTID ARTERY DISEASE

If you have carotid artery disease, you can take steps to manage the condition, reduce risk factors, and prevent complications. These steps include making heart-healthy lifestyle changes, following your treatment plan, and getting ongoing care.

Treatment Plan

Following your treatment plan may help prevent your carotid artery disease from getting worse. It also can lower your risk for stroke and other health problems.

You may need to take medicines to control certain risk factors and to prevent blood clots that could cause a stroke. Taking prescribed medicines and following a healthy lifestyle can help control carotid artery disease. However, they do not cure the disease. You will likely have to stick with your treatment plan for life.

Ongoing Care

If you have carotid artery disease, having ongoing medical care is important.

Most people who have the disease will need to have their blood pressure checked regularly and their blood sugar and blood cholesterol levels tested one or more times a year. If you have diabetes, you will need routine blood sugar tests and other tests.

Testing shows whether these conditions are under control, or whether your doctor needs to adjust your treatment for better results.

If you have had a stroke or procedures to restore blood flow in your carotid arteries, you will likely need a yearly carotid Doppler ultrasound test. This test shows how well blood flows through your carotid arteries.

Repeating this test over time will show whether the narrowing in your carotid arteries is getting worse. Results also can show how well procedures to treat your arteries have worked.

Follow up with your doctor regularly. The sooner your doctor spots problems, the sooner she or he can prescribe treatment.

Stroke Warning Signs

The signs and symptoms of stroke may include:
- Sudden weakness or numbness in the face or limbs, often on only one side of the body

- The inability to move one or more of your limbs
- Trouble speaking or understanding speech
- Sudden trouble seeing in one or both eyes
- Dizziness or loss of balance
- A sudden, severe headache with no known cause

If you are a candidate for clot-busting therapy, you have the best chance for full recovery if treatment to open a blocked artery is given within 4 hours of symptom onset. The sooner treatment occurs, the better your chances of recovery.

Make those close to you aware of stroke symptoms and the need for urgent action. Learning the signs and symptoms of a stroke will allow you to help yourself or someone close to you lower the risk of damage or death due to a stroke.

Section 16.4 | Peripheral Artery Disease and Stroke Risk

This section includes text excerpted from "Facts about Peripheral Arterial Disease (P.A.D.)" National Heart, Lung, and Blood Institute (NHLBI), August 2006. Reviewed May 2020.

FACTS ABOUT PERIPHERAL ARTERIAL DISEASE

One in every 20 Americans over 50 years of age has peripheral arterial disease (PAD), a condition that raises the risk for heart attack and stroke.

Peripheral arterial disease develops when your arteries become clogged with plaque—fatty deposits that limit blood flow to your legs. Just like clogged arteries in the heart, clogged arteries in the legs mean you are at risk for having a heart attack or stroke.

You can lower your risk for PAD. Timely detection and treatment of PAD. can improve the quality of life; help you keep your independence and mobility; and reduce your risk of heart attack, stroke, leg amputation, and even death. Taking steps to learn about PAD., including asking your healthcare provider to check your risk, can help you stay in circulation longer to enjoy your life.

WHAT CAUSES PERIPHERAL ARTERIAL DISEASE

Having a personal history of vascular disease, heart attack, or stroke causes PAD. If you have heart disease, you have a one in three chance of also having PAD.

HOW IS PERIPHERAL ARTERIAL DISEASE TREATED?

The overall goals for treating PAD are to reduce any symptoms, improve quality of life and mobility, and prevent heart attack, stroke, and amputation. There are three main approaches to treating PAD: making lifestyle changes; taking medication; and in some cases, having a special procedure or surgery. Your healthcare provider will determine the best treatment options for you, based on your medical history and the severity of your condition.

Section 16.5 | Sleep Apnea and Stroke Risk

This section includes text excerpted from "Sleep Apnea Tied to Increased Risk of Stroke," National Heart, Lung, and Blood Institute (NHLBI), April 7, 2010. Reviewed May 2020.

Obstructive sleep apnea is associated with an increased risk of stroke in middle-aged and older adults, especially men, according to results from a landmark study supported by the National Heart, Lung, and Blood Institute (NHLBI) of the National Institutes of Health (NIH). Overall, sleep apnea more than doubles the risk of stroke in men. Obstructive sleep apnea is a common disorder in which the upper airway is intermittently narrowed or blocked, disrupting sleep and breathing during sleep.

Researchers from the Sleep Heart Health Study (SHHS) report that the risk of stroke appears in men with mild sleep apnea and rises with the severity of sleep apnea. Men with moderate-to-severe sleep apnea are nearly three times more likely to have a stroke than men without sleep apnea or with mild sleep apnea. The risk from sleep apnea is independent of other risk factors such as weight, high blood pressure, race, smoking, and diabetes.

The researchers suggest that the differences between men and women might be because men are more likely to develop sleep apnea at younger ages. Therefore, they tend to have untreated sleep apnea for longer periods of time than women. It is possible that the stroke risk is related to cumulative effects of sleep apnea adversely influencing health over many years. Findings provide compelling evidence that obstructive sleep apnea is a risk factor for stroke, especially in men and overall, there is an increased risk of stroke in men with sleep apnea comparable to adding 10 years to a man's age. Importantly, it was found that increased stroke risk in men occurs even with relatively mild levels of sleep apnea.

"Research on the effects of sleep apnea not only increases our understanding of how lapses of breathing during sleep affects our health and well-being, but it can also provide important insight into how cardiovascular problems, such as stroke and high blood pressure develop," noted Michael J. Twery, Ph.D., director of the NIH National Center on Sleep Disorders Research, an office administered by the NHLBI.

The new results support earlier findings that have linked sleep apnea to stroke risk. SHHS researchers have also reported that untreated sleep apnea is associated with an increased risk of high blood pressure, heart attack, irregular heartbeats, heart failure, and death from any cause. Other studies have also linked untreated sleep apnea with overweight or obesity and diabetes. It is also linked to excessive daytime sleepiness, which lowers performance in the workplace and at school, and increases the risk of injuries and death from drowsy driving and other accidents.

More than 12 million American adults are believed to have sleep apnea, and most are not diagnosed or treated. Treatments to restore regular breathing during sleep include mouthpieces, surgery, and breathing devices, such as continuous positive airway pressure, or CPAP. In people who are overweight or obese, weight loss can also help.

These treatments can help improve breathing and reduce the severity of symptoms, such as loud snoring and excessive daytime sleepiness, thereby improving sleep-related quality of life and performance at work or in school. Randomized clinical trials to test whether treating sleep apnea lowers the risk of stroke, other cardiovascular diseases, or death are needed.

Chapter 17 | Stroke Prevention

Chapter Contents

Section 17.1 | Preventing and Managing Diabetes

This section includes text excerpted from "Diabetes—How Can I Prevent Diabetes?" Centers for Disease Control and Prevention (CDC), March 31, 2015. Reviewed May 2020.

HOW CAN I PREVENT DIABETES?

Research studies have found that moderate weight loss and exercise can prevent or delay type 2 diabetes among adults at high risk of diabetes. Find out more about the risk factors for type 2 diabetes, what it means to have prediabetes, and what you can do to prevent or delay diabetes.

WHAT ARE THE MOST IMPORTANT THINGS TO DO TO PREVENT DIABETES?

The Diabetes Prevention Program (DPP), a major federally funded study of 3,234 people at high risk for diabetes, showed that people can delay and possibly prevent the disease by losing a small amount of weight (5 to 7 percent of total body weight) through 30 minutes of physical activity 5 days a week and healthier eating.

WHEN SHOULD I BE TESTED FOR DIABETES?

Anyone 45 years of age or older should consider getting tested for diabetes, especially if you are overweight. If you are younger than 45, but are overweight and have one or more additional risk factors, you should consider getting tested.

Additional risk factors include:
- Being overweight or obese.
- Having a parent, brother, or sister with diabetes.
- Being African American, American Indian, Asian American, Pacific Islander, or Hispanic American/ Latino heritage.
- Having a prior history of gestational diabetes or birth of at least one baby weighing more than 9 pounds.
- Having high blood pressure measuring 140/90 or higher.

- Having abnormal cholesterol with high-density lipoproteins (HDL) ("good") cholesterol is 35 or lower, or triglyceride level is 250 or higher.
- Being physically inactive—exercising fewer than three times a week.

HOW DOES BODY WEIGHT AFFECT THE LIKELIHOOD OF DEVELOPING DIABETES?

Being overweight or obese is a leading risk factor for type 2 diabetes. Being overweight can keep your body from making and using insulin properly, and can also cause high blood pressure. The DPP, a major federally funded study of 3,234 people at high risk for diabetes, showed that moderate diet and exercise of about 30 minutes or more, 5 or more days per week, or of 150 or more minutes per week, resulting in a 5 percent to 7 percent weight loss can delay and possibly prevent type 2 diabetes.

WHAT IS PREDIABETES?

People with blood glucose levels that are higher than normal but not yet in the diabetic range have "prediabetes." Doctors sometimes call this condition impaired fasting glucose (IFG) or impaired glucose tolerance (IGT), depending on the test used to diagnose it. Insulin resistance and prediabetes usually have no symptoms. You may have one or both conditions for several years without noticing anything.

If you have prediabetes, you have a higher risk of developing type 2 diabetes. In addition, people with prediabetes also have a higher risk of heart disease.

Progression to diabetes among those with prediabetes is not inevitable. Studies suggest that weight loss and increased physical activity among people with prediabetes prevent or delay diabetes and may return blood glucose levels to normal.

Section 17.2 | Preventing and Managing High Blood Pressure

This section includes text excerpted from "Preventing Diseases—High Blood Pressure," National Center for Health Promotion and Disease Prevention (NCP), U.S. Department of Veterans Affairs (VA), July 25, 2018.

WHY IS HIGH BLOOD PRESSURE DANGEROUS?

If blood pressure rises and stays high over time, it is called hypertension. If it is not controlled, high blood pressure can cause:
- Stroke
- Kidney problems
- Heart failure
- Heart attack
- Eye problems

Most people with high blood pressure feel healthy and do not have symptoms. The only way to know if you have high blood pressure is to have your blood pressure checked.

HOW DO YOU GET CHECKED FOR HIGH BLOOD PRESSURE?

Checking your blood pressure is simple. Your provider places a fabric cuff around your upper arm and pumps it full of air. Your provider then listens to your heartbeat while the air lets out of the cuff.

Follow these steps to help your provider correctly measure your blood pressure:
- Wear a short-sleeved shirt or blouse.
- Empty your bladder.
- For at least 30 minutes before your appointment, do not:
  - Smoke
  - Do any vigorous activity
  - Drink caffeine (in coffee, tea or cola)
- Sit down and relax with your feet on the floor and your back supported for at least 5 minutes before your blood pressure is checked.
- Do not talk while your blood pressure is being checked.

WHAT DO YOUR BLOOD PRESSURE NUMBERS MEAN?

Blood pressure is measured by two numbers.

The first (or top) number—"systolic"—is the pressure in your blood vessels when your heartbeats. The second (or bottom) number—"diastolic"—is the pressure in your blood vessels between heartbeats.

If your blood pressure is normal, that's great! You should have it rechecked every year or so to be sure it stays within the normal range. If your blood pressure is normal, that's great! You should have it rechecked every year or so to be sure it stays within the normal range.

If your blood pressure is prehigh or high, it should be rechecked to determine whether you have hypertension. Ask your provider the following questions:

- When should I have my blood pressure checked again?
- Do I need treatment for high blood pressure?

WHAT CAN YOU DO TO PREVENT OR CONTROL HIGH BLOOD PRESSURE?

- Quit smoking and/or chewing tobacco. Ask your provider for help with quitting.
- Achieve and maintain a healthy weight. If you are overweight, ask your provider for help with a plan to lose weight.
- Be physically active.
  - "Physical activity" includes any activity that raises your heart rate, such as brisk walking, working in the house or yard, or playing sports.
  - Do activity for 10 minutes or more at a time. Aim for at least 2 hours and 30 minutes of activity each week.
- Reduce salt (sodium) in your diet.
  - Read food labels. Choose and prepare foods that are low in sodium or are sodium-free.
  - Ask to see a registered dietitian if you need help with a plan.
- Limit alcohol.
  - Men should have no more than 2 drinks per day.
  - Women should have no more than 1 drink per day.

WHAT ELSE CAN YOU DO?

Always ask your provider what your blood pressure is and write it down. Keep track of your blood pressure numbers.

Your provider may prescribe medicine to help lower your blood pressure.
- Take your medicine every day, or as directed by your provider
- If your blood pressure numbers get lower, it's because your medicine is working. Don't stop it or take a lower dose unless your provider says you should.

Here are some questions to ask your provider:
- Is my blood pressure under good control?
- How often should I have my blood pressure checked?
- What is a healthy weight for me?
- Is it safe for me to start doing regular physical activity?

Section 17.3 | Preventing and Managing High Cholesterol

This section includes text excerpted from "Preventing Diseases—High Cholesterol," National Center for Health Promotion and Disease Prevention (NCP), U.S. Department of Veterans Affairs (VA), July 25, 2018.

WHAT IS HIGH CHOLESTEROL?

Cholesterol is a fat-like material that provides structure for your body's cells. Your liver makes most of the cholesterol your body needs, but you also get some from the foods you eat. Too much cholesterol can cause a sticky substance (plaque) to build up in your blood vessels. This plaque can block blood vessels and cause heart attacks and strokes.

Most people with high cholesterol feel healthy and don't have symptoms. The only way to know if you have high cholesterol is to have your cholesterol checked.

HOW IS CHOLESTEROL CHECKED?

Cholesterol is checked with a blood test. The test works best if you don't eat or drink anything for at least 8 hours before the test.

WHAT DO THE CHOLESTEROL NUMBERS MEAN?

Your total cholesterol is made up of two types of cholesterol: LDL (low-density lipoproteins) and HDL (high-density lipoproteins).

- High levels of LDL increase your chances of heart disease. It is sometimes called the "bad cholesterol."
- High levels of HDL decrease your chances of heart disease. It is sometimes called the "good cholesterol."

Total Cholesterol Levels

Your provider will usually look at your total cholesterol first. Your total cholesterol should be under 200. If you already have heart disease or you have heart disease risk factors, such as smoking, diabetes, or high blood pressure, your provider will also look at your LDL and HDL results.

If your cholesterol is in the desirable range and you are healthy, have it checked again in 5 years.

If your cholesterol is borderline high or high, or you have heart disease, your next step depends on your LDL and HDL levels and your other conditions or risk factors.

Ask your provider these questions:

- What should my cholesterol levels be?
- Do I need treatment for my cholesterol?

WHAT CAN YOU DO TO PREVENT OR CONTROL HIGH CHOLESTEROL?

Follow a Healthy Eating Plan

- Read food labels and limit foods high in saturated fat, trans fat, and cholesterol.
- Eat plenty of fruits, vegetables, low-fat dairy foods, and whole grains.
- Ask to see a registered dietitian if you need help with a plan.

Be Physically Active

- "Physical activity" includes any activity that raises your heart rate, such as brisk walking, working in the house or yard, or playing sports.

- Do activity for 10 minutes or more at a time. Aim for at least 2 hours and 30 minutes of activity each week.

Achieve and Maintain a Healthy Weight
If you are overweight, ask your provider for help with an eating and physical activity plan to lose weight.

WHAT ELSE CAN YOU DO?
Always ask your provider what your cholesterol numbers are and write them down. Keep track with the log at the MyHealtheVet website: www.myhealth.va.gov.

Your provider may prescribe medicine to help lower your cholesterol.
- Take your medicine every day, or as directed by your provider.
- If your cholesterol numbers get lower, it's because your medicine is working. Don't stop it or take a lower dose unless your provider says you should.

Here are some questions to ask your provider:
- Is my cholesterol under good control?
- When should I have my cholesterol next checked?
- What is a healthy weight for me?
- Is it safe for me to start doing regular physical activity?

Section 17.4 | Smoking, Cardiovascular Disease, and Stroke

This section includes text excerpted from "Smoking and Heart Disease and Stroke," Centers for Disease Control and Prevention (CDC), March 23, 2020.

WHAT IS HEART DISEASE AND STROKE?
Heart disease and stroke are cardiovascular (heart and blood vessel) diseases (CVDs).

Heart disease includes several types of heart conditions. The most common type in the United States is coronary heart disease (also known as "coronary artery disease"), which is the narrowing of the blood vessels that carry blood to the heart. This can cause:
- Chest pain
- Heart attack (when blood flow to the heart becomes blocked and a section of the heart muscle is damaged or dies)
- Heart failure (when the heart cannot pump enough blood and oxygen to support other organs)
- Arrhythmia (when the heart beats too fast, too slow, or irregularly)

HOW IS SMOKING RELATED TO HEART DISEASE AND STROKE?

Smoking is a major cause of CVD and causes one in every three deaths from CVD. Smoking can:
- Raise triglycerides (a type of fat in your blood)
- Lower "good" cholesterol (HDL)
- Make blood sticky and more likely to clot, which can block blood flow to the heart and brain
- Damage cells that line the blood vessels
- Increase the buildup of plaque (fat, cholesterol, calcium, and other substances) in blood vessels
- Cause thickening and narrowing of blood vessels

HOW IS BREATHING SECONDHAND SMOKE RELATED TO HEART DISEASE AND STROKE?

Breathing secondhand smoke also harms your health. Secondhand smoke is the smoke from burning tobacco products. Secondhand smoke also is smoke breathed out by a smoker. Breathing secondhand smoke can cause coronary heart disease, including heart attack and stroke. Know the facts:
- Secondhand smoke causes nearly 34,000 early deaths from coronary heart disease each year in the United States among nonsmokers.

- Nonsmokers who breathe secondhand smoke at home or at work increase their risk of developing heart disease by 25 to 30 percent. Secondhand smoke increases the risk for stroke by 20 to 30 percent.
- Each year, secondhand smoke exposure causes more than 8,000 deaths from stroke.
- Breathing secondhand smoke interferes with the normal functioning of the heart, blood, and vascular systems in ways that increase your risk of having a heart attack.
- Even briefly breathing secondhand smoke can damage the lining of blood vessels and cause your blood to become stickier. These changes can cause a deadly heart attack.

HOW CAN HEART DISEASE AND STROKE BE PREVENTED?

Heart disease and stroke are major causes of death and disability in the United States. Many people are at high risk for these diseases and do not know it. The good news is that many risk factors for heart disease and stroke can be prevented or controlled.

The federal government's Million Hearts® initiative aimed to prevent 1 million heart attacks and strokes by 2017. It is important to know your risk for heart disease and stroke and to take action to reduce that risk. A good place to start is with the aspirin, blood pressure, cholesterol, smoking (ABCS) of heart health:

- **Aspirin.** Aspirin may help reduce your risk for heart disease and stroke. But, do not take aspirin if you think you are having a stroke. It can make some types of stroke worse. Before taking aspirin, talk to your doctor about whether aspirin is right for you.
- **Blood pressure.** Control your blood pressure.
- **Cholesterol.** Manage your cholesterol.
- **Smoking.** Quit smoking, or do not start.

In addition to your ABCS, several lifestyle choices can help protect your heart and brain health. These include the following:

129

- Avoid breathing secondhand smoke.
- Eat low-fat, low-salt foods, and fresh fruits and vegetables most of the time.
- Maintain a healthy weight.
- Exercise regularly.
- Limit alcohol use.
- Get other health conditions (such as diabetes) under control.

Section 17.5 | Role of Physical Activity in Stroke Prevention

This section contains text excerpted from the following sources: Text in this section begins with excerpts from "Relationship of Sedentary Behavior and Physical Activity to Cardiovascular Disease Risk," Centers for Disease Control and Prevention (CDC), June 19, 2019; Text under the heading "Physical Activity and Cardiovascular Disease" is excerpted from "Physical Activity," Million Hearts®, Centers for Disease Control and Prevention (CDC), October 25, 2019; Text under the heading "Working Up a Sweat May Help Reduce Stroke Risk" is excerpted from "Working Up a Sweat May Help Reduce Stroke Risk," National Institutes of Health (NIH), August 5, 2013. Reviewed May 2020; Text beginning with the heading "What Is an Inactive Lifestyle?" is excerpted from "Health Risks of an Inactive Lifestyle," MedlinePlus, National Institutes of Health (NIH), January 9, 2020.

Few studies have examined the association between sitting time and risk for cardiovascular disease (CVD), and few have looked beyond CVD mortality outcomes. The current analysis reviews CVD events (e.g., heart attack) and new cases of heart disease and stroke in relationship to sitting time and physical activity habits within a large sample. Examining the independent and joint effects of sedentary time and physical activity on the risk for CVD events in older women, the authors found that:

- Overall, a combination of low physical activity and prolonged sitting increases CVD risk. Extended sitting time was associated with increased risk for heart disease, stroke, and CVD, independent of physical activity levels. This association was strongest in women who were overweight or obese and women who were 70 years of age or older.

- Low levels of physical activity were strongly associated with increased CVD risk, independent of sitting time.
- Women who were physically inactive and spent 10 hours or more sitting each day were at 63 percent greater risk for CVD events compared with highly active women who spent 5 hours or fewer each day sitting.
- Women who met physical activity guidelines, but sat for long periods each day were still at increased CVD risk.
- White women, women who attended college, and women with higher incomes were most likely to report sitting 10 hours or more per day.
- Smokers, women with a higher body mass index, and women who reported being depressed were more likely than others to spend prolonged periods sitting and were less likely to engage in physical activity.

PHYSICAL ACTIVITY AND CARDIOVASCULAR DISEASE

To prevent cardiovascular disease, the U.S. Preventive Services Task Force (USPSTF) recommends intensive behavioral counseling to promote physical activity for people with known cardiovascular risk factors. Physical activity can also help people with cardiovascular disease manage their conditions; exercise training has been shown to have a positive effect on people with certain types of heart failure; and cardiac rehabilitation, which includes physical activity training, helps improve the health of people who have had a heart attack or bypass surgery.

Despite the substantial health benefits of physical activity, about 3 in every 10 U.S. adults report being inactive during their leisure time, and only half of U.S. adults report levels of aerobic physical activity consistent with national guidelines. There are evidence-based strategies to promote physical activity that can be put into action where people live, learn, work, and play, including behavioral counseling for adults with cardiovascular risk factors and designing safe community spaces that encourage activity.

WORKING UP A SWEAT TO HELP REDUCE STROKE RISK

Some findings suggest that breaking a sweat during regular physical activity may lower your risk of having a stroke.

To investigate the relationship between physical activity and stroke, a team led by Dr. Michelle N. McDonnell from the University of South Australia and Dr. Virginia Howard of the University of Alabama at Birmingham analyzed data from the Reasons for Geographic and Racial Differences in Stroke (REGARDS) study. The dataset included information on more than 27,000 black and white participants, both men and women, from across the country. They were at least 45 years of age at the time of recruitment and had no prior history of stroke.

The participants were asked how many times per week they exercised to the point of sweating. They were then contacted every six months to see if they had experienced a stroke or a mini-stroke known as a "transient ischemic attack." Participants were followed for an average of 5.7 years. Medical records confirmed their responses. The study was funded by the National Institutes of Health's (NIH) National Institute of Neurological Disorders and Stroke (NINDS). It appeared online on July 18, 2013, in the journal *Stroke*.

Participants who were inactive (exercising less than once a week) were 20 percent more likely to have a stroke or transient ischemic attack than those who exercised at least four times a week. After adjusting for traditional stroke risk factors (diabetes, hypertension, body mass index, alcohol use, and smoking) exercise was not a significant independent predictor of stroke risk, suggesting that the effect of physical activity is mediated through its association with obesity, hypertension, and diabetes.

"Physical inactivity is a major modifiable risk factor for stroke," Howard says. "This should be emphasized in routine physician checkups."

"Exercise reduces blood pressure, weight, and diabetes. If exercise was a pill, you would be taking one pill to treat four or five different conditions," McDonnell says.

One limitation of the study is that it included self-reported data on the frequency of exercise, but not on the duration of activity. Official guidelines recommend that healthy adults (ages 18 to 64) get at least 2.5 hours of moderate aerobic physical activity each week. Activity should be done for at least 10 minutes at a time.

WHAT IS AN INACTIVE LIFESTYLE?

Being a couch potato. Not exercising. A sedentary or inactive lifestyle. You have probably heard of all of these phrases, and they mean the same thing: a lifestyle with a lot of sitting and lying down, with very little to no exercise.

In the United States and around the world, people are spending more and more time doing sedentary activities. During your leisure time, you are often sitting: while using a computer or other device, watching TV, or playing video games. Many of your jobs have become more sedentary, with long days sitting at a desk. And the way most of them get around involves sitting—in cars, on buses, and on trains.

HOW DOES AN INACTIVE LIFESTYLE AFFECT YOUR BODY?

When you have an inactive lifestyle:
- You burn fewer calories. This makes you more likely to gain weight.
- You may lose muscle strength and endurance, because you are not using your muscles as much.
- Your bones may get weaker and lose some mineral content.
- Your metabolism may be affected, and your body may have more trouble breaking down fats and sugars.
- Your immune system may not work as well.
- You may have poorer blood circulation.
- Your body may have more inflammation.
- You may develop a hormonal imbalance.

WHAT ARE THE HEALTH RISKS OF AN INACTIVE LIFESTYLE?

Having an inactive lifestyle can be one of the causes of many chronic diseases. By not getting regular exercise, you raise your risk of:
- Obesity

- Heart diseases, including coronary artery disease and heart attack
- High blood pressure
- High cholesterol
- Stroke
- Metabolic syndrome
- Type 2 diabetes
- Certain cancers, including colon, breast, and uterine cancers
- Osteoporosis and falls
- Increased feelings of depression and anxiety

Having a sedentary lifestyle can also raise your risk of premature death. And the more sedentary you are, the higher your health risks are.

HOW CAN YOU GET STARTED WITH EXERCISE?

If you have been inactive, you may need to start slowly. You can keep adding more exercise gradually. The more you can do, the better. But, try not to feel overwhelmed, and do what you can. Getting some exercise is always better than getting none. Eventually, your goal can be to get the recommended amount of exercise for your age and health.

There are many different ways to get exercise; it is important to find the types that are best for you. You can also try to add activity to your life in smaller ways, such as at home and at work.

HOW CAN YOU BE MORE ACTIVE AROUND THE HOUSE?

There are some ways you can be active around your house:
- Housework, gardening, and yard work are all physical work. To increase the intensity, you could try doing them at a more vigorous pace.
- Keep moving while you watch TV. Lift hand weights, do some gentle yoga stretches, or pedal an exercise bike. Instead of using the TV remote, get up and change the channels yourself.

- Work out at home with a workout video (on your TV or on the Internet).
- Go for a walk in your neighborhood. It can be more fun if you walk your dog, walk your kids to school, or walk with a friend.
- Stand up when talking on the phone.
- Get some exercise equipment for your home. Treadmills and elliptical trainers are great, but not everyone has the money or space for one.
- Less expensive equipment such as yoga balls, exercise mats, stretch bands, and hand weights can help you get a workout at home too.

HOW CAN YOU BE MORE ACTIVE AT WORK?

Most of us sit when we are working, often in front of a computer. In fact, less than 20 percent of Americans have physically active jobs. It can be challenging to fit physical activity into your busy workday, but here are some tips to help you get moving:

- Get up from your chair and move around at least once an hour.
- Stand when you are talking on the phone.
- Find out whether your company can get you a stand-up or treadmill desk.
- Take the stairs instead of the elevator.
- Use your break or part of your lunch hour to walk around the building.
- Stand up and walk to a colleague's office instead of sending an e-mail.
- Have walking or standing meetings with coworkers instead of sitting in a conference room.

Section 17.6 | **Dietary Pattern and Nutritional Status in Stroke Prevention**

This section contains text excerpted from the following sources: Text in this section begins with excerpts from "How Dietary Factors Influence Disease Risk," National Institutes of Health (NIH), March 14, 2017; Text under the heading "Dietary Patterns Associated with Decreased Risk of Cardiovascular Disease" is excerpted from "Dietary Patterns and Risk of Cardiovascular Disease," U.S. Department of Agriculture (USDA), March 14, 2014. Reviewed May 2020; Text under the heading "Eating an Healthy Diet" is excerpted from "Prescribing Healthy Foods Could Bring Cost-Effective Benefits," National Institutes of Health (NIH), April 2, 2019; Text beginning with the heading "How to Lower Your Blood Pressure Using DASH?" is excerpted from "Your Guide to Lowering Your Blood Pressure with DASH," National Heart, Lung, and Blood Institute (NHLBI), August 2015. Reviewed May 2020; Text beginning with the heading "The DASH Eating Plan" is excerpted from "Facts about the DASH Eating Plan," U.S. Department of Veterans Affairs (VA), May 1, 2003. Reviewed May 2020.

Having too much sugar, salt, or fat in your diet can raise your risk for certain diseases. Healthy eating can lower your risk for heart disease, stroke, diabetes, and other health conditions. A healthy eating plan emphasizes vegetables, fruits, whole grains, and fat-free or low-fat dairy products; includes lean meats, poultry, fish, beans, eggs, and nuts; and limits saturated and trans fats, sodium, and added sugars.

The major cardiometabolic diseases—heart disease, stroke, and type 2 diabetes—pose substantial health and economic burdens on society. To better understand how different dietary components affect the risk of dying from these diseases, a research team led by Dr. Dariush Mozaffarian of Tufts University analyzed data from the Centers for Disease Control and Prevention's (CDC) National Health and Nutrition Examination Survey (NHANES) and national disease-specific mortality data. The study was supported in part by the National Institutes of Health's (NIH) National Heart, Lung, and Blood Institute (NHLBI). Results appeared on March 7, 2017, in the *Journal of the American Medical Association.*

The researchers investigated the relationships of 10 different foods and nutrients with deaths related to heart disease, stroke, and type 2 diabetes. They also compared data on participants' age, sex, ethnicity, and education. They found that nearly half of all the deaths in the United States in 2012 that were caused by cardiometabolic diseases were associated with suboptimal eating habits. Of 702,308 adult deaths due to heart disease, stroke, and type 2 diabetes, 318,656 (45%) were associated with inadequate consumption of certain foods and nutrients widely considered vital for healthy living, and over consumption of other foods that are not.

The highest percentage of cardiometabolic disease-related death (9.5%) was related to excess consumption of sodium. Not eating enough nuts and seeds (8.5%), seafood omega-3 fats (7.8%), vegetables (7.6%), fruits (7.5%), whole grains (5.9%), or polyunsaturated fats (2.3%) also increased risk of death compared with people who had an optimal intake of these foods or nutrients. Eating too much processed meat (8.2%), sugar-sweetened beverages (7.4%), and unprocessed red meat (0.4%) also raised the risk of heart disease, stroke, and type 2 diabetes-related deaths.

DIETARY PATTERNS ASSOCIATED WITH DECREASED RISK OF CARDIOVASCULAR DISEASE

Dietary patterns associated with decreased risk of cardiovascular disease were characterized by regular consumption of fruits, vegetables, whole grains, low-fat dairy, and fish, and were low in red and processed meat and sugar sweetened foods and drinks. Regular consumption of nuts and legumes and moderate consumption of alcohol were also shown to be beneficial in most studies. Additionally, research that included specific nutrients in their description of dietary patterns indicated that patterns that were low in saturated fat, cholesterol, and sodium, and rich in fiber and potassium may be beneficial for reducing cardiovascular disease risk.

EATING A HEALTHY DIET

Your diet plays an important role in your health. An unhealthy diet is one of the leading risk factors for cardiometabolic diseases such as heart disease, stroke, and diabetes.

Eating a healthy diet can lower your risk for some of these conditions. A healthy eating plan includes vegetables, fruits, whole grains, fat-free or low-fat dairy products, lean meats, poultry, fish, beans, eggs, and nuts. It also limits how much sugar, salt, and fat you eat.

Prescribing healthy foods is one potential approach to help lower heart disease and other cardiometabolic conditions. However, it has not been well established whether this would be cost-effective or help lower the disease burden.

If the fruit and the vegetable incentive was carried out over a lifetime, the model estimated that the average consumption of fruits and vegetables would increase by about 0.4 servings per day. This would prevent about 1.93 million cardiovascular disease events and save $39.7 billion in healthcare costs.

The model predicted that the general healthy foods incentive carried out over a lifetime would increase fruit and vegetable intake by the same amount. It would also increase the average consumption of whole grains by 0.2 servings per day, nuts and seeds by 0.1 servings, seafood by 0.2 servings, and plant oils by 1.5 teaspoons. This would prevent about 3.28 million cardiovascular disease events and 120,000 cases of diabetes and save $100.2 billion in healthcare costs.

HOW TO LOWER YOUR BLOOD PRESSURE USING DASH?

The DASH eating plan is rich in fruits, vegetables, fat-free or low-fat milk and milk products, whole grains, fish, poultry, beans, seeds, and nuts. It also contains less sodium; sweets, added sugars, and beverages containing sugar; fats; and red meats than the typical American diet. This heart-healthy way of eating is also lower in saturated fat, trans fat, and cholesterol and rich in nutrients that are associated with lowering blood pressure—mainly potassium, magnesium, calcium, protein, and fiber.

HOW DO YOU MAKE THE DASH?

The DASH eating plan requires no special foods and has no hard-to-follow recipes. It simply calls for a certain number of daily servings from various food groups.

The number of servings depends on the number of calories you are allowed each day. Your calorie level depends on your age and, especially, how active you are. Think of this as an energy balance system—if you want to maintain your current weight, you should take in only as many calories as you burn by being physically active. If you need to lose weight, eat fewer calories than you burn or increase your activity level to burn more calories than you eat.

What is your physical activity level? Are you mostly:
- Sedentary? You do only light physical activity that is part of your typical day-to-day routine.
- Moderately active? You do physical activity equal to walking about one to three miles a day at three to four miles per hour, plus light physical activity.
- Active? You do physical activity equal to walking more than three miles per day at three to four miles per hour, plus light physical activity.

THE DASH EATING PLAN

Research has found that diet affects the development of high blood pressure, or hypertension (the medical term). The studies showed that blood pressure can be lowered by following a particular eating plan—called the "Dietary Approaches to Stop Hypertension" eating plan—and reducing the amount of sodium consumed.

While each step alone lowers blood pressure, the combination of the eating plan and a reduced sodium intake gives the biggest benefit and may help prevent the development of high blood pressure.

The DASH research findings, tells about high blood pressure, and how to follow the DASH eating plan and reduce the amount of sodium you consume. It offers tips on how to start and stay on the eating plan, as well as a week of menus and some recipes. The menus and recipes are given for two levels of daily sodium consumption—2,400 milligrams (the upper limit recommendations by the federal government's National High Blood Pressure Education Program (NHBPEP) and the amount used to figure food labels' Nutrition Facts Daily Value) and 1,500 milligrams.

WHAT IS THE DASH EATING PLAN?

Blood pressure can be unhealthy even if it stays only slightly above the normal level of less than 120/80 mmHg. The higher blood pressure rises above normal, the greater the health risk.

139

In the past, researchers tried to find clues about what in the diet affects blood pressure by testing various single nutrients, such as calcium and magnesium. These studies were done mostly with dietary supplements and their findings were not conclusive.

Then, scientists supported by the National Heart, Lung, and Blood Institute (NHLBI) conducted two key studies. The first was called "Dietary Approaches to Stop Hypertension"(DASH), and it tested nutrients as they occur together in food. Its findings showed that blood pressures were reduced with an eating plan that is low in saturated fat, cholesterol, and total fat, and that emphasizes fruits, vegetables, and low-fat dairy foods. This eating plan—known as the "DASH eating plan"—also includes whole-grain products, fish, poultry, and nuts. It is reduced in red meat, sweets, and sugar-containing beverages. It is rich in magnesium, potassium, and calcium, as well as protein and fiber.

The DASH study involved 459 adults with systolic blood pressures of less than 160 mmHg and diastolic pressures of 80 to 95 mmHg. About 27 percent of the participants had hypertension. About 50 percent were women and 60 percent were African Americans.

DASH compared three eating plans: A plan similar in nutrients to what many Americans consume; a plan similar to what Americans consume, but higher in fruits and vegetables; and the DASH eating plan. All three plans included about 3,000 milligrams of sodium daily. None of the plans was vegetarian or used specialty foods.

Results Were Dramatic

Both the fruits and vegetables plan and the DASH eating plan reduced blood pressure. But, the DASH eating plan had the greatest effect, especially for those with high blood pressure. Furthermore, the blood pressure reductions came fast—within two weeks of starting the plan.

Results showed that reducing dietary sodium lowered blood pressure for both eating plans. At each sodium level, blood pressure was lower on the DASH eating plan than on the other eating plan. The biggest blood pressure reductions were for the DASH eating plan at the sodium intake of 1,500 milligrams per day. Those with hypertension saw the biggest reductions, but those without it also had large decreases. Those on the 1,500-milligram sodium intake eating plan, as well as those on the DASH eating plan, had fewer headaches. Other than that and blood pressure levels, there were no significant effects caused by the two eating plans or different sodium levels. DASH-Sodium shows the importance of lowering sodium intake—whatever your eating plan. But, for a true winning combination, follow the DASH eating plan and lower your intake of salt and sodium.

How to Lower Calories on the DASH Eating Plan

The DASH eating plan was not designed to promote weight loss. But, it is rich in lower-calorie foods, such as fruits and vegetables. You can make it lower in calories by replacing higher-calorie foods with more fruits and vegetables—and that also will make it easier for you to reach your DASH goals. Here are some examples:

To increase fruits:
- Eat a medium apple instead of four shortbread cookies. You will save 80 calories.
- Eat 1/4 cup of dried apricots instead of a 2-ounce bag of pork rinds. You will save 230 calories.

To increase vegetables:
- Have a hamburger that is three ounces of meat instead of 6 ounces. Add 1/2 cup serving of carrots and 1/2 cup serving of spinach. You will save more than 200 calories.
- Instead of five ounces of chicken, have a stir-fry with 2 ounces of chicken and 11/2 cups of raw vegetables. Use a small amount of vegetable oil. You will save 50 calories.

To increase low-fat or fat-free dairy products:
- Have a 1/2 cup serving of low-fat frozen yogurt instead of a 11/2-ounce milk chocolate bar. You will save about 110 calories.

And do not forget these calorie-saving tips:
- Use low fat or fat-free condiments.
- Use half as much vegetable oil, soft or liquid margarine, or salad dressing, or choose fat free versions.
- Eat smaller portions—cut back gradually. Choose low fat or fat-free dairy products to reduce total fat intake.
- Check the food labels to compare fat content in packaged foods—items marked low fat or fat free are not always lower in calories than their regular versions.
- Limit foods with lots of added sugar such as pies, flavored yogurts, candy bars, ice cream, sherbet, regular soft drinks, and fruit drinks.
- Eat fruits canned in their own juice.
- Add fruit to plain yogurt.
- Snack on fruit, vegetable sticks, unbuttered and unsalted popcorn, or bread sticks.
- Drink water or club soda.

You should be aware that the DASH eating plan has more daily servings of fruits, vegetables, and whole-grain foods than you may be used to eating. Because the plan is high in fiber, it can cause bloating and diarrhea in some people. To avoid these problems, gradually increase your intake of fruits, vegetables, and whole-grain foods. This gives menus and recipes for both 2,400 and 1,500 milligrams of daily sodium intake. Twenty-four hundred milligrams of sodium equals about six grams, or one teaspoon, of table salt (sodium chloride); 1,500 milligrams of sodium equals about 4 grams, or 2/3 teaspoon, of table salt. These amounts include all salt consumed— that in food products, used in cooking, and added to the table. Only small amounts of sodium occur naturally in food. Processed foods account for most of the salt and sodium Americans consume. So, be sure to read food labels to choose products lower in sodium. You may be surprised at many of the foods that have sodium. They include soy sauce, seasoned salts, monosodium glutamate (MSG), baking soda, and some antacids—the range is wide. Because it is rich in fruits and vegetables, which are naturally lower in sodium than many other foods, the DASH eating plan makes it easier to consume less salt and sodium.

Part 3 | Diagnosis and Treatment of Stroke

Chapter 18 | Emergency Medical Services: The First Line of Defense

Chapter Contents

Section 18.1 | Importance of Prehospital Treatment for Stroke

This section includes text excerpted from "Think It Is a Stroke? 4 Reasons It Is Better to Call 9-1-1 than Drive Yourself to the Hospital," Centers for Disease Control and Prevention (CDC), May 23, 2017.

PREHOSPITAL TREATMENT FOR STROKE

Your best chance for surviving a stroke and having a full recovery is getting to the hospital quickly. But did you know that one in three stroke patients do not call an ambulance? Instead, they may not recognize they are having a stroke, try to wait to see if their symptoms go away, or may try to drive themselves or have another person drive them to the emergency room. All of these things actually increase your risk for disability and death.

Learn why it is always best to call 911 if you think that someone is having a stroke.

- **Emergency medical services (EMS) gets you to the hospital faster.** You may think that you will get to the hospital faster if you drive yourself or have a loved one drive you during a stroke. But, the truth is, the EMS professionals on board may be able to start your treatment right away. Think of calling the doctor as bringing emergency room resources to your door. Ambulance drivers also have the right of way when they use lights and sirens.
- **EMS saves precious time once you reach the hospital.** You are more likely to be treated quicker at the hospital when you arrive by ambulance. This is because, on the way to the hospital, EMS professionals begin your treatment by:
  - Screening you for stroke symptoms
  - Monitoring your heart rate and blood pressure
  - Getting information about any medicines you take, your medical history, or other important information a medical team needs to know
  - Calling ahead to the hospital to let the medical team know a stroke patient is arriving. This gives the hospital team time to prepare equipment and medicines that you may need.

- **You can get an important drug to treat strokes if you call the doctor right away.** When it comes to stroke, time lost is brain lost. Every minute a stroke goes untreated, a patient loses nearly two million brain cells. Because stroke is often caused by a blood clot, a clot-busting drug, such as alteplase is an effective treatment if you get to the hospital in time. But, clot-busting drugs can only be given to patients within three hours of a stroke. EMS professionals responding to a call about stroke will ask the patient and any bystanders questions about when the symptoms started, giving the medical team critical information about whether the patient can be treated with the clot-busting drug. At the hospital, you are also more likely to get alteplase if you arrive by ambulance. Many stroke patients who need the drug do not get it, because they wait too long to call the doctor or get to the hospital too late for treatment.
- **EMS can get you to a hospital that specializes in stroke treatment.** When stroke happens, getting to any hospital is important. But, some hospitals are better equipped than others to treat stroke patients. Hospitals that specialize in stroke, like certified stroke centers, have developed standards of care for stroke patients and may have more staff, medicine, and equipment for treating stroke on hand. There are more than 1,000 certified stroke centers nationwide. Find a stroke center near you.

Stroke happens to nearly 800,000 Americans a year. Do not hesitate to call the doctor right away if you suspect a stroke is happening to you or someone else because that is the best chance at survival, treatment, and recovery.

Section 18.2 | EMS Stroke Field Triage Improves Outcomes

This section contains text excerpted from the following sources: Text in this section begins with excerpts from "Emergency Medical Services: The First Step to Stroke Recovery," Centers for Disease Control and Prevention (CDC), May 16, 2017; Text beginning with the heading "What and How Should EMT-Basics Be Taught?" is excerpted from "Proceedings of a National Symposium on Acute Stroke," National Institutes of Health (NIH), June 19, 2008. Reviewed May 2020.

Emergency medical services (EMS) professionals, such as paramedics and emergency technicians, are key to a stroke patient's treatment. Learn how the Coverdell program supports EMS through training and resources.

THE COVERDELL PROGRAM AND EMERGENCY MEDICAL SERVICES

The Coverdell program seeks to improve the time it takes for a stroke patient to receive the necessary treatment at the hospital. Improving the quality of care for stroke patients during EMS transport is crucial to improving health outcomes for patients with this time-sensitive condition.

Most strokes are caused by a clot in the brain, which blocks blood flow and causes brain cells to die. A common treatment for this type of stroke is a clot-busting drug, but for most patients, it must be given within three hours of having a stroke to be effective. In addition, to quickly transporting the patient to a hospital or certified stroke center, EMS professionals ask questions about stroke symptoms and when they started. This information helps the medical team at the hospital act more quickly to administer the clot-busting drug or other treatments that can save a patient's life and improve recovery time from stroke.

The Coverdell program helps support EMS in this mission. Funded states provide training and resources for hospitals and EMS agencies on collecting and sharing data and ways to improve the patient hand-off at the emergency room. The Coverdell program also helps standardize stroke performance measures across the nation to provide more opportunities for collaboration and learning.

EMERGENCY MEDICAL SERVICES SUCCESS STORIES

Partnerships with EMS agencies through the Coverdell program improve the quality of care for stroke patients in many states.

- In 2013, Georgia's Coverdell Program wrote a set of guidelines on stroke care for EMS. Just one year later, stroke patients were receiving potentially life-saving medicine eight minutes sooner, on average.
- In 2015 in New York, 7 in 10 stroke patients got a necessary clot-busting drug within one hour, compared to 6 in 10 in 2014.
- The Massachusetts Coverdell team developed a patient education program for 344 nursing home and skilled nursing facility employees on the F.A.S.T. assessment. The percentage of staff who knew the importance of acting quickly and who could accurately identify symptoms rose from 66 percent to 94 percent.

WHAT AND HOW SHOULD EMERGENCY MEDICAL TECHNICIANS-BASICS BE TAUGHT?

Emergency medical technicians (EMTs)-basics must learn to recognize the key symptoms of an acute stroke. Studies need to measure the impact of such training on the accuracy of stroke diagnosis by EMT-basics and paramedics. EMT-basics should be taught about stroke using the following objectives:

- To gain a better understanding of the etiology of stroke, including the two major types of stroke and the three conditions that cause blockages
- To describe the biochemical sequence of events that occurs during a stroke and to gain insight into why a stroke must be treated within the first three to six hours
- To identify the signs and symptoms of stroke and list the common dispatch complaints for stroke
- To understand the importance of a transient ischaemic attack (TIA)
- To obtain and interpret the key vital signs in the stroke patient

- To determine the time of symptom onset, including asking bystanders when the patient was last at baseline neurological function
- To perform a simple physical assessment including testing for aphasia ("The sky is blue in Cincinnati"), facial weakness (show teeth), and motor weakness (pronator and arm drift)
- To encourage bystanders or family members to accompany the patient to the hospital so they can provide historical information to the treating team and provide support to the patient. If bystanders cannot go to the hospital, EMT-basics should obtain a telephone number where they can be contacted
- To notify the receiving hospital about the impending arrival of an acute stroke patient

WHAT AND HOW SHOULD PARAMEDICS BE TAUGHT?

Paramedics also need to learn skills for the early identification of the stroke patient. Early notification of the receiving emergency department (ED) is an important part of this process. In addition, paramedics need to have a good understanding of the pathophysiology of stroke including the etiology. They need to be aware of the primary risk factors.

Paramedics also need to learn to recognize hypertension in the stroke patient, and literature needs to be developed to support that knowledge. They need to be made aware that thrombolytic therapy is available in hospitals. Paramedics need to understand the mechanism of action of thrombolytic therapy for stroke as well as the indications and contraindications for that treatment so they can accurately advise the receiving hospital of a potentially treatable patient.

They need to be aware of other, still experimental, therapies that may be useful in the early management of the stroke patient. Therapies, such as intra arterial thrombolytics might require that some acute stroke patients be transported to hospitals other than the closest available hospital. The development of neuroprotective agents may permit some therapy to be initiated in the prehospital setting. However, studies still need to be done to demonstrate that such therapy is safe and effective when given before hospital arrival.

Chapter 19 | After a Stroke: The First 24 Hours

Chapter Contents

Section 19.1 | Stroke Scale: Assessing Stroke Severity

This section includes text excerpted from "NIH Stroke Scale," Know Stroke, National Institute of Neurological Disorders and Stroke (NINDS), February 1, 2001. Reviewed May 2020.

Administer stroke scale items in the order listed. Record performance in each category after each subscale exam. Do not go back and change scores. Follow directions provided for each exam technique. Scores should reflect what the patient does, not what the clinician thinks the patient can do. The clinician should record answers while administering the exam and work quickly. Except where indicated, the patient should not be coached (i.e., repeated requests to the patient to make a special effort).

STROKE SCALE: 1A
Instructions—Level of Consciousness
The investigator must choose a response if a full evaluation is prevented by such obstacles as an endotracheal tube, language barrier, orotracheal trauma/bandages. A 3 is scored only if the patient makes no movement (other than reflexive posturing) in response to noxious stimulation.

Scale Definition
- 0 = Alert; keenly responsive
- 1 = Not alert; but arousable by minor stimulation to obey, answer, or respond
- 2 = Not alert; requires repeated stimulation to attend, or is obtunded and requires strong or painful stimulation to make movements (not stereotyped)
- 3 = Responds only with reflex motor or autonomic effects, or totally unresponsive, flaccid, and areflexic

STROKE SCALE: 1B
Level of Consciousness Questions
The patient is asked the month and her or his age. The answer must be correct—there is no partial credit for being close. Aphasic and

157

stuporous patients who do not comprehend the questions will score 2. Patients unable to speak because of endotracheal intubation, orotracheal trauma, severe dysarthria from any cause, language barrier, or any other problem not secondary to aphasia are given a 1. It is important that only the initial answer be graded and that the examiner not "help" the patient with verbal or nonverbal cues.

Scale Definition
- 0 = Answers both questions correctly
- 1 = Answers one question correctly
- 2 = Answers neither question correctly

STROKE SCALE: 1C
Level of Consciousness Questions
The patient is asked to open and close the eyes and then to grip and release the nonparetic hand. Substitute another one-step command if the hands cannot be used. Credit is given if an unequivocal attempt is made, but not completed due to weakness. If the patient does not respond to command, the task should be demonstrated to her or him (pantomime), and the result scored (i.e., follows none, one, or two commands). Patients with trauma, amputation, or other physical impediments should be given suitable one-step commands. Only the first attempt is scored.

Scale Definition
- 0 = Performs both tasks correctly
- 1 = Performs one task correctly
- 2 = Performs neither task correctly

STROKE SCALE: 2
Instructions
Only horizontal eye movements will be tested. Voluntary or reflexive (oculocephalic) eye movements will be scored, but caloric testing is not done. If the patient has a conjugate deviation of the eyes that can be overcome by voluntary or reflexive activity, the score

will be 1. If a patient has an isolated peripheral nerve paresis (CN III, IV, or VI), score a 1. Gaze is testable in all aphasic patients. Patients with ocular trauma, bandages, preexisting blindness, or other disorder of visual acuity or fields should be tested with reflexive movements, and a choice made by the investigator. Establishing eye contact and then moving about the patient from side to side will occasionally clarify the presence of a partial gaze palsy.

Scale Definition
- 0 = Normal
- 1 = Partial gaze palsy; gaze is abnormal in one or both eyes, but forced deviation or total gaze paresis is not present
- 2 = Forced deviation, or total gaze paresis is not overcome by the oculocephalic maneuver

STROKE SCALE: 3
Instructions
VISUAL
Visual fields (upper and lower quadrants) are tested by confrontation, using finger counting or visual threat, as appropriate. Patients may be encouraged, but if they look at the side of the moving fingers appropriately, this can be scored as normal. If there is unilateral blindness or enucleation, visual fields in the remaining eye are scored. Score 1 only if a clear-cut asymmetry, including quadrantanopia, is found. If a patient is blind from any cause, score 3. Double simultaneous stimulation is performed at this point. If there is extinction, the patient receives a 1, and the results are used to respond to item 11.

Scale Definition
- 0 = No visual loss
- 1 = Partial hemianopia
- 2 = Complete hemianopia
- 3 = Bilateral hemianopia (blind including cortical blindness)

STROKE SCALE: 4
Instructions
FACIAL PALSY

Ask or use pantomime to encourage the patient to show teeth or raise eyebrows and close eyes. Score symmetry of grimace in response to noxious stimuli in the poorly responsive or noncomprehending patient. If facial trauma/bandages, orotracheal tube, tape, or other physical barriers obscure the face, these should be removed to the extent possible.

Scale Definition

- 0 = Normal symmetrical movements
- 1 = Minor paralysis (flattened nasolabial fold, asymmetry on smiling)
- 2 = Partial paralysis (total or near-total paralysis of lower face)
- 3 = Complete paralysis of one or both sides (absence of facial movement in the upper and lower face)

STROKE SCALE: 5
Instructions
MOTOR ARM

The limb is placed in the appropriate position: extend the arms (palms down) 90 degrees (if sitting) or 45 degrees (if supine). Drift is scored if the arm falls before 10 seconds. The aphasic patient is encouraged using urgency in the voice and pantomime, but not noxious stimulation. Each limb is tested in turn, beginning with the nonparetic arm. Only in the case of amputation or joint fusion at the shoulder, the examiner should record the score as untestable (UN) and clearly write the explanation for this choice.

Scale Definition

- 0 = No drift; limb holds 90 (or 45) degrees for full 10 seconds
- 1 = Drift; limb holds 90 (or 45) degrees, but drifts down before full 10 seconds; does not hit bed or other support

- 2 = Some effort against gravity; limb cannot get to or maintain (if cued) 90 (or 45) degrees, drifts down to bed, but has some effort against gravity
- 3 = No effort against gravity; limb falls
- 4 = No movement
- UN = Amputation or joint fusion, explain

STROKE SCALE: 6
Instructions
MOTOR LEG

The limb is placed in the appropriate position: hold the leg at 30 degrees (always tested supine). Drift is scored if the leg falls before 5 seconds. The aphasic patient is encouraged using urgency in the voice and pantomime, but not noxious stimulation. Each limb is tested in turn, beginning with the nonparetic leg. Only in the case of amputation or joint fusion at the hip, the examiner should record the score as untestable (UN) and clearly write the explanation for this choice.

Scale Definition
- 0 = No drift; leg holds 30-degree position for full 5 seconds
- 1 = Drift; leg falls by the end of the 5 second period, but does not hit the bed
- 2 = Some effort against gravity; leg falls to bed by 5 seconds, but has some effort against gravity
- 3 = No effort against gravity; leg falls to bed immediately
- 4 = No movement
- UN = Amputation or joint fusion, explain

STROKE SCALE: 7
Instructions
LIMB ATAXIA

Limb Ataxia is aimed at finding evidence of a unilateral cerebellar lesion. Test with eyes open. In case of visual defect, ensure testing is done in intact visual field. The finger-nose-finger and heel-shin tests are performed on both sides, and ataxia is scored only if present out of proportion to weakness. Ataxia is absent in the patient who cannot understand or is paralyzed. Only in the case of amputation or joint fusion, the examiner should record the score as untestable (UN) and clearly write the explanation for this choice. In case of blindness, test by having the patient touch her or his nose from an extended arm position.

Scale Definition
- 0 = Absent
- 1 = Present in one limb
- 2 = Present in two limbs
- UN = Amputation or joint fusion, explain

STROKE SCALE: 8
Instructions
SENSORY

Sensation or grimace to pinprick when tested, or withdrawal from the noxious stimulus in the obtunded or aphasic patient. Only sensory loss attributed to stroke is scored as abnormal and the examiner should test as many body areas [arms (not hands), legs, trunk, face] as needed to accurately check for hemisensory loss. A score of 2, "severe or total sensory loss," should only be given when a severe or total loss of sensation can be clearly demonstrated. Stuporous and aphasic patients will, therefore, probably score 1 or 0. The patient with brainstem stroke who has bilateral loss of sensation is scored 2. If the patient does not respond and is quadriplegic, score 2. Patients in a coma (item 1a=3) are automatically given a 2 on this item.

Scale Definition
- 0 = Normal; no sensory loss
- 1 = Mild-to-moderate sensory loss; patient feels pinprick is less sharp or is dull on the affected side; or there is a loss of superficial pain with pinprick, but patient is aware of being touched

- 2 = Severe or total sensory loss; patient is not aware of being touched in the face, arm, and leg

STROKE SCALE: 9
Instructions
BEST LANGUAGE

A great deal of information about comprehension will be obtained during the preceding sections of the examination. For this scale item, the patient is asked to describe what is happening in the attached picture, to name the items on the attached naming sheet, and to read from the attached list of sentences. Comprehension is judged from responses here, as well as to all of the commands in the preceding general neurological exam. If visual loss interferes with the tests, ask the patient to identify objects placed in the hand, repeat, and produce speech. The intubated patient should be asked to write. The patient in a coma (item 1a=3) will automatically score three on this item. The examiner must choose a score for the patient with stupor or limited cooperation, but a score of three should be used only if the patient is mute and follows no one-step commands.

Scale Definition

- 0 = No aphasia; normal
- 1 = Mild-to-moderate aphasia; some obvious loss of fluency or facility of comprehension, without significant limitation on ideas expressed or form of expression. Reduction of speech and/or comprehension, however, makes conversation about provided materials difficult or impossible. For example, in conversation about provided materials, the examiner can identify picture or naming card content from the patient's response
- 2 = Severe aphasia; all communication is through fragmentary expression; great need for inference, questioning, and guessing by the listener. Range of information that can be exchanged is limited; the listener carries a burden of communication. Examiners cannot identify materials provided from patient response

- 3 = Mute, global aphasia; no usable speech or auditory comprehension

STROKE SCALE: 10
Instructions
DYSARTHRIA

If a patient is thought to be normal, an adequate sample of speech must be obtained by asking the patient to read or repeat words from the National Institutes of Health (NIH) Stroke Scale document. If the patient has severe aphasia, the clarity of articulation of spontaneous speech can be rated. Only if the patient is intubated or has other physical barriers to producing speech, the examiner should record the score as untestable (UN) and clearly write the explanation for this choice. Do not tell the patient why she or he is being tested.

Scale Definition
- 0 = Normal
- 1 = Mild-to-moderate dysarthria; patient slurs at least some words and, at worst, can be understood with some difficulty.
- 2 = Severe dysarthria; patient's speech is so slurred as to be unintelligible in the absence of or out of proportion to any dysphasia, or is mute/anarthric
- UN = Intubated or other physical barrier, explain

STROKE SCALE: 11
Instructions
EXTINCTION AND INATTENTION (FORMERLY NEGLECT)

Sufficient information to identify neglect may be obtained during the prior testing. If the patient has a severe visual loss preventing visual double simultaneous stimulation, and the cutaneous stimuli are normal, the score is normal. If the patient has aphasia, but does appear to attend to both sides, the score is normal. The presence of visual-spatial neglect or anosognosia may also be taken as evidence of abnormality. Since the abnormality is scored only if present, the item is never untestable.

Scale Definition
- 0 = No abnormality
- 1 = Visual, tactile, auditory, spatial, or personal inattention, or extinction to bilateral simultaneous stimulation in one of the sensory modalities
- 2 = Profound hemi-inattention or extinction to more than one modality; does not recognize own hand or orients to only one side of space

Section 19.2 | Stroke Treatment: An Overview

This section includes text excerpted from "Stroke Treatment," Centers for Disease Control and Prevention (CDC), November 14, 2019.

Your stroke treatment begins the moment emergency medical services (EMS) arrives to take you to the hospital. Once at the hospital, you may receive emergency care, treatment to prevent another stroke, rehabilitation to treat the side effects of stroke, or all three.

ON THE WAY TO THE HOSPITAL
If someone you know shows signs of stroke, call the doctor right away.

Do not drive to the hospital or let someone else drive you. The key to stroke treatment and recovery is getting to the hospital quickly. Yet 1 in 3 stroke patients never calls 911. Calling an ambulance means that medical staff can begin life-saving treatment on the way to the emergency room.

Stroke patients who are taken to the hospital in an ambulance may get diagnosed and treated more quickly than people who do not arrive in an ambulance. This is because emergency treatment starts on the way to the hospital. The emergency workers may take you to a specialized stroke center to ensure that you receive the quickest possible diagnosis and treatment. The emergency workers will also collect valuable information that guides treatment and alert hospital medical staff before you arrive at the emergency room, giving them time to prepare.

WHAT HAPPENS AT THE HOSPITAL

At the hospital, health professionals will ask about your medical history and about the time your symptoms started. Brain scans will show what type of stroke you had. You may also work with a neurologist who treats brain disorders, a neurosurgeon that performs surgery on the brain, or a specialist in another area of medicine.

If you get to the hospital within three hours of the first symptoms of an ischemic stroke, you may get a type of medicine called a "thrombolytic" (a "clot-busting" drug) to breakup blood clots. Tissue plasminogen activator (tPA) is a thrombolytic.

The tPA improves the chances of recovering from a stroke. Studies show that patients with ischemic strokes who receive tPA are more likely to recover fully or have less disability than patients who do not receive the drug. Patients treated with tPA are also less likely to need long-term care in a nursing home. Unfortunately, many stroke victims do not get to the hospital in time for tPA treatment. This is why it is so important to recognize the signs and symptoms of stroke right away and call the doctor.

Medicine, surgery, or other procedures may be needed to stop the bleeding and save brain tissue. For example:

- **Endovascular procedures.** Endovascular procedures may be used to treat certain hemorrhagic strokes. The doctor inserts a long tube through a major artery in the leg or arm and then guides the tube to the site of the weak spot or break in a blood vessel. The tube is then used to install a device, such as a coil, to repair the damage or prevent bleeding.
- **Surgical treatment.** Hemorrhagic strokes may be treated with surgery. If the bleeding is caused by a ruptured aneurysm, a metal clip may be put in place to stop the blood loss.

WHAT HAPPENS NEXT

If you have had a stroke, you are at high risk for another stroke:

- One in four stroke survivors has another stroke within five years.
- The risk of stroke within 90 days of a TIA may be as high as 17 percent, with the greatest risk during the first week.

That is why it is important to treat the underlying causes of stroke, including heart disease, high blood pressure, atrial fibrillation (fast, irregular heartbeat), high cholesterol, and diabetes. Your doctor may give you medications or tell you to change your diet, exercise, or adopt other healthy lifestyle habits. Surgery may also be helpful in some cases.

STROKE REHABILITATION

After a stroke, you may need rehabilitation (rehab) to help you recover. Before you are discharged from the hospital, social workers can help you find care services and caregiver support to continue your long-term recovery. It is important to work with your healthcare team to find out the reasons for your stroke and take steps to prevent another stroke.

Chapter 20 | Working with a Neurologist

Neurologists are medical doctors who specialize in diagnosing, treating, and managing disorders of the brain and nervous system, including the peripheral nerves that connect the brain to organs and muscles throughout the body. Their extensive training includes an undergraduate degree, four years of medical school, a one-year internship, and a minimum of three years of specialty training. In addition, many neurologists train in subspecialties, such as specific diseases or disorders that affect particular body systems. Because of the complexity of the brain and nervous system, which influence and control so many bodily functions, neurologists must be extremely detail-oriented and attuned to even the smallest signs of neurological problems.

WHAT DO NEUROLOGISTS DO?

Neurologists do not perform surgery but rather treat disorders through the use of medication, physical therapy, and rehabilitation. However, the neurosurgeons who do perform surgeries always work with neurologists to ensure the best possible outcome for the patient, so consulting is another important role for a neurologist. And when patients require ongoing treatment, the neurologist is often the principal care provider. Some of the disorders treated by neurologists include:

- Headaches
- Pain
- Stroke

"Working with a Neurologist," © 2017 Omnigraphics. Reviewed May 2020.

169

- Brain tumors
- Sleep disorders
- Epilepsy
- Brain and spinal cord injuries
- Parkinson disease
- Seizure disorders
- Alzheimer disease
- Multiple sclerosis
- Amyotrophic lateral sclerosis (ALS, or Lou Gehrig disease)

HOW DO NEUROLOGISTS DIAGNOSE DISORDERS?

As is the case with most doctors, the first thing a neurologist will do is perform an examination of the patient. This includes a review of the person's medical history and a discussion of the current condition, followed by a neurological exam. This will generally include an assessment of the patient's vision, hearing, reflexes, strength, and coordination. Often, additional tests will be required, such as:

- Magnetic resonance imaging (MRI)
- Computer-assisted tomography (CAT scan)
- Electroencephalogram (EEG)
- Electromyogram (EMG)
- Transcranial Doppler (TCD)
- Neurosonography
- Cerebrospinal fluid analysis
- Evoked potentials
- Sleep studies

HOW DO NEUROLOGISTS TREAT DISORDERS?

Because of the wide range of neurological disorders, treatments can vary considerably depending on the nature of the disease and the parts of the body that are affected. In the case of stroke, treatment options depend on whether the diagnosis is ischemic stroke or hemorrhagic stroke.

Ischemic strokes result from an obstruction (clot) in a vessel supplying blood to the brain.

Treatment options for ischemic stroke generally include:

- **Medication.** A drug called a "tissue plasminogen activator" (tPA) is injected into a vein in the arm to dissolve the clot that is restricting blood flow to the brain. For this treatment to be most effective, it is important for the medication to be given as soon as possible after the stroke occurs. In addition, an anticoagulant, such as heparin, may be administered to help prevent more blood clots from forming.
- **Mechanical thrombectomy.** In this procedure, a catheter is inserted into an artery leading to the brain and a wire-cage device called a "stent retriever" is used to capture and remove the clot and restore blood flow to the brain. The procedure is most beneficial if it is performed within six hours of the onset of stroke symptoms, and it can only be used on patients who have a clot in one of the large arteries in the brain.

Hemorrhagic strokes occur when a vessel ruptures and allows blood to flow into the brain where it compresses the brain tissue. Treatment options for hemorrhagic stroke usually include:

- **Emergency treatment.** Emergency care is vital for a patient with hemorrhagic stroke in order to control bleeding and reduce pressure in the brain. Medication can be used to reduce blood pressure or slow the bleeding. Patients who are taking blood thinners will likely be given drugs to counteract their effects.
- **Mechanical repair.** A catheter may be inserted through an artery in the arm or leg and guided to site of the rupture in the brain. Then the doctor places a coil or other device through the catheter to help repair the problem. In some cases, though, surgery may be required to repair the problem.

HOW TO CHOOSE A NEUROLOGIST

Obviously, in an emergency situation patients do not get to choose their doctors, but often there is time to consider which neurologist might be the best physician to work with.

Here are some tips:
- **Referrals.** Your primary care doctor will likely recommend a neurologist that she or he works with and knows to be good. Family and friends might also have recommendations.
- **Research.** Make the effort to research the neurologist's credentials, experience, and patient satisfaction surveys and ratings. This information is generally available online, as are records of malpractice claims and disciplinary actions.
- **Meet.** Request an introductory visit with the neurologist. Discuss your case and ask about her or his experience treating your condition, as well as possible treatment plans.
- **Consider.** Think about what you have learned, and take into account your impressions of the neurologist at your meeting. It is important not only that the doctor be qualified but also that you feel comfortable with her or him.
- **Do not forget the hospital.** In addition to researching the neurologist, be sure to do your homework about the hospital or treatment facility. Again, get recommendations when possible, and research the facility online, paying special attention to its neurology unit.
- **Insurance.** It is also important to be sure the neurologist, facility, and expected treatment are compatible with your insurance plan in order to incur the least out-of-pocket expense.

References

1. Caplan, Louis. "Stroke Is Best Managed by Neurologists," Stroke, November 6, 2003.
2. "How Is Stroke Treated?" National Institutes of Health (NIH), January 27, 2017.
3. "Neurologists and Neurosurgeons Explained," Lifenph.com, n.d.

4. "Quick Stroke Treatment for Saving the Brain," American Stroke Association, n.d.
5. "What Does a Neurologist do?" Sokanu.com, n.d.
6. "Working with Your Doctor," American Academy of Neurology (AAN), n.d.

Chapter 21 | **How a Stroke Is Diagnosed**

Stroke is a medical emergency. Tests for stroke usually start when you are in the ambulance before you get to the hospital. This is one reason why it is important to call 911 for a stroke, rather than have someone drive you to the hospital. The goals of the tests are to figure out whether you have had a stroke, what type of stroke you have had, and what caused the stroke. This will help your doctors plan your treatment.

PHYSICAL AND NEUROLOGICAL EXAM

After the ambulance arrives, an ambulance worker will start the stroke exam. A doctor will continue the exam at the hospital. The ambulance worker or doctor will:

- **Ask you or a family member about your symptoms and medical history**
- **Do a physical exam.** This includes taking your blood pressure and checking for mental alertness, numbness or weakness, or trouble speaking, seeing, or walking.
- **Do a neurological exam.** This test checks how well your nervous system is working to show whether you have had a stroke. In this exam, the doctor will ask you questions, test your reflexes, and ask you to do simple actions. Each part of the exam tests a different part of your brain. This test can show how serious your stroke was and were in your brain the stroke might have happened.

This chapter includes text excerpted from "How Is Stroke Diagnosed?" Office on Women's Health (OWH), U.S. Department of Health and Human Services (HHS), October 29, 2018.

IMAGING TESTS FOR STROKE

At the hospital, you will probably get at least one imaging test that allows your doctor to see inside your brain, see how much damage was done and where the stroke happened. Some imaging tests you may get include:

- **Computed tomography (CT) scan.** A CT scan uses x-rays to take pictures of the brain. A CT scan of the head is usually one of the first tests used for a stroke. A CT scan can show bleeding in the brain or damage to brain cells. The CT scan also can find other problems that can cause stroke symptoms.
- **Magnetic resonance imaging (MRI).** MRI uses a strong magnet and radio waves to make pictures of the brain. MRI shows brain changes caused by stroke sooner than a CT scan. MRI also can show any bleeding or blood flow problems. It can rule out other problems, such as tumors that can cause symptoms similar to a stroke.
- **CT or MR angiogram.** An angiogram is an x-ray movie of the blood vessels and blood flow through them. A dye is injected into the veins to show a detailed picture of the blood vessels after a stroke. A CT angiogram is used with a CT scanner, and an MR angiogram is used with an MRI.
- **Carotid ultrasound.** Carotid ultrasound is a test that uses sound waves to create pictures of your carotid arteries, which supply blood to your brain. Often used with a CT or MR angiogram, the carotid ultrasound shows whether plaque has built up in your arteries and is blocking blood flow to your brain.
- **Transcranial Doppler (TCD) ultrasound.** Doppler ultrasound is a test that uses sound waves to measure blood flow. Also used with a CT or MR angiogram, the TCD helps your doctor find out which artery in your brain is blocked.
- **Electroencephalogram (EEG).** An EEG is done less often. This test records electrical activity in the brain to be sure your stroke symptoms are not caused by a

seizure. Seizures can cause symptoms like movement problems and confusion. These can be mistaken for the symptoms of stroke or transient ischemic attack (TIA). During this test, you will have sticky electrodes placed on your head, with wires attached to a machine. The machine records the electrical signals picked up by the electrodes.

- **Electrocardiogram (ECG or EKG).** This test detects and records your heart's electrical activity. It can help your doctor find out if atrial fibrillation caused the stroke. An ECG can be done during physical activity to monitor your heart when it is working hard.

BLOOD TESTS FOR STROKE

There is no blood test that can diagnose a stroke. However, in the hospital, your doctor or nurse may do a series of blood tests to learn the cause of your stroke symptoms.

- **Complete blood count (CBC).** A CBC measures the overall health of your blood and helps diagnose infection, anemia, clotting problems, or other blood problems.
- **Serum electrolytes.** This test looks at substances in your blood that carry an electric charge, called "electrolytes." An electrolyte problem can cause stroke-like symptoms such as, confusion or muscle weakness. Electrolytes also show whether you are dehydrated, which can cause confusion or tiredness. This test can also show whether you have kidney problems, which can change the stroke tests and treatments your doctor does.
- **Blood clotting tests.** These tests measure how quickly your blood clots. It is also called a "coagulation panel." If your blood clots too quickly, your stroke may have been caused by a clot (ischemic stroke). If your blood clots too slowly, your stroke may have been caused by bleeding (hemorrhagic stroke).
- **Heart attack tests.** Your doctor may also order tests to see whether you have had a heart attack. Some women

with stroke symptoms also have heart attack symptoms. Some heart problems can lead to a stroke.

- **Thyroid tests.** Your doctor may measure your thyroid hormone levels with a blood test. Having hyperthyroidism raises your risk of atrial fibrillation, which can lead to stroke.
- **Blood glucose.** This test measures the glucose (sugar) in your blood. Low blood sugar is a common complication of diabetes treatments. Low blood sugar can cause symptoms of a stroke, even when it is not a stroke.
- **Cholesterol tests.** This test examines whether high blood cholesterol might have led to your stroke.
- **C-reactive protein test and blood protein test.** These tests look for substances in your blood that your body releases in response to swelling or inflammation. Damage to arteries is one cause of inflammation. Your doctor might order these tests to understand your stroke risk better and to determine how to treat your stroke.

Chapter 22 | Neurological Diagnostic Tests and Procedures

WHAT IS A NEUROLOGICAL EXAMINATION?

A neurological examination assesses motor and sensory skills, hearing and speech, vision, coordination, and balance. It may also test mental status, mood, and behavior. The examination uses tools such as a tuning fork, flashlight, reflex hammer, and a tool for examining the eye. The results of the neurological examination and the patient's history are used to determine a list of possibilities, known as the "differential diagnosis," that help determine which additional diagnostic tests and procedures are needed.

WHAT ARE ADDITIONAL TESTS USED TO DIAGNOSE NEUROLOGICAL DISORDERS?

The following list of procedures—in alphabetical order—describes some of the other tests used to help diagnose a neurological condition:

Angiography is a test that involves injecting dye into the arteries or veins to detect blockage or narrowing. A cerebral angiogram can show narrowing or obstruction of an artery or blood vessel in the brain, head, or neck. It can determine the location and size of an aneurysm or vascular malformation. Angiograms are used in certain strokes where there is a possibility of unblocking the artery

This chapter includes text excerpted from "Neurological Diagnostic Tests and Procedures Fact Sheet," National Institute of Neurological Disorders and Stroke (NINDS), March 16, 2020.

using a clot retriever. Angiograms can also show the blood supply of a tumor prior to surgery or embolectomy (surgical removal of a blood clot or other material that is blocking a blood vessel).

Angiograms are usually performed in a hospital outpatient or inpatient setting and may take up to three hours, followed by a six to eight hour resting period. The person, wearing a hospital or imaging gown, lies on a table that is wheeled into the imaging area. A physician anesthetizes a small area of the leg near the groin and then inserts a catheter into a major artery located there. The catheter is threaded through the body and into an artery in the neck. Dye is injected and travels through the bloodstream into the head and neck. A series of x-rays are taken. The person may feel a warm to hot sensation or slight discomfort as the dye is released. In many situations, cerebral angiograms have been replaced by specialized MRI scans, called "MR angiograms" (MRA), or "CT angiograms." A spinal angiogram is used to detect blockage of arteries or blood vessels, and malformations in the vessels to the spinal cord.

Biopsy involves the removal and examination of a small piece of tissue from the body. Muscle or nerve biopsies are used to diagnose neuromuscular disorders. A small sample of muscle or nerve is removed under local anesthetic (pain-relieving medication) and studied under a microscope. The muscle sample may be removed either surgically, through a slit made in the skin, or by needle biopsy, in which a thin hollow needle is inserted through the skin and into the muscle. A piece of the nerve may be removed through a small surgical incision near the ankle, or occasionally near the wrist. Muscle and nerve biopsies are usually performed in an outpatient testing facility. A skin biopsy can be used to measure small nerve fibers or to test for certain metabolic disorders. A small piece of skin is removed under local anesthesia, usually in an office setting. A brain biopsy, used to determine tumor type or certain infections, requires surgery to remove a small piece of the brain or tumor. A brain biopsy is an invasive procedure that carries its own risks.

Cerebrospinal fluid analysis involves the removal of a small amount of the fluid that surrounds the brain and spinal cord. The procedure is commonly called a "lumbar puncture or spinal tap."

The fluid is tested to detect evidence of brain hemorrhage, infection, multiple sclerosis, metabolic diseases, or other neurological conditions. Pressure inside the skull can be measured to detect conditions, such as a false brain tumor. The lumbar puncture may be done as an inpatient or as an outpatient procedure. During the lumbar puncture the person will either lie on one side, with knees close to the chest, or lean forward while sitting on a table, bed, or massage chair. The person's back will be cleaned and injected with a local anesthetic. The injection may cause a slight stinging sensation. Once the anesthetic has taken effect, a special needle is inserted between the vertebrae into the spinal sac and a small amount of fluid (usually about three teaspoons) is withdrawn for testing. Most people will only feel a sensation of pressure as the needle is inserted. Generally, people are asked to lie flat for an hour or two to reduce the aftereffect of headache. There is a small risk of nerve root injury or infection from a lumbar puncture. The procedure takes about 45 minutes.

Electronystagmography (ENG) describes a group of tests used to diagnose involuntary eye movement, dizziness, and balance disorders. The test is performed at a clinic or imaging center. Small electrodes are taped on the skin around the eyes to record eye movements. If infrared photography is used in place of electrodes, the person being tested wears special goggles that help record the information. Both versions of the test are painless and risk-free.

Evoked potentials, also called "evoked response," measure the electrical signals to the brain generated by hearing, touch, or sight. Evoked potentials are used to test sight and hearing (especially in infants and young children) and can help diagnose neurological conditions such as multiple sclerosis, spinal cord injury, and acoustic neuroma (small tumors of the acoustic nerve). Evoked potentials are also used to monitor brain activity among coma patients, and confirm brain death.

Testing may take place in a doctor's office or hospital setting. One set of electrodes is attached to the person's scalp with conducting paste. The electrodes measure the brain's electrical response to stimuli. A machine records the amount of time it takes for impulses generated by stimuli to reach the brain.

- *Auditory evoked potentials* (also called "brain stem auditory evoked response") can assess hearing loss and damage to the acoustic nerve and auditory pathways in the brainstem, and detect acoustic neuromas. The person being tested sits in a soundproof room and wears headphones. Clicking sounds are delivered one at a time to one ear while a masking sound is sent to the other ear. Each ear is usually tested twice, and the entire procedure takes about 45 minutes.
- *Visual evoked potentials* detect loss of vision from optic nerve damage (for example from multiple sclerosis). The person sits close to a screen and is asked to focus on the center of a shifting checkerboard pattern. One eye is tested at a time. Each eye is usually tested twice. Testing takes 30 to 45 minutes.
- *Somatosensory evoked potentials* (SSEPs) measure responses from electrical stimuli to the nerves. In addition to electrodes on the scalp, electrodes are pasted to the arms, leg, and back to measure the signal as it travels from the peripheral nerves to the brain. Tiny electrical shocks are delivered by electrodes pasted to the skin over a nerve in an arm or leg. SSEPs may be used to help diagnose multiple sclerosis, spinal cord compression or injury, and certain metabolic or degenerative diseases. SSEP tests usually take longer than an hour.

Myelography involves the injection of contrast dye into the spinal canal to enhance imaging of the spine, by CT or by x-ray. Myelograms have mostly been replaced by MRI, but may be used in special situations. For example, myelograms may be used to diagnose tumors of the spine or spinal cord, or spinal cord compression from herniated discs or fractures. The procedure takes about 60 minutes and can be performed as an outpatient procedure. Following an injection of anesthesia to a site between two vertebrae in the lower back, a small amount of the cerebrospinal fluid is removed by spinal tap. Contrast dye is injected into the spinal canal and a CT scan or a series of x-rays is taken. People may experience some pain during the spinal tap as well as headache following the spinal tap. There is a slight risk of fluid leakage or allergic reaction to the dye.

A **polysomnogram** measures brain and body activity during sleep. It is performed over one or more nights at a sleep center. Electrodes are pasted or taped to the person's scalp, eyelids, and/or chin. Throughout the night and during the various wake/ sleep cycles, the electrodes record brain waves, eye movement, breathing, leg and skeletal muscle activity, blood pressure, and heart rate. The person may be videotaped to note any movement during sleep. Results are then used to identify any characteristic patterns of sleep disorders, including restless legs syndrome, periodic limb movement disorder, insomnia, and breathing disorders such as, sleep apnea. Polysomnograms are noninvasive, painless, and risk-free.

Thermography (also known as "digital infrared thermal imaging") uses infrared sensing devices to measure small temperature changes and thermal abnormalities between the two sides of the body or within a specific organ. Some scientists question its use in diagnosing neurological disorders. It may be used to evaluate complex regional pain syndromes and certain peripheral nerve disorders, and nerve root compression. It is performed at a specialized imaging center, using infrared light recorders to take pictures of the body. The information is converted into a computer-generated two-dimensional picture of abnormally cold or hot areas indicated by color or shades of black and white. Thermography does not use radiation and is safe, risk-free, and noninvasive.

Ultrasound imaging, also called "ultrasonography," uses high-frequency sound waves to obtain images inside the body. During an ultrasound examination, the person lies on a table or reclines in an examination chair. A jelly-like lubricant is applied to the bare skin and a transducer, which both sends and receives high-frequency sound waves, is passed over the body. The sound wave echoes are recorded and displayed as a computer-generated real-time visual image of the structure or tissue being examined. Ultrasound is painless, noninvasive, and risk-free. The test is performed on an outpatient basis and takes between 15 and 30 minutes to complete.

Ultrasound can be used to assess changes in the anatomy of soft tissues, including muscle and nerve. It is more effective than an x-ray in displaying soft tissue changes, such as tears in ligaments or soft tissue masses. In pregnant women, ultrasound can suggest the diagnosis of conditions, such as chromosomal disorders in the fetus. The ultrasound creates a picture of the fetus and the placenta. Ultrasound also may be used in newborns to diagnose hydrocephalus (buildup of cerebrospinal fluid in the brain) or hemorrhage.

- *Carotid Doppler ultrasound* is used to measure blood flow in arteries and blood vessels in the neck.
- *Transcranial Doppler ultrasound* is used to view blood flow in certain arteries and blood vessels inside the skull. Carotid dopplers and transcranial dopplers are used to assess the risk of stroke.
- *Duplex ultrasound* refers to ultrasound studies that are combined with anatomical ultrasound.

X-rays of a person's chest and skull may be taken as part of a neurological work-up. X-rays can be used to view any part of the body, such as a joint or major organ system. In a conventional x-ray, a concentrated burst of low-dose ionized radiation passes through the body and onto a photographic plate. Since calcium in bones absorbs x-rays more easily than soft tissue or muscle, the bony structure appears white on the film. Any vertebral misalignment or fractures can be seen within minutes. Tissue masses, such as injured ligaments or a bulging disc are not visible on conventional x-rays. This fast, noninvasive, painless procedure is usually performed in a doctor's office or at a clinic.

- *Fluoroscopy* is a type of x-ray that uses a continuous or pulsed beam of low-dose radiation to produce continuous images of a body part in motion. The fluoroscope (x-ray tube) is focused on the area of interest and pictures are either videotaped or sent to a monitor for viewing. Fluoroscopy is used to evaluate swallowing and can be used for other procedures such as a lumbar puncture, angiogram for clot removal, or myelogram.

Chapter 23 | Medications Used to Treat Stroke

Chapter Contents

Section 23.1 | Thrombolytic Drugs

This section contains text excerpted from the following sources: Text in this section begins with excerpts from "Stroke: Challenges, Progress, and Promise," Know Stroke, National Institute of Neurological Disorders and Stroke (NINDS), February 1, 2009. Reviewed May 2020; Text under the heading "Development of Tissue Plasminogen Activator" is excerpted from "Tissue Plasminogen Activator for Acute Ischemic Stroke (Alteplase, Activase®)," National Institute of Neurological Disorders and Stroke (NINDS), March 27, 2019.

In treating acute ischemic stroke (acute meaning that the stroke has occurred within the past few hours), the immediate goal is to break apart the offending clot, a process known as "thrombolysis." The body produces its own thrombolytic proteins, and some of these have been engineered into drugs. One, called "tissue plasminogen activator" (tPA), had a proven track record for treating heart attacks. In the late 1980s, the National Institute of Neurological Disorders and Stroke (NINDS)-funded investigators laid the plans for the first placebo-controlled trial of tPA to treat acute ischemic stroke. They knew from animal studies that irreversible brain injury is likely to occur if blood flow is not restored within the first few hours after ischemic stroke. Therefore, the NINDS tPA Study Group tested the drug within a three-hour time window. Compared to individuals given placebo, those given intravenous tPA were more likely to have minimal or no disability three months after treatment—a finding that persuaded the U.S. Food and Drug Administration (FDA) to approve tPA for use against acute stroke. Trials in Europe and the United States subsequently confirmed those results. The studies attempted to identify individuals who may benefit even after three hours of stroke onset. In any case, more brain tissue will be saved the earlier the treatment is delivered.

A follow-up analysis of the NINDS trial found that, after their initial hospitalization, people who received tPA were less likely to require inpatient rehabilitation or nursing home care. The authors estimated that this lower dependency on long-term care would translate into a savings to the healthcare system of more than $4 million for every 1,000 individuals treated with tPA.

Because treatment with tPA interferes with blood clotting and has also been shown to increase leaking along the blood-brain barrier, it carries a risk of intracerebral hemorrhage. Therefore, it is not recommended for some people, such as those with a history of brain hemorrhage or significantly elevated blood pressure (greater than 185/110 mm Hg). The risk of tPA-induced hemorrhage increases over time from stroke onset, which has limited its use to the first three hours after stroke (where benefit was most clearly established in the United States trials).

DEVELOPMENT OF TISSUE PLASMINOGEN ACTIVATOR

The NINDS played a major role in the development of tPA, from funding early studies that provided a rationale for its use, to leading pivotal clinical trials that supported the treatment's FDA approval in 1996.

Discovery of a Clot-Buster

Beginning in the 1950s, investigators first began to develop clot-dissolving, or thrombolytic, interventions for heart attacks and stroke. Early agents included the bacterial enzyme streptokinase and urokinase, an enzyme produced in the kidneys. However, both carried significant risks for dangerous internal bleeding, or hemorrhage, as they prevented clotting throughout the body. While tPA had also been discovered by this time, it was not extensively studied until the late 1970s, following a fortuitous finding that certain cancer cells grown in the lab-produced large amounts of the enzyme. This allowed more thorough characterization, which showed that tPA acted preferentially at clots, a potentially major advantage over previously tested enzymes.

The first studies demonstrating the clot-busting effects of tPA were conducted in the early 1980s, in animal models of coronary artery and other blockages and in a small number of heart attack patients, though not yet in stroke patients. The 1980s also ushered in a revolution in biotechnology. Scientists could now clone genes and directly express proteins in cell cultures, and Genentech researchers began producing recombinant tPA in sufficient quantities for future commercialization. In 1984, the National Heart, Lung, and Blood Institute (NHLBI) supported the first multicenter, randomized clinical trial using recombinant tPA in heart attack patients. This trial showed successful coronary artery opening in

75 percent of patients with limited adverse bleeding. Based on positive results in additional trials, the FDA approved tPA (alteplase, Activase®) for treating heart attack in 1987.

Restoring Blood Flow to the Brain

Meanwhile, the NINDS researchers and others thought tPA might be used to treat strokes as well. Earlier failures with streptokinase and urokinase had discouraged further investigation of thrombolytic agents for stroke. However, researchers now understood that these trials had begun treatment too late to salvage oxygen-deprived brain tissue. Furthermore, since tPA carried less risk of internal bleeding, it could be given intravenously, as opposed directly to an affected artery, a process that required additional time-consuming examination. By the late 1980s, several studies supported in part by the NINDS had found that intravenous tPA could dissolve clots in animal models with limited risk of hemorrhage, but only if tPA was administered shortly after the clot-blocked blood flow.

In the early 1990s, reports of pilot trials of tPA in small numbers of stroke patients described artery opening and improved outcomes. In particular, two studies involving the NINDS support and the NINDS intramural investigators developed protocols for assessing and treating stroke patients within 90 minutes or less and three hours or less of symptom onset, based on earlier evidence of the window of opportunity to prevent irreversible damage.

These pioneering studies radically increased the speed with which stroke patients could be diagnosed and treated. They also established that the effective dose of tPA for stroke was less than the standard dose for heart attack, further decreasing the risk for dangerous bleeding. Larger randomized, placebo-controlled studies followed, including the NINDS tPA Stroke Trial. In 1995, results from this pivotal trial showed that patients treated with tPA within three hours of symptom onset were at least 30 percent more likely than placebo-treated patients to have minimal or no disability for up to three months.

Treatment with tPA was associated with a greater risk of bleeding in the brain, especially in patients with severe strokes. However, tPA treatment in such patients was still more likely than placebo to result in better outcomes, and mortality did not increase overall in tPA-treated patients.

Thanks in large part to the NINDS-supported trial, the FDA approved tPA for the treatment of ischemic stroke in 1996. Follow-up studies confirmed that tPA treatment outcomes observed in the NINDS trial persisted for up to one year, and postmarketing studies showed that community hospitals could achieve similar results with adherence to recommended protocols for rapid assessment and treatment. In addition, a study on cost benefits estimated $4 million in savings for every 1,000 patients treated with tPA, due to improved outcomes and reduced long-term care costs.

Building on tPA's Benefits

The implementation of rapid treatment protocols transformed acute stroke care in the United States, even beyond contributing to the success of tPA. Hundreds of hospitals developed organized stroke teams and resources to become primary stroke centers for tPA treatment. On the heels of tPA's approval, the NINDS launched a public awareness and education campaign to help people recognize the signs and symptoms of stroke and understand the importance of getting to the hospital quickly. This successful Know Stroke campaign has reached millions through a variety of media and community programs, including programs for Spanish-speaking and minority communities.

The NINDS and others have continued to support efforts to increase the use of tPA in eligible patients and improve treatment outcomes, including research on ways to mitigate the risk of bleeding in the brain and extend the time window for treatment. Moreover, the success of tPA motivated the search for additional acute stroke treatments, including interventions to remove large clots resistant to the clot-busting drug. In 2015, multiple clinical trials demonstrated the benefit of clot-retrieval devices as compared to tPA alone for the treatment of severe strokes affecting large arteries to the brain, prompting the FDA to expand approval for such devices. Subsequent clinical trials sponsored by industry and the NINDS showed that the time window for effective treatment with these devices can be extended to 16 hours or more in patients determined by brain imaging to have salvageable brain tissue.

Section 23.2 | Antiplatelet Drugs and Anticoagulants

This section includes text excerpted from "Stroke: Challenges, Progress, and Promise," Know Stroke, National Institute of Neurological Disorders and Stroke (NINDS), February 1, 2009. Reviewed May 2020.

Blood-thinning medications fall into two classes: antiplatelet drugs and anticoagulants. Antiplatelet drugs inhibit the activity of cells called "platelets," which stick to damaged areas inside blood vessels and lay the foundation for blood clots. The most common antiplatelet drug is aspirin. Anticoagulants, such as heparin (produced by inflammatory cells in the body) and warfarin (found in plants and also known by the trade name Coumadin©), inhibit proteins in the blood that stimulate clotting.

Antiplatelet drugs and anticoagulants can help prevent a variety of potentially life-threatening conditions such as myocardial infarction, pulmonary embolism, and deep vein thrombosis—which are caused by clots in the heart, lungs, and deep veins of the legs, respectively, for which individuals with stroke are at risk. In these years, the value of these drugs in treating and preventing stroke itself has been more closely scrutinized.

One focus of this research has been to determine if there is any benefit in giving antiplatelet drugs or anticoagulants during an acute ischemic stroke, as an adjunct to tPA, or as an alternative for people ineligible to receive tPA. In an international trial coordinated by researchers in the United Kingdom in the late 1990s, individuals received aspirin, subcutaneous heparin injections, or neither treatment within 48 hours of an ischemic stroke. Aspirin significantly reduced the risk of a recurrent ischemic stroke at two weeks. A similar benefit from heparin was offset by an increased risk of hemorrhagic stroke. Around the same time, the National Institute of Neurological Disorders and Stroke (NINDS)-funded researchers tested whether acute stroke could be treated with intravenous Org 10172, a form of heparin considered less likely to cause bleeding. This study, Trial of Org 10172 in Acute Stroke Treatment (TOAST), found that Org 10172 produced no significant benefit. The study authors also developed the TOAST criteria, a set of guidelines for classifying different subtypes of ischemic stroke that are now widely used in other studies.

Another issue is whether individuals at risk for ischemic stroke should be placed on a daily maintenance program of aspirin or anticoagulants. For many years, aspirin and warfarin were used as a means of stroke prevention in individuals with atrial fibrillation (AF), but this practice was based more on anecdotal evidence than on scientific data. A systematic analysis of warfarin's benefits was especially important since it is an expensive drug and, like heparin, is associated with an increased risk of hemorrhagic stroke. The NINDS Boston Area Anticoagulation Trial for Atrial Fibrillation (BAATAF) and the Stroke Prevention in Atrial Fibrillation (SPAF) trials showed that daily warfarin is best for people with AF who are over 65 years of age or who have additional vascular risk factors. Daily aspirin provides adequate protection against stroke among young people with AF.

The two other NINDS-sponsored trials compared the effectiveness of daily warfarin and aspirin for individuals who did not have AF, but who had experienced a prior stroke—and thus were at risk for another. The Warfarin versus Aspirin Recurrent Stroke Study (WARSS) showed that aspirin was as effective as warfarin in preventing recurrent stroke in people with no history of AF or other cardioembolic causes of stroke. The Warfarin-Aspirin Symptomatic Intracranial Disease (WASID) trial focused more narrowly on individuals with stenosis of arteries in the brain and was terminated early because of a high rate of adverse events in participants treated with warfarin. Both trials concluded that aspirin is equivalent to warfarin for reducing the risk of stroke in people without AF.

Section 23.3 | Medication for Subarachnoid Hemorrhage

This section contains text excerpted from the following sources: Text in this section begins with excerpts from "Stroke: Challenges, Progress, and Promise," Know Stroke, National Institute of Neurological Disorders and Stroke (NINDS), February 1, 2009. Reviewed May 2020; Text beginning with the heading "Safety Announcement" is excerpted from "The FDA Drug Safety Communication: Serious Medication Errors from Intravenous Administration of Nimodipine Oral Capsules," U.S. Food and Drug Administration (FDA), August 3, 2017.

The drug nimodipine is used to treat cerebral vasospasm, a complication that sometimes follows subarachnoid hemorrhage. This refers to a constriction of blood vessels in the brain that can significantly reduce blood flow, leading to ischemia and infarction. Although its precise origins are unclear, cerebral vasospasm is thought to be triggered in part by an influx of calcium into the smooth muscles that control blood vessel diameter. Nimodipine is a calcium antagonist, meaning that it works by blocking the entry of calcium into cells. Nimodipine has been shown to reduce infarction and improve outcome in individuals with subarachnoid hemorrhage.

SAFETY ANNOUNCEMENT

The U.S. Food and Drug Administration (FDA) has alerted healthcare professionals that nimodipine capsules should be given ONLY by mouth or through a feeding tube (nasogastric tube). This oral medication should NEVER be given by intravenous administration. The FDA continues to receive reports of intravenous nimodipine use, with serious, sometimes fatal, consequences. Intravenous injection of nimodipine can result in death, cardiac arrest, severe falls in blood pressure, and other heart-related complications.

Nimodipine is a medication intended to be given in a critical care setting to treat neurologic complications from subarachnoid hemorrhage (ruptured blood vessels in the brain) and is only available as a capsule.

In 2006, the FDA added a Boxed Warning and made other revisions to the prescribing information to warn against intravenous use of nimodipine. The prescribing information also provides clear instructions on how to remove the liquid contents from the capsules for nasogastric tube administration in patients who are unable to swallow. The instructions recommend that the syringe used for withdrawal of capsule contents be labeled with "Not for IV Use."

The FDA continues to work with the manufacturers of nimodipine and with outside groups to evaluate and implement additional ways to prevent medication errors with this product.

ADDITIONAL INFORMATION FOR PATIENTS

- The FDA encourages all patients to talk to their healthcare professional if they have concerns about any treatment they are receiving.
- Report any side effects from the use of medication to the FDA MedWatch program, using the information in the "Contact Us" box at the bottom of the page.

ADDITIONAL INFORMATION FOR HEALTHCARE PROFESSIONALS

- Be aware that nimodipine should be administered ONLY by the oral route or via nasogastric tube. It should NEVER be administered intravenously.
- If the nimodipine capsule cannot be swallowed, e.g., at the time of surgery, or if the patient is unconscious, a hole should be made in both ends of the capsule with an 18 gauge needle, and the contents of the capsule extracted into a syringe. To help minimize administration errors, it is recommended that the syringe be labeled "Not for IV Use." The needle should be removed from the syringe and the contents should then be emptied into the patient's in situ nasogastric tube and washed down the tube with 30 mL of normal saline (0.9%).
- Report adverse events or medication errors involving nimodipine capsules to the FDA MedWatch program using the information in the "Contact Us" box at the bottom of this page.

ACTIONS BY THE U.S. FOOD AND DRUG ADMINISTRATION

Since the approval of nimodipine in 1988, the FDA has taken several actions intended to reduce the occurrence of inappropriate intravenous use of this drug. In 1996, a bolded statement was added to the prescribing information to warn against incorrect administration of nimodipine. In 2006, the FDA added both a Boxed Warning and a warning to the nimodipine labeling to alert practitioners not to administer nimodipine intravenously or by other parenteral routes, and described the potential for fatal and life-threatening adverse effects following erroneous parenteral nimodipine administration. The FDA also revised the Dosage and Administration section regarding administration of the capsule contents to patients who are unable to swallow.

The FDA identified 31 cases of medication errors associated with the use of nimodipine that were reported to the FDA's Adverse Event Reporting System (AERS), the Pennsylvania Patient Safety Reporting System (PA-PSRS), the Institute for Safe Medication Practices' (ISMP) Quantros MEDMARX database, and the Council for International Organizations of Medical Sciences (CIOMS) II database, and published in the medical literature between 1989 (initial marketing of nimodipine) and 2009. Of the 31 medication errors, 25 involved erroneous intravenous nimodipine prescribing or administration. Four of the patients who mistakenly received nimodipine intravenously died; five patients were characterized as having near-death events; and one patient was characterized as having suffered permanent harm as a result of the inadvertent intravenous administration of nimodipine.

Based on the FDA's review of these reports, the following factors have been identified as contributing to this preventable medication error:

- Since some patients receiving nimodipine cannot swallow the capsules, they must receive the liquid from the capsules through a feeding tube. The nimodipine prescribing information has instructions for using a needle to make a hole in both ends of the capsule to remove the liquid contents with a syringe and then empty the contents into the feeding tube. Because a

195

standard needle will not fit on an oral syringe, the needle must be attached to an intravenous syringe. The use of intravenous syringes to deliver nimodipine increases the chance that the medication will be given intravenously instead of by mouth or nasogastric tube.

- Most patients receiving nimodipine are hospitalized in critical care units and are already receiving intravenous medications.

Section 23.4 | The Scoop on Statins: What Do You Need to Know

This section includes text excerpted from "The Scoop on Statins: What Do You Need to Know?" U.S. Department of Health and Human Services (HHS), December 1, 2018.

WHY IS IT IMPORTANT TO UNDERSTAND THE BENEFITS AND RISKS OF STATINS?

Most heart attacks and strokes are preventable by practicing a healthy lifestyle, and when necessary, taking medications to lower blood pressure or cholesterol or to help quit smoking. Statins, when used as indicated, can dramatically reduce a person's risk of having a heart attack or stroke, but millions of people are missing that opportunity. Some clinicians may miss prescribing a statin to a person who can benefit. Many times, individuals stop or do not start taking a statin due to concerns about side effects. The good news is that understanding your individual benefits and risks and working through your concerns with your clinician can help you prevent heart attacks and strokes and enjoy a longer, healthier life.

WHAT IS A STATIN AND HOW DOES IT WORK?

Statins are a class of medicines used to lower cholesterol. While some of the cholesterol in your blood comes from food, most is made by the liver. Statins work by reducing the amount of cholesterol made by the liver and helping the liver remove cholesterol that is already in the blood. Statins may also reduce inflammation in the artery walls. This inflammation can lead to blockages that damage organs, such as the heart and brain.

WHAT ARE THE BENEFITS OF STATINS?

Scientific studies and years of use all over the world have proven that statins, when used as indicated, reduce a person's chances of having a heart attack or stroke; needing surgery, angioplasty, or stenting to improve blood flow in an artery; and dying from a heart attack. The higher a person's risk of having a heart attack or stroke, the stronger the benefit of the statin. The benefit increases the longer the statin is taken. In general, taking a statin can cut a person's risk of a heart attack or stroke in half.

WHAT ARE THE RISKS OF TAKING A STATIN?

Serious risks are rare. Studies involving thousands of people show no differences in muscle aches, liver abnormalities, dementia, memory problems, or cancer between those taking a statin and those on an inactive pill. Despite these findings, just over one in four people (29%) taking a statin describes some symptoms, most commonly muscle aches or weakness. It is important to note that muscle-related symptoms are also common with aging and inactive adults who are not on statins. Very uncommon risks associated with statins include a type of stroke caused by bleeding, muscle damage that can usually be detected with a blood test, and increased blood sugar levels or new-onset diabetes in those who are prone to developing diabetes. The large benefit of taking statins to prevent heart attacks and strokes likely outweighs the small risk associated with an elevated blood sugar level.

HOW CAN SIDE EFFECTS BE MANAGED WHEN TAKING A STATIN?

Side effects from statins can frequently be managed by adjustments in the dose or by choosing a different statin drug. Before stopping or changing your medication, please discuss your concerns with your clinician who can help determine the likelihood that symptoms are related to the statin. Together you can map out a practical plan to keep you safe from heart attack and stroke. Who should consider taking a statin? People who have had a heart attack or stroke, who have diabetes or very high "bad" cholesterol levels, and who are at high risk for heart disease or stroke due to other factors like high blood pressure will live healthier and longer lives by taking a statin. Because the degree of the benefit from a statin varies with your chances of having a heart attack or stroke, it is important to discuss your individual risks and preferences with your clinician. Together you can make a good decision for your healthiest future.

Chapter 24 | Surgical Interventions for Stroke Prevention

Chapter Contents

Section 24.1 | Brain Aneurysm Repair

This section includes text excerpted from "Cerebral Arteriosclerosis Information Page," National Institute of Neurological Disorders and Stroke (NINDS), January 6, 2020.

WHAT IS CEREBRAL ARTERIOSCLEROSIS?

Cerebral arteriosclerosis is the result of thickening and hardening of the walls of the arteries in the brain. Symptoms of cerebral arteriosclerosis include headache, facial pain, and impaired vision.

Cerebral arteriosclerosis can cause serious health problems. If the walls of an artery are too thick, or a blood clot becomes caught in the narrow passage, blood flow to the brain can become blocked and cause an ischemic stroke. When the thickening and hardening is uneven, arterial walls can develop bulges (called "aneurysms"). If a bulge ruptures, bleeding in the brain can cause a hemorrhagic stroke. Both types of stroke can be fatal.

Cerebral arteriosclerosis is also related to a condition known as "vascular dementia," in which small, symptom-free strokes cause cumulative damage and death to neurons (nerve cells) in the brain. Personality changes in the elderly such as apathy, weeping, transient befuddlement, or irritability, might indicate that cerebral arteriosclerosis is present in the brain. Computed tomography (CT) and magnetic resonance imaging (MRI) of the brain can help reveal the presence of cerebral arteriosclerosis before ischemic strokes, hemorrhagic strokes, or vascular dementia develop.

TREATMENT FOR CEREBRAL ARTERIOSCLEROSIS

Treatment for cerebral arteriosclerosis can include medications or surgery. Physicians also may recommend treatments to help people control high blood pressure, quit cigarette smoking, and reduce cholesterol levels, all of which are risk factors for cerebral arteriosclerosis.

PROGNOSIS OF CEREBRAL ARTERIOSCLEROSIS

Cerebral arteriosclerosis can lead to life-threatening health events, such as ischemic or hemorrhagic strokes. People who survive stroke may have long-term neurological and motor impairments.

Section 24.2 | Carotid Artery Angioplasty and Stent Placement

This section includes text excerpted from "Medicare Expands Coverage of Carotid Artery Stenting for Patients at High Risk for Surgery," Centers for Medicare & Medicaid Services (CMS), May 17, 2005. Reviewed May 2020.

MEDICARE EXPANDS COVERAGE OF CAROTID ARTERY STENTING FOR PATIENTS AT HIGH RISK FOR SURGERY

The Centers for Medicare & Medicaid Services (CMS) announced it was expanding coverage of percutaneous transluminal angioplasty (PTA) of the carotid artery concurrent with stent placement to patients who were at high risk for carotid surgery—also known as "carotid endarterectomy" or "CEA." The coverage expansion reflected the latest evidence on the effective use of stenting, and included support for development of better evidence in additional uses.

"CMS is committed to providing broader access to appropriate and innovative care to our beneficiaries in the management of their carotid artery disease," said CMS Administrator Mark B. McClellan, M.D., Ph.D. "We are working with health professionals and product developers to reduce the occurrence of stroke in our population, and getting the maximum health improvements possible by soliciting and responding to public comments on the most effective way to provide improved coverage."

The national coverage determination (NCD) issued in 2005 expanded Medicare coverage for carotid artery stenting to high-risk patients with symptomatic narrowing of carotid artery of 70 percent or more.

Medicare also covers patients who meet the U.S. Food and Drug Administration (FDA) labeled criteria for carotid stents (who are at high risk for CEA and have symptomatic carotid artery stenosis between 50 percent and 70 percent and asymptomatic high-risk patients with carotid artery stenosis of 80% or more) in Category B IDE clinical trials, as a routine cost under the clinical trials policy, or in postapproval studies.

Under previous policy, CMS only covered carotid artery stenting in clinical trials being conducted prior to FDA approval (so-called "Category B Investigational Device Exemption" [IDE] clinical trial) and more recently in FDA required postapproval studies.

Centers for Medicare & Medicaid Services and Guidant Corporation has worked with the FDA to expand the scope of postapproval studies and increase the number of participating facilities and study enrollees. Guidant Corporation is currently the only company with an FDA approved carotid stent and an ongoing postapproval study.

Carotid endarterectomy is a surgical procedure used to prevent stroke in which the surgeon removes fatty deposits or plaques from the carotid arteries, the two main arteries in the neck supplying blood to the brain. Carotid artery stenting is a less invasive, alternative procedure to CEA, in which a catheter is used to place the stent that will widen the narrowed artery.

To help ensure optimal patient outcomes and to evaluate and monitor provider and facility performance, Medicare has limited the use of carotid stenting to facilities and providers who have been determined to be competent in performing the evaluation, procedure, and necessary follow-up care.

Competency is based on published clinical guidelines that outline physician training and facility support requirements for carotid artery stenting. Facilities must also meet CMS' minimum standards in performing carotid artery stenting.

These standards outlined in the coverage determination include physician training criteria, facility support requirements, and data collection to evaluate outcomes during a required reevaluation. Facilities can provide a written affidavit to CMS attesting that the facility has met these standards.

Each year about 700,000 people experience a new or recurrent stroke. More than 70 percent of stroke victims are over 65 years of age and eligible for Medicare.

Obstructive lesions in the carotid arteries have the potential to cause stroke, leading to substantial morbidity, mortality, and long-term disability. Stroke prevention includes the following measures:

- Treating hypertension and diabetes
- Smoking cessation
- Limiting alcohol intake
- Controlling diet and obesity

Some medical conditions or anatomical risk factors that increase the risk for CEA include congestive heart failure (CHF), unstable angina, and recent heart attack (myocardial infarction).

"The evidence on carotid artery stenting demonstrates its effectiveness in improving net health outcomes for certain patients." said CMS chief medical officer Sean Tunis MD, MSc. "By requiring hospitals to certify their competency, CMS can help ensure patient safety and quality care for those undergoing this procedure."

Section 24.3 | Carotid Endarterectomy

This section includes text excerpted from "Questions and Answers about Carotid Endarterectomy," National Institute of Neurological Disorders and Stroke (NINDS), August 13, 2019.

WHAT IS A CAROTID ENDARTERECTOMY?

A carotid endarterectomy is a surgical procedure in which a doctor removes fatty deposits blocking one of the two carotid arteries, the main supply of blood to the brain. Carotid artery problems become more common as people age. The disease process that causes the buildup of fat and other material inside the artery walls is called "atherosclerosis," popularly known as "hardening of the arteries." The fatty deposit is called "plaque;" the narrowing of the artery is called "stenosis." The degree of stenosis is usually expressed as a percentage of the normal diameter of the opening.

WHY IS SURGERY PERFORMED?

Carotid endarterectomy is performed to prevent stroke. Two large clinical trials supported by the National Institute of Neurological Disorders and Stroke (NINDS) identified specific individuals for whom the surgery is beneficial when performed by surgeons and in institutions that can match the standards set in those studies. The surgery has been found highly beneficial for people who have already had a stroke or experienced the symptoms of a stroke and have a severe stenosis of 70 to 99 percent. In this group, surgery reduced the estimated 2-year risk of stroke or death by more than 80 percent, from greater than 1 in 4 to less than 1 in 10.

For patients who have already had transient or mild stroke symptoms due to moderate carotid stenosis (50 to 69 percent), surgery reduces the 5-year risk of stroke or death by 6.5 percent. The failure rate for ipsilateral stroke or death for the medical group is 22.2 percent, and for the surgery group is 15.7 percent from greater than 1 in 4 to less than 1 in 7. Individuals who have already had stroke symptoms, and who have carotid stenosis greater than 50 percent, may wish to consider surgery to prevent future stroke. Based on findings of the North American Symptomatic Carotid Endarterectomy Trial (NASCET), patients with moderate (50 to 69 percent) stenosis are now better able to make more informed decisions.

In another trial (Asymptomatic Carotid Atherosclerosis Study, or ACAS), the procedure has also been found highly beneficial for people who are symptom-free but have a carotid stenosis of 60 to 99 percent. In this group, the surgery reduces the estimated 5-year risk of stroke by more than one-half, from about 1 in 10 to less than 1 in 20.

The Carotid Revascularization Endarterectomy vs. Stenting Trial (CREST) compared carotid endarterectomy surgery to carotid artery stenting and found no significance between the procedures regarding the 4-year rate of stroke or death in patients with or without a previous stroke. The pivotal differences were the lower rate of stroke following surgery and the lower rate of heart attack following stenting. The study also found that the age of the patient made a difference—the younger the age of the patient—the larger the benefit for stenting. At 69 years of age and younger, stenting results were slightly better. Conversely, for patients older than 70 years of age, surgical benefits were slightly superior to stenting—the larger the benefits for surgery.

HOW IMPORTANT IS A BLOCKAGE AS A CAUSE OF STROKE?

A blockage of a blood vessel is the most frequent cause of stroke and is responsible for about 80 percent of the approximately 700,000 strokes in the United States each year. With nearly 150,000 stroke deaths each year, stroke ranks as the fourth leading killer in the United States. Stroke is the leading cause of adult disability in the United States with 2 million of the 3 million Americans who have survived a stroke sustaining some permanent disability. The overall cost of stroke to the nation is $40 billion a year.

HOW MANY CAROTID ENDARTERECTOMIES WERE PERFORMED EACH YEAR?

An estimated 140,000 carotid endarterectomies were performed in the United States in 2009, according to the National Hospital Discharge Survey. The procedure was first described in the mid-1950s. It began to be used increasingly as a stroke prevention measure in the 1960s and 1970s. Its use peaked in the mid-1980s when more than 100,000 operations were performed each year. At that time, several authorities began to question the trend and the risk-benefit ratio for some groups, and the use of the procedure dropped precipitously. The NINDS-supported NASCET and ACAS trials were launched in the mid-1980s to identify the specific groups of people with carotid artery disease who would clearly benefit from the procedure.

WHAT ARE THE RISK FACTORS AND HOW RISKY IS THE SURGERY?

Important risk factors in addition to the degree of stenosis include, gender, diabetes, the type of stroke symptoms, and blockage of the carotid artery on the opposite side. Without other complicating illnesses, age alone is not a worrisome risk factor. Risk factors can affect patients in two ways. They can, particularly in combination, greatly increase a person's risk of having a stroke. In addition, these risk factors can increase the likelihood of surgical complications.

HOW IS CAROTID ARTERY DISEASE DIAGNOSED?

In some cases, the disease can be detected during a normal checkup by a physician. In other cases, further testing is needed. Some of the tests a physician can use or order include ultrasound imaging, arteriography, and magnetic resonance angiography (MRA). Frequently these procedures are carried out in a stepwise fashion:

from a doctor's evaluation of signs and symptoms to ultrasound, MRA, and arteriography for increasingly difficult cases.

- **History and physical exam.** A doctor will ask about symptoms of a stroke such as numbness or muscle weakness, speech or vision difficulties, or lightheadedness. Using a stethoscope, a doctor may hear a rushing sound, called a "bruit," in the carotid artery. Unfortunately, dangerous levels of disease sometimes fail to make a sound, and some blockages with a low risk can make the same sound.
- **Ultrasound imaging.** This is a painless, noninvasive test in which sound waves above the range of human hearing are sent into the neck. Echoes bounce off the moving blood and the tissue in the artery and can be formed into an image. Ultrasound is fast, risk-free, relatively inexpensive, and painless procedure compared to MRA and arteriography.
- **Arteriography.** This procedure can be used to confirm the findings of ultrasound imaging which can be uncertain in some cases. Arteriography is an x-ray of the carotid artery taken when a special dye is injected into the artery. A burning sensation may be felt when the dye is injected. An arteriogram is more expensive and carries its own small risk of causing a stroke.
- **Magnetic resonance angiography (MRA).** This is a new imaging technique that avoids most of the risks associated with arteriography. An MRA is a type of image that uses magnetism instead of x-rays to create an image of the carotid arteries.

WHAT IS THE "BEST MEDICAL THERAPY" FOR STROKE PREVENTION?

The mainstay of stroke prevention is risk factor management: smoking cessation, treatment of high blood pressure, and control of blood sugar levels among people with diabetes. Additionally, physicians may prescribe aspirin, warfarin, or ticlopidine for some individuals.

The NINDS health-related material is provided for information purposes only and does not necessarily represent endorsement by or an official position of the National Institute of Neurological Disorders and Stroke or any other federal agency. Advice on the treatment or care of an individual patient should be obtained through consultation with a physician who has examined that patient or is familiar with that patient's medical history.

Chapter 25 | Advances in Stroke Care and Research

Chapter Contents

Section 25.1 | Advances in Stroke Research Priorities

This section contains text excerpted from the following sources: Text in this section begins with excerpts from "Stroke: Research Activities and Scientific Advances," *Eunice Kennedy Shriver* National Institute of Child Health and Human Development (NICHD), December 1, 2016. Reviewed May 2020; Text beginning with the heading "Stroke Research Priorities" is excerpted from "Stroke Research Priorities Meeting 2012," National Institute of Neurological Disorders and Stroke (NINDS), August 13, 2019.

Stroke is a leading cause of serious disability and death in the United States. Although the majority of individuals who sustain a stroke survive, a significant proportion of survivors require rehabilitation, and nearly one-third have some type of permanent disability. Among those who survive stroke, 50 percent are alive more than 5 years after the event, which means that rehabilitation needs to continue well after the initial event. The *Eunice Kennedy Shriver* National Institute of Child Health and Human Development (NICHD) supports and conducts research to better understand stroke, its prevention, treatment, and methods for rehabilitation.

INSTITUTE ACTIVITIES AND ADVANCES

The NICHD supports and conducts research to better understand stroke, its prevention, treatment, and methods for rehabilitation through several organizational units. NICHD-supported research covers multiple effects of stroke including motor, cognitive, swallowing, and communication deficits.

- National Center for Medical Rehabilitation Research (NCMRR)
  - Projects within the Traumatic Brain Injury (TBI) and Stroke Rehabilitation (TSR) Program involve studying how to improve recovery of abilities that can be affected by stroke including movement, mobility, and language, as well as investigating potential treatments for other side effects of stroke, such as mental-health problems.
  - The Behavioral Sciences and Rehabilitation Technologies (BSRT) Program supports clinical studies of interventions that promote development of emotional, cognitive, and physical attributes. The

211

program also supports basic behavioral studies on factors, such as plasticity.
- The Biological Sciences and Career Development (BSCD) Program supports basic research on substrate responses to injury and on strategies to promote regeneration, recovery, plasticity, adaptation, and recovery.
- One of the longstanding program project grants supported by the Intellectual and Developmental Disabilities Branch (IDDB) focuses on the natural history of a large cohort of individuals with Mitochondrial Encephalopathy, Lactic Acidosis, and Stroke-like Episodes (MELAS) syndrome. Researchers involved with this project have examined treatments for this and related disorders as well as genes that may be involved.
- Division of Intramural Research (DIR)
  - The section on Cellular and Synaptic Physiology studies the development and regulation of excitability in the brain's cortex.
  - The section on Neurophysiology and Biophysics studies how dysfunction of ionotropic glutamate receptor (iGluR) activity mediates several neurological and psychiatric diseases and damage during stroke. This group analyzes iGluR function at the molecular level.
  - The aim of the section on Tissue Biophysics and Biomimetics is developing novel next-generation in vivo imaging methods to gain a better understanding of brain function and organization and to improve the diagnosis of neurological and developmental disorders, including stroke.
  - The section on Vertebrate Organogenesis research group studies zebrafish vasculature. Projects include a genetic screen to identify hemorrhagic stroke—susceptibility genes and molecular analysis of the formation and maintenance of vertebrate vasculature.

STROKE RESEARCH PRIORITIES

In 2011, the National Institute of Neurological Disorders and Stroke (NINDS) began a two-phase planning process in order to identify the highest priority research areas in stroke to address over the next five to ten years. In Phase 1, the NINDS asked the Stroke Progress Review Group (SPRG) to conduct a final review of the stroke research landscape, ten years after the first SPRG established research priorities for the field. The resulting report, published in January, 2012, recognized 48 priority areas.

Phase 2 of the stroke planning process was designed to build on the comprehensive analysis of the SPRG, identifying a smaller number of areas that represent the most promising opportunities in stroke research. This process was guided by a working group of the NINDS Council chaired by Drs. Tom Brott and Barbara Vickrey. It capitalized on the expertise of three working groups of external scientists representing prevention, treatment, and recovery. To solicit potential research priorities for Phase 2, the NINDS released a request for information (RFI) in May, 2012. The RFI called for broad input from the public and research community to identify opportunities for which significant, community-based effort and focus could lead to major advances in stroke research over the next five to ten years. In advance of a planning meeting, members of the three working groups—prevention, treatment, and recovery—rated over 180 RFI responses on impact, feasibility, need for targeted NINDS investment, and overall merit.

Top priorities were identified and strengthened at the Stroke Research Priorities Meeting held on August 29 and 30, 2012. Premeeting scores were used to identify which proposals were discussed and further optimized, and after discussions, individuals in each working group re-rated the proposals. The top proposals for each group were identified through further discussion and voting within the working groups. To encourage input from all working group participants, discussions were led by an impartial moderator, and ratings were done anonymously. The top proposals from each group were then further refined and presented to the Steering Committee, the NINDS staff, and other attendees.

Through this process, each of the working groups developed two or three proposals, as well as one joint proposal (cross-cutting), that represent combined, modified, and optimized versions of the best ideas presented in the RFI proposals. Each research opportunity identified by the working groups is presented below with a description of the goals, impact, feasibility, barriers, rationale, relevant ongoing efforts, and potential approaches.

TOP SCIENTIFIC RESEARCH OPPORTUNITIES FROM WORKGROUPS ON STROKE PREVENTION, TREATMENT, AND RECOVERY RESEARCH
Cross-Cutting
ACCELERATING THE TRANSLATION OF STROKE RESEARCH IN PRECLINICAL ANIMAL MODELS INTO CLINICAL STUDIES OF HIGHLY PROMISING TREATMENTS

Systematic, evidence-based criteria are needed to inform decisions to proceed from preclinical to clinical studies. Scientific milestones at each stage should ensure that only therapies with robust and repeatable results move forward. Potentially, this would greatly accelerate the development of novel and effective strategies for prevention, treatment, and recovery. With systematic, evidence-based progression along the translational pathway, identification and translation of one or more positive, highly vetted candidates into human studies would be feasible within the next decade.

Prevention
PREVENTION OF VASCULAR COGNITIVE IMPAIRMENT

The prevalence of vascular cognitive impairment (VCI) is greater than all clinical strokes combined. The underlying small vessel and white matter biology is incompletely understood, and there are no targeted therapies that exist for small vessel disease. The contribution of vascular pathology to the biology of Alzheimer disease is also incompletely understood. Prevention of vascular cognitive impairment thus represents both a huge public-health challenge and a major opportunity. This initiative would address both preclinical and clinical scientific opportunities, by (1) identifying key biological pathways that promote small vessel disease underlying VCI and agents that interfere with them, as well as (2) developing pilot clinical trials of targeted therapies using imaging biomarker outcomes.

IMAGING BIOMARKERS IN STROKE PREVENTION: FROM BENCH TO BEDSIDE

Imaging is one approach to the development of biomarkers, which are measurable indicators of disease risk, onset, progression, and response to therapy. The potential applications of biomarkers are to guide early neuroprotective and reperfusion interventions, to monitor neuroplasticity in stroke recovery, and to expedite therapy development. These applications can be applied to both large vessel occlusive and small vessel disease. Developing biomarkers highly predictive of stroke risk or occurrence could leverage more investment from industry to develop therapies for neurological disorders. Highly valid biomarkers could potentially revolutionize therapy development and preventive stroke care.

EXPEDITING HIGH PRIORITY COMPARATIVE EFFECTIVENESS TRIALS IN STROKE PREVENTION

Many stroke therapies in clinical practice are not guided by a strong evidence base. Some have associated risks and some are costly. Without a strong and comprehensive body of evidence, effective stroke prevention therapies may be unknowingly under-utilized, and/or less effective treatments may be over-utilized. Inappropriate treatment choices based on this lack of knowledge may increase the risk of medical and surgical complications and excess healthcare costs. As a result, CMS (the Centers for Medicaid and Medicare Services) and other insurers may not have the necessary data to make informed payment decisions. In addition to generating evidence on the most effective interventions overall, a closely related and important goal is to understand which treatments work for which patients and under which circumstances (i.e., personalized medicine). The current evidence base for stroke prevention therapies is based on aggregate effects in a population that likely includes those who benefit, those who do not benefit, and those who are harmed. Identifying which sub-populations benefit from specific interventions would allow for more targeted, effective, and efficient use of available therapies.

Treatment
EXPAND AND INTEGRATE EXISTING STROKE TRIAL NETWORKS TO ACCELERATE TRANSLATION

The NINDS established several complementary network/consortia aimed at improving treatment and care for individuals who experience a stroke. The Specialized Program of Translational Research in Acute Stroke (SPOTRIAS) helps move experimental therapies for acute stroke from the lab into early-phase clinical studies. The Neurological Emergencies Treatment Trials (NETT) network creates a similar collaborative framework among neurologists, neurosurgeons, and emergency medicine physicians to facilitate phase III clinical trials that can be initiated in the emergency room. More recently, the NINDS established the Network for Excellence in Neuroscience Clinical Trials (NeuroNEXT) which has been created to more broadly conduct early or phase II studies of promising treatments across all neurological diseases through partnerships with academia, private foundations, and industry.

Enhancing these networks ensures that the NINDS can support trials that span the prehospital setting, emergency department, catheterization lab, operating room, and intensive care unit. Conducting research in these settings poses many logistic challenges, especially when multiple studies are being conducted simultaneously. Efficient coordination allows priorities to be established and managed to facilitate the completion of NINDS trials in a timely and efficient manner.

PRECLINICAL AND CLINICAL STUDIES TO IMPROVE EARLY REPERFUSION THERAPY AND ESTABLISH THE LIMITATIONS OF LATE REPERFUSION THERAPY (REPERFUSE)

Improvements in lytic drugs, in imaging selection of patients for treatment, and in catheter-based approaches to reopening blocked arteries all represent promising scientific opportunities to improve reperfusion therapy. Over the last decade, there have been significant technology developments for intravascular approaches, including devices that can aid in the retrieval or removal of large occlusions causing an ischemic stroke. A number of devices have now been cleared by the FDA for use in reopening blocked arteries. However, despite some evidence that they can effectively open blocked arteries, these emerging endovascular therapies are limited by incomplete evidence of whether they improve final clinical outcome, which patients are most likely to benefit, how to limit hemorrhagic complications, and when recanalization attempts are futile and likely harmful. Thus, with the limitations of currently available reperfusion therapies, there remains an urgent need to improve early reperfusion and establish the therapeutic window of late reperfusion therapy.

PRECLINICAL AND CLINICAL STUDIES TO ACHIEVE ROBUST BRAIN PROTECTION

The scientific initiative that is proposed is a focused effort to promote studies to evaluate various therapeutic agents for neuroprotection after stroke, their potential combinations, and treatment windows for administration, through rigorous preclinical and clinical trials. Further efforts would focus on enhancing early administration, enhancing cytoprotection (glial as well as neural protection), and investigating synergies with reperfusion therapy.

Recovery
TRANSLATIONAL RESEARCH USING NEURAL INTERFACE DEVICES FOR STROKE AND OTHER NEUROLOGIC DISORDERS

For several decades, NIH investment in fundamental systems neuroscience and neural engineering, initiated through the early Neural Prosthesis Program, has led to creation of a few early-stage devices that can either be implanted in the brain or used relatively noninvasively to restore lost function. These neural interfaces have the potential to allow people to control computer cursers or prosthetic limbs, and they also have the potential to serve as rehabilitation training aids. In the last year, 'proof-of-concept' studies of both brain-computer interfaces (BCIs) that allow control of a robotic limb and intracortical technologies that detect brain signals to allow people to move a mouse curser have demonstrated utility of these devices in humans.

PROGRAM FOR TRANSLATIONAL RESEARCH TARGETING EARLY RECOVERY AFTER STROKE IN HUMANS

Most patients who survive a stroke experience some spontaneous return of neurologic function in the following months, but the degree of recovery is variable and often less than desired. Understanding how to manipulate the biology of recovery to improve functional outcome is a relatively unexplored scientific area with great potential public-health benefit given there are 7 million stroke survivors in the United States annually.

Section 25.2 | Optimizing Endovascular Therapy for Ischemic Stroke

This section includes text excerpted from "Optimizing Endovascular Therapy for Ischemic Stroke," National Institutes of Health (NIH), August 14, 2019.

Nearly 800,000 people in the United States. have a stroke each year. Most of these strokes are ischemic strokes, caused when a clot in a brain artery blocks blood flow, leading to permanent impairment if blood flow is not restored promptly. The clot-busting drug tPA (tissue plasminogen activator) was the first treatment approved for acute ischemic stroke and is an important frontline therapy. However, intravenous (IV) tPA must be given within four and a half hours after stroke onset, and it has limited effectiveness in patients with strokes due to clots in large brain arteries, which account for over a third of ischemic strokes and a disproportionately larger fraction of stroke-related death and disability.

With major contributions from the National Institute of Neurological Disorders and Stroke (NINDS)-supported research, a procedure called "endovascular thrombectomy" now offers another way to restore blood flow and save at-risk brain tissue in people with strokes due to blockages in large brain arteries. In a typical version of the procedure, a catheter is threaded through an artery at the groin, up to the neck, and to the site of a clot in a brain artery. A device called a "stent-retriever" is guided via the catheter to the clot. There, the surgeon opens the stent and retrieves the clot into the catheter to restore blood flow. Several endovascular thrombectomy devices are cleared by the U.S. Food and Drug Administration (FDA) for removing clots from the brain, and clinical guidelines provide criteria for their use in carefully selected patients up to 24 hours after stroke symptom onset.

Endovascular thrombectomy has developed alongside advances in brain imaging methods that help physicians determine which patients are most likely to benefit from this treatment. The NINDS-supported research was essential to understanding stroke injury progression, developing the first device approved for endovascular thrombectomy, applying novel imaging methods to acute stroke evaluation, and defining brain imaging profiles that, together with time since symptom onset, guide treatment decisions for acute stroke. Urgent medical attention remains imperative for stroke, as increasing numbers of neurons die in every minute of blocked blood flow. However, endovascular devices and sophisticated brain imaging enable good outcomes for more stroke patients and at later times after stroke onset than was once thought possible.

UNDERSTANDING INJURY PROGRESSION IN STROKE

When an artery supplying blood to the brain is blocked, as in ischemic stroke, the tissue served by that artery does not get the oxygen and nutrients it needs. In the 1970s and 1980s, researchers with NINDS and other support used experimental animal models of stroke to understand what levels of blood flow were required for brain tissue to function and survive. They began to distinguish a region of irreversible damage after stroke (the infarct or core lesion) from a surrounding zone they called the "penumbra," an area with reduced blood flow where tissue is functionally impaired but surviving. The core lesion inevitably expands into the penumbra over time without restored blood flow, but studies in animal models and later research in stroke patients suggested that the rate of injury expansion differs across individuals. Although brain cells quickly die if their blood supply remains blocked, other blood vessels in the region, called "collaterals," can compensate to varying degrees. In some studies, viable brain tissue remained in the penumbra for 17 hours or more after stroke onset. Identifying and then saving at-risk tissue in the penumbra by restoring blood flow became a primary goal for stroke treatment.

ENDOVASCULAR THERAPIES FOR LARGE ARTERY STROKES

Multiple studies supported by the NINDS and other sources assessed the benefit of administering clot-busting drugs via catheter directly to blockages inside blood vessels in the brain. This intra-arterial approach was based on the idea that direct delivery would allow higher drug concentrations at the blockage site than IV delivery, and in turn to more successful degradation of offending clots in large arteries. In the 1950s, case reports began to describe another intuitively attractive alternative: the surgical removal of blockages. Early attempts used devices designed for other types of surgery, but later devices were designed specifically for removing stroke-causing clots through a procedure called "endovascular thrombectomy." The Mechanical Embolus Removal in Cerebral Ischemia (MERCI) device (Concentric Medical, California, USA), developed in part with the NINDS support, was the first such device cleared by the FDA in 2004, for use in stroke patients who cannot receive or fail to benefit from intravenous tPA. Additional improved devices followed, including stent-retrievers, which both open affected vessels and remove clots. Clinical trials showed that these devices successfully restored blood flow in patients with strokes due to LAO, but they did not compare clinical outcomes versus medical therapy alone.

In 2013, a group of clinical trials, including the NINDS-supported Interventional Management of Stroke III trial (IMS III), failed to show that endovascular or intra-arterial therapies led to better outcomes than standard medical therapy, including intravenous tPA. Although disappointing, understanding why the trials failed provided valuable lessons. Only some of the trials used brain imaging to confirm blockages in large arteries, for which endovascular therapies were presumed to be most effective. In addition, over the course of the trials, thrombectomy devices had continued to improve, yet the trials included older versions ultimately shown to be less effective. By the time the negative trials were completed, new trials addressing these and other concerns were already underway. Just two years later, five major trials together established the superiority of endovascular thrombectomy over medical therapy alone for stroke patients with LAO treated within six hours of symptom onset. Based on these trials, the American Heart Association (AHA)/American Stroke Association (ASA) added endovascular thrombectomy using stent-retrievers to clinical guidelines for the early management of acute ischemic stroke.

Section 25.3 | Modified Stem Cells Boost Regeneration after Stroke

This section includes text excerpted from "Modified Stem Cells Boost Regeneration after Stroke," National Institutes of Health (NIH), May 14, 2019.

NEW TECHNIQUE OVERCOMES MAJOR OBSTACLE TO STEM-CELL-BASED TREATMENTS

Your brain cells need plenty of oxygen and nutrients to survive—that is unless you are a hibernating ground squirrel. By tapping into the cellular process that keeps these animals' brains healthy during the long winter months, IRP scientists have discovered a way to increase the survival of neuron-producing stem cells implanted into the brain after a stroke, a development that could one day dramatically improve stroke treatment.

An ischemic stroke cuts off blood flow to part of the brain, depriving the cells there of life-sustaining substances. While clinicians can reduce the damage by restoring blood flow as quickly as possible, there is not yet a way to help patients regenerate lost neurons. One promising approach is to implant neural stem cells into the damaged area, which would then develop into new neurons and establish connections with nearby cells to restore function. Unfortunately, like an oil spill that makes a patch of ocean

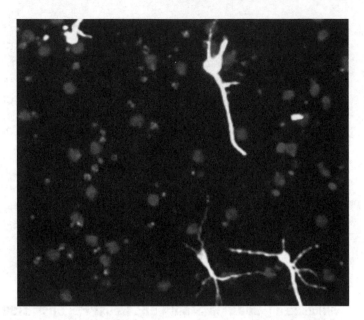

Figure 25.1. Neurons

Boosting a cellular process called "SUMOylation" helped neural stem cells survive hostile conditions similar to those in the poststroke brain and encouraged them to develop into neurons (white).

uninhabitable, a stroke creates conditions that make it difficult for stem cells to survive.

In an attempt to overcome this obstacle, the lab of IRP senior investigator John Hallenbeck, M.D., has spent more than a decade studying a process called "SUMOylation" that the group discovered helps brain cells survive the lack of blood flow that occurs when a certain species of squirrel hibernates. SUMOylation alters the activity and cellular location of proteins by attaching chemical tags called "small ubiquitin-like modifiers" (SUMOs) to them. In theory, revving up SUMOylation in stem cells could help them survive in the hostile environment of a poststroke brain.

"Stroke therapy is a field ripe for innovation," says Dr. Joshua Bernstock, who led the new study as part of his graduate research in Dr. Hallenbeck's lab. "Stem cells are really dynamic molecular medicines that can react in real-time to the conditions in the focal diseased environment, so they are kind of like living drugs."

In the new study, Dr. Bernstock and his colleagues utilized transgenic mice that had more of the enzyme that attaches SUMO tags to other proteins. They found that neural stem cells from the brains of these mice had higher levels of SUMOylation and less activity in genes involved in cell death. Moreover, when placed in a petri dish, the cells consumed less oxygen than neural stem cells from normal mice and more frequently developed into neurons rather than other types of brain cells.

Next, the scientists placed the transgenic stem cells and neurons that grew from them into a petri dish that lacked oxygen and nutrients. After five hours, the cells were re-exposed to those life-sustaining substances. Compared to stem cells and neurons with typical levels of SUMOylation, significantly more of the transgenic stem cells and neurons survived this experiment, which approximates the conditions in the brain caused by an ischemic stroke.

Finally, the research team examined the survival and behavior of neural stem cells implanted into the brains of mouse models of ischemic stroke. Once again, more of the transgenic cells survived the hostile conditions of the poststroke brain. In addition, those cells produced more neurons than did normal stem cells, and those neurons formed more connections with neighboring cells.

"The same phenomenon that we had seen in the petri dish played out in the brains of the mice," Dr. Bernstock explains. "That's very promising when you think about how to engineer a cell that you would ultimately hope to use in the context of regenerative medicine."

Future studies will need to examine how grafts of neural stem cells with greater SUMOylation affect functional recovery in mouse models of stroke. Scientists might also look into methods of boosting SUMOylation that do not involve manipulating genes. Ultimately, if the approach is proven to be safe and effective in animals, clinicians may one day implant neural stem cells with increased SUMOylation into the brains of stroke patients to help them regenerate lost neurons.

"As a physician-scientist, it Is always exciting to be working on an experimental therapeutic that has clinical implications," Dr. Bernstock says. "As we continue to refine these techniques and define the mechanisms by which stem cells help protect and repair the brain, I am incredibly optimistic that these sorts of preclinical studies will advance from the bench to the bedside."

Section 25.4 | Gene Therapy for Brain Tissue Repair in Stroke

This section includes text excerpted from "Gene Therapy Shows Promise Repairing Brain Tissue Damaged by Stroke," National Institute on Aging (NIA), National Institutes of Health (NIH), September 26, 2019.

GENE THERAPY

It is a race against time when someone suffers a stroke caused by a blockage of a blood vessel supplying the brain. Unless clot-busting treatment is given within a few hours after symptoms appear, vast numbers of the brain's neurons die, often leading to paralysis or other disabilities. It would be great to have a way to replace those lost neurons. Thanks to gene therapy, some encouraging strides are now being made.

In a recent study in *Molecular Therapy*, researchers reported that, in their mouse and rat models of ischemic stroke, gene therapy could actually convert the brain's support cells into new, fully functional neurons. Even better, after gaining the new neurons, the animals had improved motor and memory skills.

For the team led by Gong Chen, Penn State, University Park, the quest to replace lost neurons in the brain began about a decade ago. While searching for the right approach, Chen noticed other groups had learned to reprogram fibroblasts into stem cells and make replacement neural cells.

As innovative as this work was at the time, it was performed mostly in lab petri dishes. Chen and his colleagues thought, why not reprogram cells already in the brain?

They turned their attention to the brain's billions of supportive glial cells. Unlike neurons, glial cells divide and replicate. They also are known to survive and activate following a brain injury, remaining at the wound, and ultimately forming a scar. This same process had also been observed in the brain following many types of injury, including stroke and neurodegenerative conditions, such as Alzheimer disease.

To Chen's National Institutes of Health (NIH)-supported team, it looked like glial cells might be a perfect target for gene therapies to replace lost neurons. As reported about five years ago, the researchers were on the right track.

The Chen team showed it was possible to reprogram glial cells in the brain into functional neurons. They succeeded in using a genetically engineered retrovirus that delivered a single protein called "NeuroD1." It is a neural transcription factor that switches genes on and off in neural cells and helps to determine their cell fate. The newly generated neurons were also capable of integrating into brain circuits to repair damaged tissue.

There was one major hitch: the NeuroD1 retroviral vector only reprogrammed actively dividing glial cells. That suggested their strategy likely could not generate the large numbers of new cells needed to repair damaged brain tissue following a stroke.

Fast-forward a couple of years, and improved adeno-associated viral vectors (AAV) have emerged as a major alternative to retroviruses for gene therapy applications. This was exactly the breakthrough that the Chen team needed. The AAVs can reprogram glial cells whether they are dividing or not.

In the new study, Chen's team, led by post doc Yu-Chen Chen, put this new gene therapy system to work, and the results are quite remarkable. In a mouse model of ischemic stroke, the researchers showed the treatment could regenerate about a third of the total lost neurons by preferentially targeting reactive, scar-forming glial cells. The conversion of those reactive glial cells into neurons also protected another third of the neurons from injury.

Studies in brain slices showed that the replacement neurons were fully functional and appeared to have made the needed neural connections in the brain. Importantly, their studies also showed that the NeuroD1 gene therapy led to marked improvements in the functional recovery of the mice after a stroke.

In fact, several tests of their ability to make fine movements with their forelimbs showed about a 60 percent improvement within 20 to 60 days of receiving the NeuroD1 therapy. Together with study collaborator and NIH grantee Gregory Quirk, University of Puerto Rico, San Juan, they went on to show similar improvements in the ability of rats to recover from stroke-related deficits in memory.

While further study is needed, the findings in rodents offer encouraging evidence that treatments to repair the brain after a stroke or other injury may be on the horizon. In the meantime, the best strategy for limiting the number of neurons lost due to stroke is to recognize the signs and get to a well-equipped hospital or call 911 right away if you or a loved one experience them. Those signs include: sudden numbness or weakness of one side of the body; confusion; difficulty speaking, seeing, or walking; and a sudden, severe headache with unknown causes. Getting treatment for this kind of "brain attack" within four hours of the onset of symptoms can make all the difference in recovery.

Section 25.5 | Neuroplasticity in Stroke Rehabilitation

This section contains text excerpted from the following sources: Text beginning with the heading "Neuroplasticity and Rehabilitation" is excerpted from "Guest Editorial—Neuroplasticity and Rehabilitation," Rehabilitation Research & Development Service (RR&D), U.S. Department of Veterans Affairs (VA), November 17, 2005. Reviewed May 2020; Text beginning with the heading "Neuroplasticity Is Important to Survival and Functioning in Our Daily Lives" is excerpted from "Intro-to-Neuroplasticity," U.S. Department of Veterans Affairs (VA), February 20, 2018.

NEUROPLASTICITY AND REHABILITATION

Neuroplasticity is the ability of the central nervous system to remodel itself. In the last few decades, neuroplasticity is not only possible but that it is also constantly occurring; the brain is always changing. Neuroplasticity is how humans adapt to changing conditions, learn new facts, and develop new skills. If the brain is injured, it tries to repair itself with these normal mechanisms. If all goes well, spontaneous recovery can be excellent. Of course, the natural scope of these plastic processes is limited, and sometimes the end point of the remodeling is problematic itself. The job for those interested in rehabilitation is to promote plasticity in the right direction and, sometimes, to correct it if it has taken a wrong turn. Humans must, therefore, understand neuroplasticity and learn to control it. Fortunately, this is an active area for current research.

MECHANISMS OF NEUROPLASTICITY

Neuroplasticity can be understood at several levels. The first level is that of the individual neuron and the events responsible for remodeling that occur within the cell. The second level is that of groups of neurons and their functions that can change to alter behavior. At the cellular level, multiple processes can occur both in parallel and serially. Generally speaking, some processes are quick, but transient, and can allow for rapid adaptations. Others take longer, but are then more permanent.

One principle appears to be that the more persistent an early change is, the more likely it is that it will be permanent. The fastest type of change is a simple modulation of neuronal traffic that leads to a change in the amount of excitation and inhibition. Apparently many neural networks are chronically and largely inactive because of tonic inhibition. Release of this inhibition will allow the networks to function; a process sometimes called "unmasking." Unmasking can be demonstrated in animal models with local delivery of gamma-amino-butyric acid antagonists, which immediately opens new functional networks.

Another relatively rapid change involves alteration of the strength of specific synapses. The magnitude of the response of the synapses changes as a function of the pattern of activity that they experience, both at the individual synapse and at the temporal conjunction of two or more synapses on the same cell. The most well-known of these processes are long-term potentiation (LTP), which is an increase in synaptic strength, and long term depression (LTD), which is a decrease in synaptic strength. After only minutes of synaptic activity, there can be changes that last hours or are relatively permanent.

The molecular and cellular biologies of LTP and LTD are being intensively studied, and a fascinating set of cellular processes have been discovered, which are triggered and regulated by the influx of calcium at the active synapses. It is important to recognize as well that a decrease in inhibition will facilitate changes in synaptic strength, and this links unmasking to LTP and LTD. Another type of cellular change is anatomical and involves remodeling the dendritic spines of neurons and their resultant connectivity. Some spines appear to come and go relatively quickly.

Of course, when there are more long-lasting anatomical changes, a plastic process is more secure. Basic processes of neuroplasticity can be studied noninvasively in humans, but the correlations between the cellular mechanisms and the results from human studies are uncertain. One method for studying unmasking is acute deafferentation, which can be induced by peripheral ischemia. When employing this method, it is commonly used as a blood pressure cuff inflated over a subject's elbow; within minutes, nerve traffic begins to lessen, and it disappears completely within 20 to 30 min.

This deafferentation appears to cause a decrease in inhibition in the local region of the motor cortex, where the neurons are located that innervate the deafferented part of the body and its adjacent parts. Researchers can readily study this response by observing the rapid increase in excitability of the cortical motor representations* that control adjacent body parts with the application of transcranial magnetic stimulation (TMS). Using microneurography, researchers demonstrated that the deafferented area itself shows an increase in excitability.

When there is peripheral deafferentation for longer periods, as is seen with amputation or spinal cord injury, other mechanisms are triggered that cause more permanent changes. However, these more permanent changes can go awry, as seen by the phenomenon of phantom pain. A number of human models are being used for the study of long-term neuroplastic changes, which may be the result of changes in synaptic strength or synaptic remodeling. Motor learning can be modeled (or "studied") with the use of a variety of motor tasks from simple pinching to moving the thumb in one direction to more complex skills, such as movement sequences. The early events focus on the motor cortex, where increases in metabolic activity are measured with neuroimaging and changes

228

in muscle excitability with TMS. Motor learning can have some permanence, and some aspects of it are similar to LTP and LTD.

Another set of models for long-term changes are those that artificially modulate neuronal traffic to regions, such as the motor cortex. Repetitive TMS at rates of ≥ 5 Hz lead to increases in excitability, while rates of ≤ 1 Hz can lead to loss of inhibition. Use of the theta-burst stimulation technique to pattern the stimuli may be even more effective. The application of direct current to the brain with a technique called "direct current transcranial stimulation" can also lead to increases and decreases in excitability, depending on whether the anode or cathode is placed over the motor cortex. Additionally, paired stimuli at the motor cortex, such as a median nerve stimulus combined with TMS (a technique called "paired afferent stimulation"), can lead to excitation or inhibition, depending on the interval between the stimuli.

PRINCIPLES OF REHABILITATION

Understanding neuroplastic mechanisms allows humans to recognize how the brain tries to repair itself. Several important principles emerge:

1. Body parts can compete for representation in the brain and use of a body part can enhance its representation.

Representation areas increase or decrease depending on use. A good example is Braille readers who use their fingers many hours a day in the skilled task of interpreting Braille characters. In this situation, the first dorsal interosseus (FDI) is used for reading, while the abductor digiti minimi (ADM) is largely passive. Using TMS mapping, researchers did not find significant differences between the motor representations of right and left FDI and ADM in control subjects. However, in proficient Braille readers, the representation of the FDI in the reading hand was significantly larger than that in the nonreading hand, or in either hand of the control subjects. Conversely, the representation of the ADM in the reading hand was significantly smaller than that in the nonreading hand, or in either hand of the control subjects. These results suggest that the cortical representation of the reading finger in proficient Braille readers is enlarged at the expense of the representation of other fingers. Conversely, if a body part is not used, its representation area shrinks. For example, the representation area of the tibialis anterior is smaller after the ankle is immobilized in a cast for several weeks. In case of a stroke that damages a body part representation in the primary motor cortex, plasticity permits some reorganization that will restore a representation. This process must be competitive with all the body parts.

2. The premotor cortex can substitute for the motor cortex to control motion.

While the primary motor cortex has the largest and most powerful contribution to the function of the corticospinal tract, the premotor cortex also contributes. We know, from both anatomical and physiological studies, that there are contributions of the premotor cortex to the function of the corticospinal tract, but stimulation thresholds of the premotor cortex are higher than that of the primary motor cortex. So, while the main output of the premotor cortex is ordinarily to the primary motor cortex, the premotor cortex can also be the source of supraspinal control signals.

3. The contralesional hemisphere can take over motor control if everything else fails.

Although rather weak in humans, there are ipsilateral, corticospinal neural pathways. Although these pathways innervate many more proximal than distal muscles, they can be documented in normal humans, even in distal muscles, with the use of TMS. Such pathways are necessarily involved in recovery of patients with hemispherectomy. Although controversial, these pathways may possibly be relevant in stroke recovery. Another possible role of the undamaged hemisphere could be its interactions with the damaged hemisphere; there are transcallosal connections that are not completely characterized. Some of these transcallosal connections are inhibitory, and improvement might occur if these connections were themselves inhibited. Functional magnetic resonance imaging studies show that the damaged hemisphere has increased blood flow when bilateral movements are made; these data are consistent with the idea that activity of the undamaged hemisphere might support the damaged hemisphere. Another possibility is that the ipsilateral hemisphere helps with activity of the premotor cortex rather than the motor cortex itself.

4. Neuroplastic mechanisms can be facilitated and this is a good basis for intervention.

Intensive, focused physical therapy should help restore motor function, and evidence shows that the earlier and more intensive the therapy, the better the outcome. This concept has been most fully demonstrated by the multiple successes of constraint induced (CI) movement therapy. This method forces patients to use the hemiplegic limb by constraining the good limb. In a number of clinical trials, patients have shown behavioral improvement with the use of CI, even those with chronic and apparently stable deficits. TMS maps of the weakened muscles increase in size in these circumstances, which shows that the expected cortical changes appear to be occurring.

Other techniques such as neuromuscular electrical stimulation, robot-enhanced training, and virtual reality training likely use the same principle. Bilateral symmetrical arm movement training appears helpful; this might be due to facilitation of the contralesional hemisphere. One example is repetitive bilateral arm training with rhythmic auditory cueing; patients showed significant improvements that were largely sustained at 8 weeks after this training concluded. A prolonged period of peripheral nerve stimulation will increase the excitability of related TMS muscle representations in the motor cortex, and this suggests that sensory stimulation could be a useful rehabilitation tool. Sensory stimulation can be applied in a number of ways from passive movement to cutaneous stimulation with transcutaneous electrical nerve stimulation and even to acupuncture.

Stimulation of the pharynx may improve swallowing function. Another method for improving rehabilitation is the combined use of drug therapy and physical therapy. In general, studies indicate that the combination is important; drugs by themselves seem not to be efficacious. The most fully documented improvements are with amphetamine and related noradrenergic agents. Drug therapy was first demonstrated to be valuable in a rat model; now several clinical trials show that amphetamine, together with physical therapy, is better than physical therapy alone. The mechanism for this drug action is not completely clear. While it is possible that it

231

works by relieving diaschisis, amphetamine also enhances plastic changes in motor learning in both animals and humans. Evidence has also been found for enhanced neural sprouting and synaptogenesis. Now other agents such as fluoxetine, methylphenidate, and levodopa, have been shown to be of use.

OTHER INNOVATIVE METHODS

For the future, a variety of innovative methods may well emerge that take advantage of plastic processes. An example is a technique that researchers have been exploring that uses exercise together with local anesthesia. After a hemiplegic stroke, significant function is often lost in the hand, while strength is retained in the proximal arm muscles. Since competition exists between body parts for representation in the motor cortex, it is possible that use of the proximal muscles makes it difficult for hand muscles to increase their representation. Researchers know that peripheral deafferentation increases the excitability of proximal muscles, and recently the researchers have demonstrated that this increase is magnified by exercise of the proximal muscles during the peripheral block. Researchers reasoned that anesthesia of proximal muscles and exercise of the hand might increase cortical representation of the hand and concomitantly improve hand function. Preliminary results suggest that this may indeed occur. Other techniques may utilize brain stimulation methods to improve rehabilitation.

NEUROPLASTICITY IS IMPORTANT FOR SURVIVAL AND FUNCTIONING OF DAILY LIVES

Everyday habits you develop are an example of "neuroplasticity."
- You can drive home without having to remember all the steps, streets, or dirt roads along the way.
- Neuroplasticity means that you can travel to a good friend's house almost on 'autopilot', without having to think about every turn you make.
- You can learn phone numbers by frequent use.

232

The two sides of the plasticity coin:
- There can be downsides to neuroplasticity too and chronic pain is a good example. Here, neuroplasticity results in parts of the nervous system becoming over excitable and this means that normal everyday tasks can cause pain when they should not.

What does this mean as a person with persistent pain?
- In cases of persistent pain, the nervous system becomes very excitable. This super excitable nervous system behavior is called "central sensitization." Central sensitization is a key factor in persistent pain. Here are some of the common aspects of persistent pain:
  - Very easy to trigger a lot of pain from normal everyday activities (bending, lifting, sitting, running, playing sport, working)
  - Painful inputs that would normally hurt, are exaggerated (if you over-stretch an already sensitive low back pain, it can REALLY hurt)

Negative health effects of central sensitization include moving away from valued activities, poor sleep, low energy, low mood, negative and unhelpful thoughts, loss of control, exaggerated stress responses, and being less able to care for yourself or your family and friends.

All these changes can result in the experience of more pain sensations even though the initial tissue injury has long resolved. It is almost like pain has a mind of its own. In acute pain, the brain initially uses pain as an alarm signal to protect and warn people of a potential threat. Humans are very sensitive to things that might threaten their survival and this is good biologic design! However, chronic pain signals are like a car alarm that goes off all the time rather than serving as a signal for danger.

Pain itself can soon become a major and unwelcome focus of people's attention. The more concerned and distressed humans are about pain, especially if they interpret the pain as harmful, the more pain dominates the thinking. It is almost as if the more people do not want pain, the more the brain calls attention to pain.

WHAT CAN YOU DO?

1. Learning ways to manage the stress response and reduce the focus on pain helps you manage and function better.
2. Movement, exercise, activity done in a sensibly paced way can also help to normalize this heightened pain sensitivity.
3. Nonopioid pain medicines may also help to decrease sensitization in your system.
4. New creative hobbies or practices (like photography or meditation) help to use the positive aspects of neuroplasticity to calm and 're-wire' NONpainful nervous system connections.
5. Learning to reduce this distress response and reduce the focus on pain, especially with persistent pain, is vital to improving your function and returning to normal activities at work and with family.
6. In persistent pain, improving your function may require you to retrain the way in which your mind and body interpret and respond to pain.

Part 4 | **Poststroke Complications and Rehabilitation**

Chapter 26 | Early Complications of Stroke

Chapter Contents

Section 26.1 | Cerebral Edema after Ischemic Stroke

"Cerebral Edema after Ischemic Stroke," © 2020 Omnigraphics. Reviewed May 2020.

Cerebral edema (brain swelling) is a life-threatening condition that causes fluid to develop in the brain. This fluid increases the intracranial pressure (ICP) that is present inside of the skull. Increased ICP can reduce blood flow to the brain and decrease the oxygen level received by the brain. Cerebral edema can be caused by an ischemic stroke (occurs due to blood clot near the brain), which leads to the death of brain cells and causes the brain to swell. Cerebral edema after ischemic stroke is rare and occurs only in about 10 to 20 percent of stroke survivors. The edema (swelling) becomes severe in approximately 72 to 96 hours after the primary onset of stroke. People at a higher risk of cerebral edema include women, patients with hypertension, and people suffering from diabetes.

SYMPTOMS OF CEREBRAL EDEMA

Cerebral edema symptoms vary, depending on the severity and the cause. They usually manifest suddenly without any prior warning, and may include the following:
- Headache
- Neck pain or stiffness
- Nausea
- Dizziness
- Breathing trouble
- Vision loss or changes
- Memory loss
- Inability to walk
- Difficulty speaking
- Stupor
- Seizures
- Loss of consciousness

DIAGNOSIS OF CEREBRAL EDEMA

Diagnosing cerebral edema can be challenging since the symptoms may vary significantly. A few common procedures used to diagnose cerebral edema include:

- Physical exam of the head and neck
- CT scan or MRI of the head to check the location and extent of the swelling
- Blood tests to diagnose cause of the swelling
- Neurological exams to test brain function

TREATMENT OF CEREBRAL EDEMA AFTER ISCHEMIC STROKE

Treatment options for cerebral edema aim to restore blood flow and oxygen to the brain while reducing the swelling. It is also necessary to treat the underlying cause to prevent any further damage. These are the most common treatment options.

Medications

Depending on the severity of the condition and the primary cause, drugs may be prescribed to help reduce swelling and prevent blood clots. Medications for reducing edema and intracranial pressure in stroke patients include diuretics (removes excess water), corticosteroids (reduces swelling), and barbiturates (sedatives).

Osmotic Therapy

Osmotic therapy is a technique that drains water out of the brain using osmotic agents such as mannitol, or high-salt saline. It also helps improve blood circulation, which results in reduced swelling and ICP in the skull.

Hyperventilation

Controlled hyperventilation can be used to help lower the ICP and hence, reduce the symptoms of cerebral edema. Hyperventilation causes a person to exhale more than inhale, thus lowering the amount of carbon dioxide in the bloodstream. Proper blood flow in the brain is dependent upon carbon dioxide, and controlling this process reduces the blood flow in the brain and decreases ICP. However, prolonged and aggressive hyperventilation can cause cerebral ischemia (lack of blood flow to brain) in patients with brain injury and is usually used as a last resort.

Hypothermia

Inducing hypothermia (lowering body temperature) decreases metabolism (chemical process) in the brain and can also reduce swelling.

Surgery

Ventriculostomy is an invasive procedure that involves draining fluid from the brain. A surgeon makes a small incision in the skull and inserts a tube as a drain to relieve the ICP pressure. In more severe cases of cerebral edema, surgical decompression can also be used to create space to accommodate the increased volume created by the swollen brain. This is done by removing a part of the skull (cranial vault) and dura (membrane around the brain), or by extracting nonessential brain tissue.

References

1. Anthony, Kiara. "Cerebral Edema," Healthline, December 1, 2017.
2. "Brain Swelling," WebMD, September 16, 2018.
3. "Critical Care for Patients with Massive Ischemic Stroke," Journal of Stroke (JOS), September 30, 2014.

Section 26.2 | **Stroke and Pneumonia**

"Stroke and Pneumonia," © 2020 Omnigraphics. Reviewed May 2020.

The highest priority of a doctor treating a stroke patient is to prevent further complications that can occur as a result of the stroke and also to prevent another stroke. Some incidents of stroke arise as a direct consequence of brain damage. Others are due to a change in capabilities. Following a stroke, cognitive disabilities and sensory impairments are common. Up to 90 percent of stroke survivors will experience some paralysis or motor deficiency measurements. The swallowing process involves more than 30 muscles and about half of people with strokes suffer from trouble when swallowing, or dysphagia.

STROKE SURVIVOR'S RISK OF PNEUMONIA

Pneumonia is an infection that causes inflammation in the air sacs of one or both the lungs. The air sacs often get filled with fluid or pus, making it difficult to breathe.

Aspiration pneumonia is the most significant acute complication of the dysphagia associated with strokes. Pneumonia is a significant source of poststroke morbidity and mortality. According to the Pneumonia in Stroke Consensus (PISCES) Group, stroke-associated pneumonia (SAP) describes the continuum of low respiratory tract infections in the first week that complicate stroke. Patients with severe stroke symptoms and high disability are at particular risk of SAP. While the precise root cause of stroke-related dysphagia is not well known, it associates difficulty swallowing with brain stem injury or stroke-related lesions. The muscles used in swallowing are found on both sides of the brain.

Individuals who have experienced a stroke in their primary swallowing area are expected to be at an elevated risk for dysphagia. Swallowing trouble, poor speech, lack of gag reflex, drooling, decreased function of the mouth, vomiting, and coughing when swallowing foods and liquids, etc. are the typical symptoms of dysphagia. It is usually also referred to as trouble with feeding, drinking, breathing, and taking medicine.

Usually, if foreign substances (solid or liquid) penetrate the airway, an involuntary cough would be induced to avoid these contaminants from reaching the lungs. Dysphagia also decreases these impulses and a patient with a stroke does not cough as a reaction, resulting in the intrusion or expulsion of certain foreign substances into the lungs. This is known as a "silent aspiration" since a patient is unaware of this aspiration and will not cough out. Sadly, almost all of the survivors of stroke suffer from quiet coughing, and one percent of the survivors of stroke ultimately develop pneumonia.

RECOVERY FROM STROKE-RELATED PNEUMONIA

Occupational therapy, speech therapy, and physical therapy are among the few methods of the recovery process for those struggling with dysphagia.

Every year, 15 million individuals across the globe experience a stroke and as a result, about half of all acute stroke patients tend to be affected by dysphagia. Unfortunately, this disease raises a person's chance of contracting aspiration pneumonia by seven times. There are various approaches and changes to the lifestyle that will help patients deal with dysphagia, sustain a healthy diet, and reduce their chance of contracting pneumonia.

Every stroke is different and so for optimal outcomes, every stroke treatment program should be designed for each patient in a specific way. Now, the average quality of life of a stroke patient can be improved and problems including pneumonia can be avoided with a safe, diligent, and personally customized recovery program.

A wide range of products are available that combine evidence-based rehabilitation techniques with cutting-edge technology to treat the patients and survivors.

References

1. Hoffman, Henry. "What Is the Relationship Between Stroke and Pneumonia?" Saebo, November 26, 2018.
2. "Stroke Associated Pneumonia: Better Safe than Sorry," European Stroke Organisation, August 24, 2018.

Section 26.3 | Seizures after Stroke

This section includes text excerpted from "Strokes May Lead to Epilepsy," Centers for Disease Control and Prevention (CDC), July 9, 2019.

STROKES CAN CAUSE SEIZURES AND EPILEPSY

Epilepsy is a broad term used for a brain disorder that causes repeated seizures. There are many types of epilepsy, and there are also many different kinds of seizures.

A single seizure may happen soon after a stroke. You do not necessarily have epilepsy, or will develop epilepsy, if you have just one seizure. Certain types of strokes, such as ones that cause bleeding, and more severe strokes may be more likely to cause epilepsy.

One study found that among those who had strokes, 5 percent had one seizure and 7 percent developed epilepsy in the thirty months afterward.

Epilepsy caused by strokes can usually be controlled with anti-seizure medicines. It is important to take medicine as prescribed to keep seizures under control.

OLDER ADULTS ARE MORE AT RISK

Epilepsy is more likely to develop in older adults than younger adults. Stroke causes up to half of new epilepsy cases in older adults for which a cause can be identified. This makes stroke one of the most common reasons people develop epilepsy as they age.

Seizures may be hard to recognize in older adults and may be overlooked. For instance, trouble with memory, confusion, falls, dizziness, or numbness may be viewed as "normal" aging problems. However, these can actually be symptoms of seizures and are not normal. Older adults who have had a stroke, and their caregivers, should watch for these symptoms.

Section 26.4 | Deep Vein Thrombosis after Stroke

This section includes text excerpted from "How to Spot and Prevent Deep Vein Thrombosis," *NIH News in Health*, National Institutes of Health (NIH), January 3, 2017.

Lots of things can cause pain and swelling in your leg. But, if your symptoms stem from a blood clot deep in your leg, it can be dangerous. Blood clots can happen to anyone, anytime. But, some people are at increased risk. Taking steps to reduce your chances of a blood clot forming in your veins can help you avoid potentially serious problems.

Blood clots can arise anywhere in your body. They develop when blood thickens and clumps together. When a clot forms in a vein deep in the body, it is known as "deep vein thrombosis." Deep vein blood clots typically occur in the lower leg or thigh.

Deep vein thrombosis (DVT) has classic symptoms such as swelling, pain, warmth, and redness on the leg but about 30 to 40 percent of cases go unnoticed since they do not have typical symptoms. In fact, some people do not realize they have a deep vein clot until it causes a more serious condition.

Deep vein clots—especially those in the thigh—can break off and travel through the bloodstream. If a clot lodges in an artery in the lungs, it can block blood flow and lead to a sometimes-deadly condition called "pulmonary embolism." This disorder can damage the lungs and reduce blood-oxygen levels, which can harm other organs as well.

Some people are more at risk for DVT than others. Usually, people who develop DVT have some level of thrombophilia, which means their blood clots more rapidly or easily. Getting a blood clot is usually the first sign of this condition because it is hard to notice otherwise. In these cases, lifestyle can contribute to a blood clot forming—if you do not move enough, for example. Your risk is higher if you have recently had surgery or broken a bone if you are ill and in bed for a long time, or if you are traveling for a long time (such as during long car or airplane rides).

Having other diseases or conditions can also raise your chances of a blood clot. These include a stroke, paralysis (an inability to move), chronic heart disease, high blood pressure, surgical procedure, or having been recently treated for cancer. Women who take hormone therapy pills or birth control pills, are pregnant, or within the first 6 weeks after giving birth are also at higher risk. So are those who smoke or who are older than 60 years of age. But, deep vein thrombosis can happen at any age.

You can take simple steps to lower your chances of a blood clot. Exercise your lower leg muscles if you sit for a long time while traveling. Get out of bed and move around as soon as you are able after having surgery or being ill. The more active you are, the better your chance of avoiding a blood clot. Take any medicines your doctor prescribes to prevent clots after some types of surgery.

Prompt diagnosis and proper treatment can help prevent the complications of blood clots. See your doctor immediately if you have any signs or symptoms of deep vein thrombosis or pulmonary embolism. A physical exam and other tests can help doctors determine whether you have got a blood clot.

There are many ways to treat DVT. Therapies aim to stop the blood clot from getting bigger, prevent the clot from breaking off and moving to your lungs, or reduce your chance of having another blood clot. The NIH scientists continue to on research new medicines and better treatment options.

Chapter 27 | Functional Impairments and Disabilities Following Poststroke Complications

Chapter Contents

Section 27.1 | Physical Complications after Stroke

This section includes text excerpted from documents published by two public domain sources. Text under the headings marked 1 are excerpted from "Poststroke Rehabilitation," Know Stroke, National Institute of Neurological Disorders and Stroke (NINDS), September 1, 2014. Reviewed May 2020; Text under the headings marked 2 are excerpted from "Foot Drop Information Page," National Institute of Neurological Disorders and Stroke (NINDS), March 27, 2019.

PARALYSIS OR PROBLEMS CONTROLLING MOVEMENT[1]

Paralysis is one of the most common disabilities resulting from a stroke. The paralysis is usually on the side of the body opposite the side of the brain damaged by stroke and may affect the face, an arm, a leg, or the entire side of the body. This one-sided paralysis is called "hemiplegia" if it involves complete inability to move, or hemiparesis if it is less than total weakness. Stroke patients with hemiparesis or hemiplegia may have difficulty with everyday activities such as walking or grasping objects. Some stroke patients have problems with swallowing, called "dysphagia," due to damage to the part of the brain that controls the muscles for swallowing. Damage to a lower part of the brain, the cerebellum, can affect the body's ability to coordinate movement—a disability called "ataxia"—leading to problems with body posture, walking, and balance.

WHAT IS FOOT DROP?[2]

Foot drop describes the inability to raise the front part of the foot due to weakness or paralysis of the muscles that lift the foot. As a result, individuals with foot drop, scuff their toes along the ground or bend their knees to lift their foot higher than usual to avoid the scuffing, which causes what is called a "steppage" gait. Foot drop can be unilateral (affecting one foot) or bilateral (affecting both feet). Foot drop is a symptom of an underlying problem and is either temporary or permanent, depending on the cause. Causes include neurodegenerative disorders of the brain that cause muscular problems such as multiple sclerosis, stroke, and cerebral palsy; motor neuron disorders such as polio, some forms of spinal muscular atrophy, and amyotrophic lateral sclerosis (commonly known as "Lou Gehrig disease"); injury to the nerve roots, such as in spinal stenosis; peripheral nerve disorders, such as Charcot-Marie-Tooth disease or acquired peripheral neuropathy; local compression or damage to the peroneal nerve as it passes across the fibular bone below the knee; and muscle disorders, such as muscular dystrophy or myositis.

TREATMENT OF FOOT DROP[2]

Treatment depends on the specific cause of foot drop. The most common treatment is to support the foot with light-weight leg braces and shoe inserts, called "ankle-foot orthotics." Exercise therapy to strengthen the muscles and maintain joint motion also helps to improve gait. Devices that electrically stimulate the peroneal nerve during footfall are appropriate for a small number of individuals with foot drop. In cases with permanent loss of movement, a surgery that fuses the foot and ankle joint or that transfers tendons from stronger leg muscles is occasionally performed.

PROGNOSIS OF FOOT DROP[2]

The prognosis for foot drop depends on the cause. Foot drop caused by trauma or nerve damage usually shows partial or even complete recovery. For progressive neurological disorders, foot drop will be a symptom that is likely to continue as a lifelong disability. People with foot drop are more likely to fall, and falls, particularly in the elderly, may result in increased morbidity.

SENSORY DISTURBANCES INCLUDING PAIN[1]

Stroke patients may lose the ability to feel touch, pain, temperature, or position. Sensory deficits also may hinder the ability to recognize objects that patients are holding and can even be severe enough to cause loss of recognition of one's own limb. Some stroke patients experience pain, numbness, or odd sensations of tingling or prickling in paralyzed or weakened limbs—a symptom known as "paresthesias." The loss of urinary continence is fairly common immediately after a stroke and often results from a combination of sensory and motor deficits. Stroke survivors may lose the ability to sense the need to urinate or the ability to control bladder muscles.

Some may lack enough mobility to reach a toilet in time. Loss of bowel control or constipation also may occur. Permanent incontinence after a stroke is uncommon, but even a temporary loss of bowel or bladder control can be emotionally difficult for stroke survivors. Stroke survivors frequently have a variety of chronic pain syndromes resulting from stroke-induced damage to the nervous system (neuropathic pain).

In some stroke patients, pathways for sensation in the brain are damaged, causing the transmission of false signals that result in the sensation of pain in a limb or side of the body that has the sensory deficit. The most common of these pain syndromes is called "thalamic pain syndrome" (caused by a stroke to the thalamus, which processes sensory information from the body to the brain), which can be difficult to treat even with medications. Finally, some pain that occurs after stroke is not due to nervous system damage, but rather due to mechanical problems caused by the weakness of the stroke.

Patients who have a seriously weakened or paralyzed arm commonly experience moderate-to-severe pain that radiates outward from the shoulder. Most often, the pain results from lack of movement in a joint that has been immobilized for a prolonged period of time (such as having your arm or shoulder in a cast for weeks) and the tendons and ligaments around the joint become fixed in one position. This is commonly called a "frozen joint;" passive movement (the joint is gently moved or flexed by a therapist or caregiver rather than by the individual) at the joint in a paralyzed limb is essential to prevent painful "freezing" and to allow easy movement if and when voluntary motor strength returns.

Section 27.2 | Cognitive Impairment after Stroke

This section contains text excerpted from the following sources: Text beginning with the heading "What Is Agnosia?" is excerpted from "Agnosia," Genetic and Rare Diseases Information Center (GARD), National Center for Advancing Translational Sciences (NCATS), April 22, 2011. Reviewed May 2020; Text under the heading "Poststroke Vascular Dementia" is excerpted from "Vascular Dementia," National Heart, Lung, and Blood Institute (NHLBI), January 20, 2018; Text under the heading "Poststroke Multi-Infarct Dementia " is excerpted from "Multi-Infarct Dementia Information Page," National Institute of Neurological Disorders and Stroke (NINDS), March 27, 2019; Text beginning with the heading "Memory Problems After a Stroke" is excerpted from "Memory Problems," U.S. Department of Veterans Affairs (VA), January 5, 2011. Reviewed May 2020; Text under the heading "Unilateral Spatial Neglect" is excerpted from "VA/DoD Clinical Practice Guideline for the Management of Stroke Rehabilitation," U.S. Department of Veterans Affairs (VA), July 2019; Text under the heading "Speech and Language Impairment" is excerpted from "Aphasia," National Institute on Deafness and Other Communication Disorders (NIDCD), March 6, 2017; Text under the heading "Dysarthria and Apraxia" is excerpted from "Speech and Communication," U.S. Department of Veterans Affairs (VA), January 5, 2011. Reviewed May 2020.

WHAT IS AGNOSIA?

Agnosia is characterized by an inability to recognize and identify objects and/or persons. Symptoms may vary, according to the area of the brain that is affected. It can be limited to one sensory modality, such as vision or hearing; for example, a person may have difficulty in recognizing an object as a cup or identifying a sound like a cough. Agnosia can result from strokes, traumatic brain injury, dementia, a tumor, developmental disorders, overexposure to environmental toxins (e.g., carbon monoxide poisoning), or other neurological conditions. Visual agnosia may also occur in association with other underlying disorders. People with agnosia may retain their cognitive abilities in other areas. Treatment of primary agnosia is symptomatic and supportive; when it is caused by an underlying disorder, treatment of the disorder may reduce symptoms and help prevent further brain damage.

CAUSES OF AGNOSIA

Primary visual agnosia occurs as a result of damage to the brain. Symptoms develop due to the inability to retrieve information from those damaged areas that are associated with visual memory. Lesions may occur as a result of traumatic brain injury, stroke, tumor, or overexposure to dangerous environmental toxins (e.g., carbon monoxide poisoning). In some cases, the cause of the brain damage may not be known. Symptoms may vary, according to the area of the brain that is affected.

Visual agnosia may also occur in association with other underlying disorders (secondary visual agnosia) such as Alzheimer disease, agenesis of the corpus callosum, MELAS, and other diseases that result in progressive dementia. Disorders that may precede the development of primary visual agnosia (and may be useful in identifying an underlying cause of some forms of this disorder) include Alzheimer disease, Pick's disease, and a rare disorder known as "Balint syndrome."

POSTSTROKE VASCULAR DEMENTIA

Vascular dementia is the second most common form of dementia, after Alzheimer disease, affecting almost a third of people over 70 years of age. Dementia causes a decline in brain function, or cognitive abilities, beyond what is expected from the normal aging process. Dementia causes problems with memory, thinking, behavior, language skills, and decision making.

Vascular dementia is caused by conditions that damage the blood vessels in the brain, depriving the brain of oxygen. This oxygen shortage inhibits the brain's ability to work as well as it should. For example, stroke blocks blood flow to the brain, decreasing oxygen. However, high blood pressure, high cholesterol, and smoking also increases the risk of vascular dementia. Vascular dementia in patients can occur alone or with Alzheimer disease.

To diagnose cognitive impairment and dementia, your doctor will ask about problems you may in carrying out daily activities. Your doctor will give you brief memory or thinking tests and may ask to speak with a relative or friend who knows you well. To determine whether vascular dementia is the cause of any cognitive impairment or dementia that you may have, your doctor will consider your medical history and your lifestyle (such as your eating patterns, physical activity level, sleep health, and whether you are or have been a smoker), and order imaging tests. Diagnosis can take time. This is because it is often difficult to tell whether symptoms are a result of problems with the blood vessels, as is the case with vascular dementia, or whether they are from Alzheimer disease.

If your doctor diagnoses you with vascular dementia, your treatment plan may include taking medicine or using medical devices to manage other conditions such as high blood pressure, atherosclerosis, or sleep apnea, that may cause your vascular dementia to worsen. Your doctor may also recommend that you adopt heart-healthy lifestyle changes, such as heart-healthy eating, which includes limiting alcohol, getting regular physical activity, aiming for a healthy weight, quitting smoking, and managing stress.

POSTSTROKE MULTI-INFARCT DEMENTIA

Multi-infarct dementia (MID) is a common cause of memory loss in the elderly. MID is caused by multiple strokes (disruption of blood flow to the brain). Disruption of blood flow leads to damaged brain tissue. Some of these strokes may occur without noticeable clinical symptoms. Doctors refer to these as "silent strokes." An individual having a silent stroke may not even know it is happening, but over time, as more areas of the brain are damaged and more small blood vessels are blocked, the symptoms of MID begin to appear. MID can be diagnosed by an MRI or CT scan of the brain, along with a neurological examination. Symptoms include confusion or problems with short-term memory; wandering or getting lost in familiar places; walking with rapid, shuffling steps; losing bladder or bowel control; laughing or crying inappropriately; having difficulty following instructions, and having problems.

Treatment of Multi-Infarct Dementia

There is no treatment available to reverse brain damage that has been caused by a stroke. Treatment focuses on preventing future strokes by controlling or avoiding the diseases and medical conditions that put people at high risk for stroke: high blood pressure, diabetes, high cholesterol, and cardiovascular disease. The best treatment for MID is prevention and early intervention in life—eating a healthy diet, exercising, not smoking, moderately using alcohol, and maintaining a healthy weight.

Prognosis of Multi-Infarct Dementia

The prognosis for individuals with MID is generally poor. The symptoms of the disorder may begin suddenly, often in a stepwise pattern after each small stroke. Some people with MID may even appear to improve for short periods of time, then decline after having more silent strokes. The disorder generally takes a downward course with intermittent periods of rapid deterioration. Death may occur from stroke, heart disease, pneumonia, or other infection.

MEMORY PROBLEMS AFTER A STROKE

Most people have some memory problems after a stroke. The severity of the problems depends on how much brain damage occurred. People with less severe strokes naturally recover their memory over weeks or months. For others, there are medical treatments and things you can do to help.

Why Is It Important to Get Help?

Discuss your loved one's memory problems with your healthcare team. They can do a physical exam and basic memory tests. Certain medicines and health problems can worsen memory loss. For some people, there are helpful treatments.

How Can You Find Help for Your Loved One?

Talk with a social worker or your healthcare team. Ask about a referral to a memory clinic or for other services. Below is a list of healthcare providers who can help:
- Neurologists or cognitive neurologists diagnose and treat memory problems.
- Neuropsychologists conduct tests and work with neurologists to treat problems.
- Occupational therapists and specialist memory nurses suggest practical tips. They provide care in the office or the patient's home.

Your local stroke associations can provide information.

What Do You Need to Know?

Strokes affect people in different ways. Many stroke survivors remember things more slowly. They often forget to do tasks like taking their medicines. People with strokes often have trouble with short-term memory or recalling things that just happened. Learning new names and telephone numbers is often hard. Most stroke survivors retain their long-term memory. For example, they remember events that occurred in the past.

What Are the Common Types of Memory Problems after Stroke?

The type of memory loss depends on the part of the brain that was damaged.

People whose stroke affected the right side of the body often have problems with verbal memory. Verbal memory includes remembering names, stories, or information related to language or words.

Visual memory is often impaired in people whose stroke affected the left side of the body. Visual memory includes remembering faces, shapes, or things you see.

How Can You Use Memory Aids to Help Your Loved One?

- Place an easy-to-read digital clock on a bedside table.
- Hang a big calendar on the wall.
- Post emergency and important phone numbers in large letters near the phone.
- Place a notepad in a handy place to jot down things to remember.
- Use a pillbox to sort the pills that need to be taken each day.

How Can You Support Your Loved One?

- Make a memory book of favorite photos of people and places.
- Talk about the past. Share memories.
- Allow your loved one time to find the right words.

- Work at being understanding. It is normal to get frustrated. Keep in mind this is not your loved one's fault.
- Join a stroke support group. Other stroke caregivers can give you ideas for dealing with memory loss.

How Can You Help Your Loved One Stay Mentally Active?

The following activities may help improve memory:
- Crossword puzzles and word games
- Cards, dominoes, and board games
- Computer games that are made to improve memory

Helpful Tips

- Help your loved one focus on one thing at a time. Avoid noise and lots of people.
- Keep information simple. Break down activities into small steps.
- Have a daily routine. Do tasks at the same time each day.
- Label drawers with pictures or words to describe their contents.
- Leave reminder notes around the house. For example, leave a note to turn off the stove or lock the door.

Remember

- Problems with memory are common after stroke. They affect each stroke survivor in different ways.
- There are things you can do to help your loved one. Examples include reminder notes and making a memory book.
- Support your loved one. Remember that memory problems are not your loved one's fault.

UNILATERAL SPATIAL NEGLECT

Unilateral spatial neglect (USN) is defined as a failure to report, respond, or orient to novel or meaningful stimuli presented to the side opposite the brain lesion. USN affects two-thirds of patients with acute right hemispheric stroke. Because of the profound lack of awareness for the contralesional hemispace, patients with USN are severely functionally impaired. Traditional therapy for USN includes compensatory strategies directed towards the side of the deficit, including verbal cueing, visual scanning, full head turn (proprioceptive), anchoring techniques, limb activation aids, and environmental adaptations. Hemi-field eye patching has been used in addition to traditional therapy for patients with USN following stroke. Hemi-field eye patching may be regarded as a remedial visual-type of constraint-induced (forced use) therapy. For an individual with a right hemisphereic stroke resulting in left visual field loss and/ or left neglect, typically the right half of eyeglasses are patched with dark nontranslucent tape. Hemi-field eye patching has been suggested to work by reducing stimulation of the left hemisphere, thereby stimulating the right hemisphere and leading to interhemispheric rebalance.

SPEECH AND LANGUAGE IMPAIRMENT
What Is Aphasia?

Aphasia is a disorder that results from damage to portions of the brain that are responsible for language. For most people, these areas are on the left side of the brain. Aphasia usually occurs suddenly, often following a stroke or head injury, but it may also develop slowly, as the result of a brain tumor or a progressive neurological disease. The disorder impairs the expression and understanding of language as well as reading and writing. Aphasia may co-occur with speech disorders, such as dysarthria or apraxia of speech, which also result from brain damage.

Who Can Acquire Aphasia?

Most people who have aphasia are middle-aged or older, but anyone can acquire it, including young children. About one million people in the United States had aphasia, and nearly 180,000 Americans acquire it each year, according to the National Aphasia Association (NAA).

What Causes Aphasia

Aphasia is caused by damage to one or more of the language areas of the brain. Most often, the cause of the brain injury is a stroke. A stroke occurs when a blood clot or a leaking or burst vessel cuts off blood flow to part of the brain. Brain cells die when they do not receive their normal supply of blood, which carries oxygen and important nutrients. Other causes of brain injury are severe blows to the head, brain tumors, gunshot wounds, brain infections, and progressive neurological disorders, such as Alzheimer disease.

What Types of Aphasia Are There?

There are two broad categories of aphasia: fluent and nonfluent, and there are several types within these groups.

Damage to the temporal lobe of the brain may result in Wernicke aphasia, the most common type of fluent aphasia. People with Wernicke aphasia may speak in long, complete sentences that have no meaning, adding unnecessary words and even creating made-up words.

For example, someone with Wernicke aphasia may say, "You know that smoodle pinkard and that I want to get him round and take care of him as you want before."

As a result, it is often difficult to follow what the person is trying to say. People with Wernicke aphasia are often unaware of their spoken mistakes. Another hallmark of this type of aphasia is difficulty understanding speech.

The most common type of nonfluent aphasia is Broca aphasia. People with Broca aphasia have damage that primarily affects the frontal lobe of the brain. They often have right-sided weakness or paralysis of the arm and leg because the frontal lobe is also important for motor movements. People with Broca aphasia may understand speech and know what they want to say, but they frequently speak in short phrases that are produced with great effort. They often omit small words, such as "is," "and," and "the."

For example, a person with Broca aphasia may say, "Walk dog," meaning, "I will take the dog for a walk," or "book book two table," for "There are two books on the table." People with Broca aphasia typically understand the speech of others fairly well. Because of this, they are often aware of their difficulties and can become easily frustrated.

Another type of aphasia, global aphasia, results from damage to extensive portions of the language areas of the brain. Individuals with global aphasia have severe communication difficulties and may be extremely limited in their ability to speak or comprehend language. They may be unable to say even a few words or may repeat the same words or phrases over and over again. They may have trouble understanding even simple words and sentences.

There are other types of aphasia, each of which results from damage to different language areas in the brain. Some people may have difficulty repeating words and sentences even though they understand them and can speak fluently (conduction aphasia). Others may have difficulty naming objects even though they know what the object is and what it may be used for (anomic aphasia).

Sometimes, blood flow to the brain is temporarily interrupted and quickly restored. When this type of injury occurs, which is called a "transient ischemic attack," language abilities may return in a few hours or days.

How Is Aphasia Diagnosed?

Aphasia is usually first recognized by the physician who treats the person for her or his brain injury. Most individuals will undergo a magnetic resonance imaging (MRI) or computed tomography (CT) scan to confirm the presence of a brain injury and to identify its precise location. The physician also typically tests the person's ability to understand and produce language, such as following commands, answering questions, naming objects, and carrying on a conversation.

If the physician suspects aphasia, the patient is usually referred to a speech-language pathologist, who performs a comprehensive examination of the person's communication abilities. The person's ability to speak, express ideas, converse socially, understand language, and read and write are all assessed in detail.

How Is Aphasia Treated?

Following a brain injury, tremendous changes occur in the brain, which helps it to recover. As a result, people with aphasia often see dramatic improvements in their language and communication abilities in the first few months, even without treatment. But, in many cases, some aphasia remains following this initial recovery period. In these instances, speech-language therapy is used to help patients regain their ability to communicate.

Research has shown that language and communication abilities can continue to improve for many years and are sometimes accompanied by new activity in brain tissue near the damaged area. Some of the factors that may influence the amount of improvement include the cause of the brain injury, the area of the brain that was damaged and its extent, and the age and health of the individual.

Aphasia therapy aims to improve a person's ability to communicate by helping her or him to use remaining language abilities, restore language abilities as much as possible, and learn other ways of communicating such as gestures, pictures, or use of electronic devices. Individual therapy focuses on the specific needs of the person, while group therapy offers the opportunity to use new communication skills in a small-group setting.

The technologies have provided new tools for people with aphasia. "Virtual" speech pathologists provide patients with the flexibility and convenience of getting therapy in their homes through a computer. The use of speech-generating applications on mobile devices like tablets can also provide an alternative way to communicate for people who have difficulty using spoken language.

Increasingly, patients with aphasia participate in activities such as book clubs, technology groups, and art and drama clubs. Such experiences help patients regain their confidence and social self-esteem, in addition to improving their communication skills. Stroke clubs, regional support groups formed by people who have had a stroke, are available in most major cities. These clubs can help a person and her or his family adjust to the life changes that accompany stroke and aphasia.

Family involvement is often a crucial component of aphasia treatment because it enables family members to learn the best way to communicate with their loved ones. Family members are encouraged to:

- Participate in therapy sessions, if possible.
- Simplify language by using short, uncomplicated sentences.
- Repeat the content words or write down keywords to clarify meaning as needed.
- Maintain a natural conversational manner appropriate for an adult.
- Minimize distractions, such as a loud radio or TV, whenever possible.
- Include the person with aphasia in conversations.
- Ask for and value the opinion of the person with aphasia, especially regarding family matters.
- Encourage any type of communication, whether it is speech, gesture, pointing, or drawing.
- Avoid correcting the person's speech.
- Allow the person plenty of time to talk.
- Help the person become involved outside the home. Seek out support groups, such as stroke clubs.

What Research Is Being Done for Aphasia?

Researchers are testing new types of speech-language therapy in people with both recent and chronic aphasia to see if new methods can better help them recover word retrieval, grammar, prosody (tone), and other aspects of speech.

Some of these methods involve improving cognitive abilities that support the processing of language, such as short-term memory and attention. Others involve activities that stimulate the mental representations of sounds, words, and sentences, making them easier to access and retrieve.

Researchers are also exploring drug therapy as an experimental approach to treating aphasia. Some studies are testing whether drugs that affect the chemical neurotransmitters in the brain can be used in combination with speech-language therapy to improve the recovery of various language functions.

Other research is focused on using advanced imaging methods, such as functional magnetic resonance imaging (fMRI), to explore how language is processed in the normal and damaged brain and to understand recovery processes. This type of research may advance your knowledge of how the areas involved in speech and understanding language reorganize after a brain injury. The results could have implications for the diagnosis and treatment of aphasia and other neurological disorders.

A relatively new area of interest in aphasia research is noninvasive brain stimulation in combination with speech-language therapy. Two such brain stimulation techniques, transcranial magnetic stimulation (TMS) and transcranial direct current stimulation (tDCS), temporarily alter normal brain activity in the region being stimulated.

Researchers originally used these techniques to help them understand the parts of the brain that plays a role in language and recovery after a stroke. The scientists are studying if this temporary alteration of brain activity might help people relearn language use. Several clinical trials funded by the National Institute on Deafness and Other Communication Disorders (NIDCD) are testing these technologies.

Strokes can hurt parts of the brain and muscles used for listening, speaking, and understanding words.

DYSARTHRIA AND APRAXIA
Dysarthria
Dysarthria results from damage to the part of the brain that produces speech. As a result, speech may sound slurred. People with dysarthria may have problems saying sounds correctly.

Apraxia
Apraxia is a problem finding the "right" sounds to use when speaking. The speech may sound "flat." The person's tone may not change. She or he may only say one syllable at a time. Aphasia and apraxia of speech almost always occur at the same time.

263

Why Is It Important to Get Help?

People who have trouble talking and understanding what others say may become depressed. Stroke survivors with communication problems are often angry and get frustrated easily. Sometimes these problems last for just a short time. Most stroke survivors take a long time to regain their speech and language. You and your loved one will need to learn new ways to communicate with each other. The good news is that treatments and tips can improve communication.

What Treatments Should You Discuss with Your Healthcare Team?

Talk to your loved one's healthcare provider right away about treatments and referrals. Licensed speech-language pathologists can help stroke survivors regain speech and language skills. They can teach survivors how to learn and use writing, gestures, and other forms of communication. Some health insurance policies cover speech therapy if a healthcare provider states that it is needed.

How Can You Help Your Loved One Communicate?

- Look for changes in your survivor's speech after the stroke. Talk to your healthcare provider right away about the changes.
- Give your loved one a card to carry that states the speech problem is a medical condition.
- Let your loved one try to speak for themselves.
- Remove noise distractions like the radio. This will help your loved one focus on your words.
- Involve your loved one in family plans and meetings. Help others to look at and speak to your loved one. Give the survivor a chance to respond. A survivor who speaks differently after the stroke may still have thoughts to share.

Helpful Tips for Talking with Your Loved One

- Talk to your loved one with respect. Avoid "talking down."
- Face your loved one and keep eye contact when you talk.

- Speak slowly with simple words and phrases your loved one can understand.
- Use gestures (nods or hand signals), pictures, signs, or keywords in writing.
- Ask your loved one to repeat things that are not clear. However, avoid asking them to repeat things many times.
- Ask your loved one questions with "yes" or "no" answers.

Remember
- Talk with your healthcare provider about changes in your loved one's speech. Discuss possible therapies.
- Continue to talk and involve your loved one in social gatherings. Allow your loved one time to speak and find the right words.
- Be patient. Remember that speech recovery can be a slow process.

Chapter 28 | Poststroke Mood and Emotional Changes

Chapter Contents

Section 28.1 | Depression and Anxiety

This section includes text excerpted from "Depression after Stroke," U.S. Department of Veterans Affairs (VA), January 5, 2011. Reviewed May 2020.

After a stroke, your loved one may have many negative feelings. Your loved one may think that things will never get better. This is not true—help is available! Almost half of all stroke survivors have depression. Depression is a normal response to the losses that occur from a stroke.

WHAT ARE THE SIGNS AND SYMPTOMS OF DEPRESSION?

Here is a list of the signs and symptoms of depression. Five or more of these signs or symptoms that last more than two weeks are warning signals for depression.

- Sadness or an "empty" mood
- Feeling guilty, worthless, or helpless
- Problems concentrating, remembering, or making decisions
- Appetite and/or weight changes
- Feeling hopeless
- Lack of energy or feeling tired and "slowed down"
- Problems with sleep such as trouble getting to sleep, staying asleep, or sleeping too much
- Feeling restless or irritable
- Loss of interest or pleasure in hobbies and activities, including sex, that was once enjoyed

Red Flag: Suicidal Thoughts

If the stroke survivor talks about suicide, has thoughts of suicide, or attempts suicide, get help right away. Call emergency services or your healthcare provider as this is a serious problem.

WHAT DO YOU NEED TO KNOW?

- **Depression is real**–People need help when they have depression.

269

- **Physical and emotional changes are common after a stroke**–Accept your loved one's changes.
- **Expect improvements over time**–Things often get better.

WHY IS IT IMPORTANT TO GET HELP?

Treatment of depression will help the stroke survivor recover faster. It will make your job as a caregiver easier. For instance, treating depression helps with:
- Thinking skills and memory
- Physical recovery and rehabilitation
- Language and speech
- Emotions and motivation

WHAT TREATMENTS SHOULD YOU DISCUSS WITH YOUR HEALTHCARE TEAM?

Get help from your healthcare team quickly. The stroke survivor and family members may explain away the person's depression. Make sure that the stroke survivor receives treatment.
- Medicines, such as antidepressants, improve symptoms.
- Psychotherapy (talk therapy) is used along with medicines. Talk therapy gives your loved one a safe place to talk about feelings.
- Support groups provide help from other stroke survivors and caregivers. They know what you and your loved one are going through. There are support groups for stroke survivors and caregivers like you.

HELPFUL TIPS

- Know the warning signals of depression. Watch for the signs and symptoms of depression. Get help quickly.
- Be patient with your loved one. After a stroke, it will take time for your loved one to understand the changes.
- Help your loved one exercise and take part in fun activities.
- Encourage friends and your family to visit and talk with your loved one.

- Have a good attitude. Focus on how much your stroke survivor can do. Smile and relax about things you cannot change.

REMEMBER
- Depression is real and should be treated.
- You are the key person to watch for the warning signals of depression.
- Get help quickly if you think your loved one has depression.

Section 28.2 | Personality Changes

This section includes text excerpted from "Rescue Fact Sheet—Personality Changes," U.S. Department of Veterans Affairs (VA), January 5, 2011. Reviewed May 2020.

After a stroke, your loved one may act like a different person. This is because injury to the brain can affect personality.

WHAT ARE PERSONALITY CHANGES?
A personality change is a difference in someone's normal character. The person's thinking and behavior change. If a change is minor, it may go unnoticed. Major changes can affect relationships with others.

WHAT DO YOU NEED TO KNOW?
Changes in personality are common after stroke. They are also among the hardest to deal with. Not all changes are permanent. Some may disappear over time. Personality changes to watch for include self-centered attitude, emotional lability, apathy, and depression. You may also notice behavior problems. For instance, your loved one may get angry or easily frustrated. They may have

271

impulsive behaviors. Your loved one may even get physically aggressive.

WHY IS IT IMPORTANT TO GET HELP?

Personality changes are hard for caregivers to handle. Talk with your healthcare team. They can suggest treatments or ways to deal with personality changes. Think about joining a support group. Talking with other caregivers is often helpful.

WHAT IS EMOTIONAL LABILITY?

Emotional lability is used to describe someone with strong emotions. These emotions are close to the surface and difficult to control. The person becomes upset or cries more easily. Stroke survivors often have intense mood swings. They may be happy and sad in only a few minutes. They may react to everyday events in unexpected ways.

- Be patient. Your loved one cannot help behaving this way. Explain to your loved one that her or his emotions are part of the disease.
- Talk with other family members. Help them understand that stroke survivors have problems controlling their feelings.
- Treat the behavior as a minor problem. Continue what you were doing.
- Change the subject or lead your loved one in a new direction.

WHAT IS A SELF-CENTERED ATTITUDE?

Many survivors become mainly concerned with their own interests. They may lack empathy, or the ability to understand another's feelings.

- Kindly help your loved one know when they are not being thoughtful
- Gently remind your loved one to practice polite behavior
- Praise your loved one for doing thoughtful things for others

WHAT IS APATHY?

Apathy is a lack of motivation. Apathy is different than being tired or depressed. A person with apathy shows little emotion or feeling. There is often a loss of interest in the activities.

WHAT ARE BEHAVIOR CHANGES?

Stroke survivors often have problems with impulsive behaviors, frustration, anger, and aggression. Changes in your loved one's behavior are hard to deal with.

HELPFUL TIPS

- Personality changes are hard to deal with. Remember, this is part of the stroke injury. Try not to take it personally.
- Avoid comparing your loved one to the way they used to be.
- Seek counseling or join a support group. Talking about your anxieties can help.
- Keep up your own schedule to avoid caregiver burnout.
- Discuss personality changes with your healthcare provider. Ask for an assessment when needed.
- Try to accept the changes you see in your loved one. Avoid comparing your loved one to the way they used to be. Some of the changes may be permanent. Others will disappear over time.
- Be patient and understanding. Your loved one is facing many changes. Your support is important.

Section 28.3 | Pseudobulbar Affect or Emotional Lability

This section includes text excerpted from "VA/DoD Clinical Practice Guideline for the Management of Stroke Rehabilitation," U.S. Department of Veterans Affairs (VA), July 2019.

Pseudobulbar affect (PBA) (also known as "emotionalism," "pathological crying or laughing," "emotional incontinence," or "emotional lability") is characterized by involuntary, sudden, and frequent episodes of crying and/or laughing which may or may not be associated with a precipitant. In a 2016 SR and metaanalysis of over 3,000 patients with stroke, PBA was found to affect 17 percent of patients less than one-month poststroke, 20 percent of patients one to six months poststroke, and 12 percent of patients greater than six months poststroke. This condition may be socially disabling and interfere with the rehabilitation process. It can be potentially dangerous if it occurs during eating in a patient with dysphagia.

Medical treatment for PBA with SSRIs is widely available, inexpensive, and benefits of PBA treatment outweigh potential harms. Medical treatment is often desired by the patient and loved ones for this disabling condition, though some individuals prefer no pharmacological therapy. Medical treatment for PBA with TCA is not recommended for the elderly by the Work Group due to the known adverse effects of TCA, including anticholinergic side effects.

Of note, in 2010, the FDA approved dextromethorphan/quinidine for the treatment of PBA. This is the only FDA approved medication for the treatment of this condition at this time. However, dextromethorphan/quinidine is a costly medication (greater than $1,000 per month). Dextromethorphan/quinidine is generally well tolerated and has a wide safety margin when used at therapeutically approved doses.

Chapter 29 | What Is Poststroke Rehabilitation?

Rehabilitation helps stroke survivors relearn skills that are lost when part of the brain is damaged. For example, these skills can include coordinating leg movements in order to walk or carrying out the steps involved in any complex activity. Rehabilitation also teaches survivors new ways of performing tasks to circumvent or compensate for any residual disabilities. Individuals may need to learn how to bathe and dress using only one hand, or how to communicate effectively when their ability to use language has been compromised. There is a strong consensus among rehabilitation experts that the most important element in any rehabilitation program is carefully directed, well-focused, repetitive practice—the same kind of practice used by all people when they learn a new skill, such as playing the piano or pitching a baseball.

Rehabilitative therapy begins in the acute-care hospital after the person's overall condition has been stabilized, often within 24 to 48 hours after the stroke. The first steps involve promoting independent movement because many individuals are paralyzed or seriously weakened. Patients are prompted to change positions frequently while lying in bed and to engage in passive or active range of motion exercises to strengthen their stroke-impaired limbs. ("Passive" range-of-motion exercises are those in which the therapist actively helps the patient move a limb repeatedly,

This chapter includes text excerpted from "Poststroke Rehabilitation Fact Sheet," National Institute of Neurological Disorders and Stroke (NINDS), March 17, 2020.

whereas "active" exercises are performed by the patient with no physical assistance from the therapist.) Depending on many factors—including the extent of the initial injury—patients may progress from sitting up and being moved between the bed and a chair to standing, bearing their own weight, and walking, with or without assistance. Rehabilitation nurses and therapists help patients who are able to perform progressively more complex and demanding tasks such as bathing, dressing, and using a toilet, and they encourage patients to begin using their stroke-impaired limbs while engaging in those tasks. Beginning to reacquire the ability to carry out these basic activities of daily living represents the first stage in a stroke survivor's return to independence.

For some stroke survivors, rehabilitation will be an ongoing process to maintain and refine skills and could involve working with specialists for months or years after the stroke.

Chapter 30 | Rehabilitation of Motor Function

Stroke is the number one cause of serious adult disability in the United States. Stroke disability is devastating to the stroke patient and family, but therapies are available to help rehabilitate patients after stroke.

For most stroke patients, rehabilitation mainly involves physical therapy. The aim of physical therapy is to have the stroke patient relearn simple motor activities such as walking, sitting, standing, lying down, and the process of switching from one type of movement to another.

Another type of therapy to help patients relearn daily activities is occupational therapy. This type of therapy also involves exercise and training. Its goal is to help the stroke patient relearn everyday activities such as eating, drinking and swallowing, dressing, bathing, cooking, reading, and writing, and using the toilet. Occupational therapists seek to help the patient become independent or semi-independent.

UPPER AND LOWER LIMBS REHABILITATION
Task-Specific Practice

Task-specific practice involves the practice of a whole task or pretask movements for a whole limb or limb segment such as grasp,

This chapter contains text excerpted from the following sources: Text in this chapter begins with excerpts from "Rehabilitation after Stroke," National Institute on Aging (NIA), National Institutes of Health (NIH), June 24, 2017; Text beginning with the heading "Upper and Lower Limbs Rehabilitation" is excerpted from "VA/DoD Clinical Practice Guideline for the Management of Stroke Rehabilitation," U.S. Department of Veterans Affairs (VA), July 2019.

grip, or movement in a trajectory to facilitate activities of daily living (ADL) or mobility.

These movements can include upper and lower limb movements, balance activities in a sitting or standing position, transfers, and functional mobility (e.g., stairs, household ambulation). The approach typically includes the application of motor learning principles in regard to feedback, practice schedules, task variation, and the challenge of the activity. With task-specific training, the benefits appear to outweigh the harms. There were significant gains in many areas that were maintained for at least six months.

A potential risk for falls was the main concern; however, the risk for falls is no greater than for other therapeutic interventions. This intervention can be performed in any environment (e.g., hospital room, clinics, home, community settings). Caregivers and patients can be educated on how to carry out this intervention at home. This approach does not require additional equipment not routinely found in therapy clinics or home settings. This intervention tends to be more engaging, as it can be tailored to the patient's preferences and individual goals. Those who are severely impaired may require increased staff or the use of technology to assist with the safe performance of tasks.

Cardiovascular Exercise

Cardiovascular exercise and/or training (e.g., walking, aquatics, and rowing) has been found to improve the maximum walking speed in patients poststroke. Cardiovascular exercise is also a component for the management of several comorbidities commonly found in stroke survivors.

For patients who may have preexisting cardiorespiratory conditions, cognitive deficits, or risk for falls, providers should consider these conditions prior to recommending cardiovascular exercise interventions. Considerations should also be made for patient preferences, access to exercise facilities and equipment, neighborhood setting/safety, and local climate.

There appeared to be an overall benefit for improving the maximum walking speed with potential additional benefits of improving common comorbidities that are well-established modifiable risk factors for stroke (e.g., obesity, diabetes, dyslipidemia, hypertension).

Body-Weight Support Treadmill Training

Body-weight support treadmill training (BWSTT) is a task-specific technique for improving gait. The patient is partially suspended using a body harness from the ceiling or a frame in order to reduce (offload) the relative weight of the patient and provide postural support while walking on a treadmill.

The amount of offloading can gradually be decreased as indicated by improved control of posture and gait by the patient. When BWSTT was compared to conventional treadmill training, there was a slight trend favoring the use of the BWSTT. The most significant adverse effects associated with BWSTT compared to other gait interventions are musculoskeletal problems, skin abrasion/breakdown, and anxiety.

One notable consideration with BWSTT is the correct application of the harness to prevent increased pressure through the groin and avoid skin breakdown. Other concerns associated with gait training interventions are falls and cardiac issues (dizziness, fainting, and heart rate regulation). These also apply to BWSTT and may lead to greater risk in this population. Other considerations for the use of this modality are the costs of the equipment and the need for trained staff.

Rhythmic Auditory Cueing

The use of rhythmic auditory cueing during gait training helps to coordinate movement with timing, to stimulate and incorporate overlapping brain areas, and to improve walking speed. This therapeutic modality has been used in persons with stroke and other movement disorders. As benefits outweigh harms for using rhythmic auditory cueing to improve walking speed, it is suggested that this modality be offered as an adjunctive treatment to conventional gait training while considering comorbid diagnoses which may decrease the effectiveness of this intervention (e.g., cognitive impairments, stress disorders, hearing impairments).

Constraint-Induced Movement Therapy

Constraint-Induced Movement Therapy (CIMT) and modified Constraint-Induced Movement Therapy (mCIMT) are multi-component interventions designed to help patients overcome learned nonuse of a paretic upper extremity and increase motor function. CIMT is a neurorehabilitation technique consisting of three components: (1) immobilization of the nonparetic upper extremity to prevent its use in daily activities, (2) task-specific practice of the paretic upper extremity with frequent repetitions for about six hours per day, and (3) instruction in transfer of skills from the clinical setting to the home environment in the performance of ADLs and instrumental ADLs (IADLs). The main difference between CIMT and mCIMT is the number of hours of therapy per day, with CIMT requiring more than three hours per day, and mCIMT requiring three hours or less of therapy per day.

High-intensity CIMT may make the patient anxious, and restricting the nonparetic side for a long duration may make the rehabilitation experience less satisfactory for the patient. However, in the patient whose paretic upper extremity also happens to be her or his dominant hand, there may be strong internal motivation to be compliant with the intensity of this intervention.

Mirror Therapy

Mirror therapy uses a mirror that reflects the movement of the nonparetic limb back to the patient, creating a visual illusion that the paretic limb is moving. The paretic limb is typically hidden by the mirror. The concept behind this therapy is that cortical activation in the lesioned hemisphere may be induced by both the perception of movement in the paretic limb and stimulation from the nonparetic limb through interhemispheric communication.

This therapy could be considered as a treatment technique to add variety to a treatment program or to increase patient engagement. There is some variation between patient suitability, as those with vision impairments, neglect, or cognitive deficits will not be able to perform or will require additional assistance to trial mirror therapy. Patients are usually seated for this activity, which places them at low risk for falls. This therapy can easily be performed at home or on the ward outside of skilled therapies if the patient does not have visual or cognitive impairments.

TECHNOLOGY-ASSISTED PHYSICAL REHABILITATION

Electrical stimulation for muscle reeducation involves the application of electrical current to a targeted muscle or muscle group. This results in the activation of the targeted muscles. For patients with foot drop, either electrical stimulation or traditional ankle-foot orthoses to improve gait speed, are equally effective. The use of ankle-foot orthoses is currently considered the standard of care in the United States to treat foot drop. Electrical stimulation is also used, but less frequently. However, it has been found to be effective as an adjunctive treatment to improve upper and lower extremity motor function.

ROBOTIC-ASSISTED DEVICES

There has been an increase in the number of robotic-assisted devices available for use in stroke rehabilitation. The majority of these systems focus on improving the strength and functional activity of the upper extremity or improving walking speed and independence with ambulation.

Most of the available devices can be programmed to perform the passive motion, active-assist with movement, or resistance to the patient's movement, and some are able to adapt automatically based on the patient's ability. These devices are often combined with some type of augmented feedback, such as a video screen, most commonly in a game-like format for visual feedback or tone adjustment for auditory feedback.

The rationale use of robotics is that the patient can practice the movement in a more natural pattern and increase the amount of task-specific practice of the pattern or activity. The device can assist the movement when there is a lack of motor recruitment to perform the movement, and allow for more controlled movement earlier than standard therapies, and potentially decrease the number of staff needed for safety with movement. Transfers to the device may be difficult due to the patient's abilities and/or suboptimal location of the device within the clinic, as robotic devices can be large and require a significant area in the clinic for safe use.

VIRTUAL REALITY

Virtual reality (VR) is a computer-based, interactive, multisensory environment that occurs in real-time. Nonetheless, there are vast differences in the types of VR. For instance, VR can be nonimmersive with primarily visual and auditory sensory input, such as a person interacting with a computer screen (e.g., simple computer games). Alternatively, VR can involve a completely immersive environment, in which the person has the sense that she or he is within the VR environment. This may include the addition of haptic information through a haptic interface device, such as a glove or exoskeleton, increasing a patient's perception that she or he is actually present in and able to control the simulated environment. Regardless of the type of VR, when it is used as part of a rehabilitation intervention, a person's interaction with the virtual environment is designed so that the person can carry out task-specific practice to facilitate motor learning in a more engaging manner.

PHARMACOLOGICAL TREATMENT IN MOTOR THERAPY
Selective Serotonin Reuptake Inhibitors

Selective serotonin reuptake inhibitors (SSRIs) have been studied to try determining if they improve functional outcomes in patients with recent stroke. Since SSRIs have been used for other indications for many years, their side effect profiles are well understood. In recent years, increased bleeding risk has been shown among patients taking both SSRIs and oral anticoagulants, specifically warfarin.

This is of particular relevance in patients with stroke as one of the most common causes of ischemic stroke is atrial fibrillation, which is often best managed with oral anticoagulation to reduce the risk of stroke. Thus, in patients with motor deficits after stroke who require oral anticoagulation, especially warfarin, it may be reasonable to avoid the use of SSRIs unless there is another clinical indication or at least avoid the SSRIs with relatively potent serotonin reuptake inhibition (i.e., fluoxetine, paroxetine, or sertraline).

Botulinum Toxin

The use of botulinum toxin has been found to decrease spasticity in patients with a history of stroke. Since the publication of the 2010 *Stroke Rehabilitation Clinical Practice Guideline*, the use of botulinum toxin for poststroke spasticity has become standard care. Botulinum toxin is recommended for those patients with focal spasticity that is painful, impairs function, reduces the ability to participate in rehabilitation, or compromises proper positioning or skincare. In some patients, however, treatment of focal spasticity may actually worsen function (e.g., a patient who utilizes lower limb extensor spasticity to aid with standing, transfers, or ambulation).

Aside from some initial injection site discomfort, botulinum toxin injections are felt to have many advantages over medications for spasticity that are taken orally. The advantages include the ability to be placed directly into the muscles affected—allowing for higher dosing without limiting the function of other muscles, long duration of effect (approximately three months), and lack of sedation or other systemic side effects typical of oral antispasticity treatments. These advantages make botulinum toxin injections a highly desirable treatment option for both patients poststroke and their providers.

Intrathecal Baclofen Treatments

The use of intrathecal baclofen in patients with chronic stroke has been shown to reduce lower extremity spasticity. There is a potential for harm associated with baclofen pump use including surgical complications during device implantation or possibly superficial abdominal injury during attempted pump refill. Most concerning is the risk of baclofen withdrawal or overdose due to pump or catheter malfunction, improper refilling of the reservoir, or improper pump programming. Such cases have been reported in the literature and can be life-threatening, but are felt to be rare. Intrathecal baclofen requires the implantation of a baclofen pump—an expensive and invasive procedure. The patient must also undergo subsequent injections through the skin approximately every three to six months in order for the pump to be refilled.

Chapter 31 | Management of Poststroke Cognitive Impairment

Stroke is one of the leading causes of long-term disability in the United States and around the world. A stroke can affect the way the brain processes, organizes, and stores information. Cognitive impairment, a major impact of stroke, is referred to as "poststroke cognitive impairment" (PSCI). Different parts of the brain control various functions, and if a stroke damages one of the parts that control cognition, it can affect an individual's ability to perform certain tasks. Even minor strokes affect daily functioning, cognition, and executive functions, gradually impacting participation, quality of life, and return to work.

A cognitive assessment will be able to present more details about the problems being experienced by a PSCI patient. They are usually done by a doctor, occupational therapist, or psychologist.

EFFECTS OF POSTSTROKE COGNITIVE IMPAIRMENT

Stroke and cognitive impairment are common among older people, with around one in three having different degrees of cognitive impairment within several months after stroke. When cognition is affected, the following aftereffects are usually experienced by stroke survivors.

"Management of Poststroke Cognitive Impairment," © 2020 Omnigraphics. Reviewed May 2020.

DIFFICULTY IN CONCENTRATION

Concentration problems are especially common in the early stages following a stroke. If it is hard to focus on something, then it will be difficult to respond or remember it later. A few symptoms of stroke that can affect concentration other than cognitive impairment include tiredness, pain, or emotional problems like depression.

Managing Concentration Problems

It is essential to keep activities confined to a maximum of half an hour, or however, long it can be managed. If an activity is going to take longer, take a break and come back to it later.

When working on something that requires concentration (going to an appointment or expecting a visitor), then plan to have a rest immediately prior to the appointment.

It may be quite hard to follow a whole TV program; however, watching the news, sports, or cookery programs will probably be easier to keep up with than dramas or documentaries, which require a longer attention span.

MEMORY LOSS

Information is stored in the memory in different ways, and for varying lengths of time. Memory damaged due to cognitive impairment can improve over time, either spontaneously or through rehabilitation, but the symptoms can last for years.

Brain retraining techniques (mental exercises) are designed to improve thinking and memory after a stroke. The training can help improve alertness and attention and it can be done in person as well as with the help of computer programs and applications. To stimulate the brain and improve memory and cognitive ability, new hobbies that involve both the mind and body can be undertaken. Fitness exercises are also known to help the overall physical and mental health of stroke patients.

Managing Memory Loss

- Have a place for everything and put things away where they belong—for example, hanging keys on a hook close to the door.

- Set daily routines in the same specific sequence every day, such as bedtime tasks.
- Post both special events and daily activities on a large calendar.
- Keep a notebook of important information handy and organize it into sections such as appointments, phone numbers, and medications.
- Put up notes in prominent places and leave written directions on how to use everyday household items next to those items, including phones and microwaves.
- Memory cues help remember specific tasks or information. For example, connecting a task or piece of information to something relevant such as an image, a familiar name, or a song.
- When failing to recall what someone said, ask them to repeat as often as necessary.

PROBLEMS WITH EXECUTIVE FUNCTION

Executive function is defined as the mental process that enables a person to focus attention, plan, remember, and perform multiple tasks simultaneously.

If a stroke affects an individual's executive function, they may not be able to:

- **Figure out how to do specific tasks**—This could be something simple like changing the channel using the remote control, or it could be more complicated, like making a meal.
- **Plan how to complete a task**—May not be able to think of all the steps that are needed to do something, such as making a cup of tea or putting things in the correct order.
- **Begin or finish a task on their own**—Unable to realize that they need to do something, like getting dressed, until someone tells them to, or may need help throughout an entire task.
- **Solve problems on their own**—Not being able to figure out what action to take if something goes wrong.

287

- **Multitasking**—Finding it hard to switch between tasks, and unable to remember the point where each task had ended.

Managing Problems with Executive Functions

Executive functions, such as planning and problem solving can eventually be improved with practice. The occupational therapist or clinical neuropsychologist can help decide what activities to focus on, as it will be different for each patient. The following steps can be taken to effectively manage executive functions:

- Once a task has been mastered, like making a sandwich, move on to more difficult ones, like cooking a meal.
- Dressing in the same order every day will make it easier to relearn the steps and spot a problem, when a step is missed.
- A daily timetable with prompts and reminders may also be especially helpful if a person has problems getting motivated, also known as "apathy," which is common after a stroke.
- Write out instructions or checklists to be followed when doing something.
- Put up notes around the house to remind of things that may be forgotten, like brushing the teeth or taking medications.
- Prompts can either be written or pictures and recordings can be used as well.

OTHER COGNITIVE PROBLEMS

A few other cognitive problems like dysarthria (speech disorder), apraxia (problems moving or controlling the body), or agnosia (inability to recognize and identify objects or people) will be diagnosed by the doctors or therapists while in the hospital. If these problems are not identified, and a patient starts to notice signs of cognitive problems, they are recommended to go back to the general practitioner to get it properly diagnosed and assessed. The patient is then referred to an occupational therapist who works with the patient to find ways to help them cope with the effects of cognitive impairment and suggest aids and equipment that can be of help.

Cognitive problems can take a long time to improve; therefore, if a person needs to go back to work, an occupational therapist can advise about the best time to get back to work and can also talk to the employer about how they can support the person when they resume their work.

References

1. "A Complete Guide to Cognitive Problems after Stroke," Stroke Association, April 23, 2015.
2. "Memory Loss," American Heart Association (AHA), March 15, 2019.
3. "Post Stroke Cognitive Impairment: Mechanism and Therapy," Gantome, February 13, 2019.

Chapter 32 | Mental-Health Rehabilitation after Stroke

POSTSTROKE DEPRESSION[1]

Many people who survive a stroke feel fear, anxiety, frustration, anger, sadness, and a sense of grief for their physical and mental losses. These feelings are a natural response to the psychological trauma of stroke. Some emotional disturbances and personality changes are caused by the physical effects of brain damage. Clinical depression, which is a sense of hopelessness that disrupts an individual's ability to function, appears to be the emotional disorder most commonly experienced by stroke survivors. Signs of clinical depression include sleep disturbances, a radical change in eating patterns that may lead to sudden weight loss or gain, lethargy, social withdrawal, irritability, fatigue, self-loathing, and suicidal thoughts. Poststroke depression can be treated with antidepressant medications and psychological counseling.

TREATMENT AND THERAPIES[2]

Depression, even the most severe cases, can be treated. The earlier that treatment can begin, the more effective it is. Depression is usually treated with medications, psychotherapy, or a combination

This chapter includes text excerpted from documents published by three public domain sources. Text under the heading marked 1 is excerpted from "Poststroke Rehabilitation," Know Stroke, National Institute of Neurological Disorders and Stroke (NINDS), September 2014. Reviewed May 2020; Text under the headings marked 2 are excerpted from "Depression," National Institute of Mental Health (NIMH), February 2018; Text under the heading marked 3 is excerpted from "VA/DoD Clinical Practice Guideline for the Management of Stroke Rehabilitation," U.S. Department of Veterans Affairs (VA), July 2019.

of the two. If these treatments do not reduce symptoms, electro-convulsive therapy (ECT) and other brain stimulation therapies may be options to explore.

MEDICATIONS[2]

Antidepressants are medicines that treat depression. They may help improve the way your brain uses certain chemicals that control mood or stress. You may need to try several different antidepressant medicines before finding the one that improves your symptoms and has manageable side effects. A medication that has helped you or a close family member in the past will often be considered.

Antidepressants take time—usually two to four weeks—to work, and often, symptoms such as sleep, appetite, and concentration problems improve before mood lifts, so it is important to give medication a chance before reaching a conclusion about its effectiveness. If you begin taking antidepressants, do not stop taking them without the help of a doctor. Sometimes people taking antidepressants feel better and then stop taking the medication on their own, and the depression returns. When you and your doctor have decided it is time to stop the medication, usually after a course of 6 to 12 months, the doctor will help you slowly and safely decrease your dose. Stopping them abruptly can cause withdrawal symptoms.

PSYCHOTHERAPIES[2]

Several types of psychotherapy (also called "talk therapy" or, in a less specific form, "counseling") can help people with depression. Examples of evidence-based approaches specific to the treatment of depression include cognitive-behavioral therapy (CBT), interpersonal therapy (IPT), and problem-solving therapy.

COGNITIVE-BEHAVIORAL THERAPY[3]

CBT was the only type of psychotherapy that yielded evidence for use with the stroke population. CBT is a short-term, structured form of psychotherapy that focuses on solving current problems by teaching patients to identify, challenge, and change unhelpful thoughts and patterns of behavior. It is a collaborative approach aimed at developing and practicing problem-solving and coping skills.

Given the relatively large overall benefit of CBT on decreasing symptoms of poststroke depression and the low risk of CBT, particularly in comparison to the potential risks of pharmacotherapy in the elderly or the risks of untreated depression, the benefits of CBT likely outweigh the harms.

Despite general consistency in the evidence supporting CBT, there is some variability in provider and patient preferences regarding this treatment. Some patients wish to avoid the stigma of a mental-health diagnosis and may not accept CBT. Other patients may not be willing to commit the time and effort that CBT requires (homework assignments, practice, introspection). Although stroke-related cognitive-linguistic impairments may impede engagement in psychotherapy, CBT is well suited for adaptation and utilizes methods that support involvement for those with cognitive challenges. The present-focused approach of CBT and its organized structure with worksheets and other concrete methods make it appropriate for many patients with stroke. CBT is administered by a licensed mental-health practitioner and, when conducted in a one-on-one setting, can be somewhat resourced intensive. CBT is a widely available form of treatment for depression and is generally well regarded among medical care providers.

BRAIN STIMULATION THERAPIES[2]

If medications do not reduce the symptoms of depression, electroconvulsive therapy (ECT) may be an option to explore. Based on the latest research:

- ECT can provide relief for people with severe depression who have not been able to feel better with other treatments.
- Electroconvulsive therapy can be an effective treatment for depression. In some severe cases where a rapid response is necessary or medications cannot be used safely, ECT can even be a first-line intervention.

293

- Once strictly an inpatient procedure, today ECT is often performed on an outpatient basis. The treatment consists of a series of sessions, typically three times a week, for two to four weeks.
- ECT may cause some side effects including confusion, disorientation, and memory loss. Usually, these side effects are short-term, but sometimes memory problems can linger, especially for the months around the time of the treatment course. Advances in ECT devices and methods have made modern ECT safe and effective for the vast majority of patients. Talk to your doctor and make sure you understand the potential benefits and risks of the treatment before giving your informed consent to undergoing ECT.
- ECT is not painful, and you cannot feel the electrical impulses. Before ECT begins, a patient is put under brief anesthesia and given a muscle relaxant. Within one hour after the treatment session, which takes only a few minutes, the patient is awake and alert.

Other more recently introduced types of brain stimulation therapies used to treat medicine-resistant depression include repetitive transcranial magnetic stimulation (rTMS) and vagus nerve stimulation (VNS). Other types of brain stimulation treatments are under study.

BEYOND TREATMENT: THINGS YOU CAN DO[2]
Here are other tips that may help you or a loved one during treatment for depression:
- Try to be active and exercise.
- Set realistic goals for yourself.
- Try to spend time with other people and confide in a trusted friend or relative.
- Try not to isolate yourself, and let others help you.
- Expect your mood to improve gradually, not immediately.

- Postpone important decisions, such as getting married or divorced, or changing jobs until you feel better. Discuss decisions with others who know you well and have a more objective view of your situation.
- Continue to educate yourself about depression.

Chapter 33 | Multidisciplinary Rehabilitation Team

WHAT MEDICAL PROFESSIONALS SPECIALIZE IN POSTSTROKE REHABILITATION?

Poststroke rehabilitation involves physicians; rehabilitation nurses; physical, occupational, recreational, speech-language, and vocational therapists; and mental-health professionals.

Physicians

Physicians have the primary responsibility for managing and coordinating the long-term care of stroke survivors, including recommending which rehabilitation programs will best address individual needs. Physicians also are responsible for caring for the stroke survivor's general health and providing guidance aimed at preventing a second stroke, such as controlling high blood pressure or diabetes and eliminating risk factors such as cigarette smoking, excessive weight, a high-cholesterol diet, and high alcohol consumption.

Neurologists usually lead to acute-care stroke teams and direct patient care during hospitalization. They sometimes participate in the long-term rehabilitation team. Other subspecialists often lead the rehabilitation stage of care, especially physiatrists, who specialize in physical medicine and rehabilitation.

This chapter includes text excerpted from "Poststroke Rehabilitation Fact Sheet," National Institute of Neurological Disorders and Stroke (NINDS), March 17, 2020.

Rehabilitation Nurses

Nurses specializing in rehabilitation help survivors relearn how to carry out the basic activities of daily living. They also educate survivors about routine healthcare such as how to follow a medication schedule, how to care for the skin, how to move out of a bed and into a wheelchair, and special needs for people with diabetes. Rehabilitation nurses also work with survivors to reduce risk factors that may lead to a second stroke, and provide training for caregivers.

Nurses are closely involved in helping stroke survivors manage personal care issues, such as bathing and controlling incontinence. Most stroke survivors regain their ability to maintain continence, often with the help of strategies learned during rehabilitation. These strategies include strengthening pelvic muscles through special exercises and following a timed voiding schedule. If problems with incontinence continue, nurses can help caregivers learn to insert and manage catheters and to take special hygienic measures to prevent other incontinence-related health problems from developing.

Physical Therapists

Physical therapists specialize in treating disabilities related to motor and sensory impairments. They are trained in all aspects of anatomy and physiology related to normal function, with an emphasis on movement. They assess the stroke survivor's strength, endurance, range of motion, gait abnormalities, and sensory deficits to design individualized rehabilitation programs aimed at regaining control over motor functions.

Physical therapists help survivors regain the use of stroke-impaired limbs, teach compensatory strategies to reduce the effect of remaining deficits, and establish ongoing exercise programs to help people retain their newly learned skills. Disabled people tend to avoid using impaired limbs, a behavior called "learned nonuse." However, the repetitive use of impaired limbs encourages brain plasticity and helps reduce disabilities.

Strategies used by physical therapists to encourage the use of impaired limbs include selective sensory stimulation such as tapping or stroking, active and passive range-of-motion exercises, and temporary restraint of healthy limbs while practicing motor tasks.

In general, physical therapy emphasizes practicing isolated movements, repeatedly changing from one kind of movement to another, and rehearsing complex movements that require a great deal of coordination and balance, such as walking up or downstairs or moving safely between obstacles. People too weak to bear their own weight can still practice repetitive movements during hydrotherapy (in which water provides sensory stimulation as well as weight support) or while being partially supported by a harness. A recent trend in physical therapy emphasizes the effectiveness of engaging in goal-directed activities, such as playing games, to promote coordination. Physical therapists frequently employ selective sensory stimulation to encourage the use of impaired limbs and to help survivors with neglect regain awareness of stimuli on the neglected side of the body.

Occupational and Recreational Therapists

Like physical therapists, occupational therapists are concerned with improving motor and sensory abilities and ensuring patient safety in the poststroke period. They help survivors relearn skills needed for performing self-directed activities (also known as "occupations") such as personal grooming, preparing meals, and house cleaning. Therapists can teach some survivors how to adapt to driving and provide on-road training. They often teach people to divide a complex activity into its component parts, practice each part, and then perform the whole sequence of actions. This strategy can improve coordination and may help people with apraxia relearn how to carry out planned actions.

Occupational therapists also teach people how to develop compensatory strategies and change elements of their environment that limit activities of daily living. For example, people with the use of only one hand can substitute hook and loop fasteners (such as Velcro) for buttons on clothing. Occupational therapists also help people make changes in their homes to increase safety, remove barriers, and facilitate physical functioning, such as installing grab bars in bathrooms.

Recreational therapists help people with a variety of disabilities to develop and use their leisure time to enhance their health, independence, and quality of life (QOL).

Speech-Language Pathologists

Speech-language pathologists help stroke survivors with aphasia relearn how to use language or develop alternative means of communication. They also help people improve their ability to swallow, and they work with patients to develop problem-solving and social skills needed to cope with the aftereffects of a stroke.

Many specialized therapeutic techniques have been developed to assist people with aphasia. Some forms of short-term therapy can improve comprehension rapidly. Intensive exercises such as repeating the therapist's words, practicing following directions, and doing reading or writing exercises form the cornerstone of language rehabilitation. Conversational coaching and rehearsal, as well as the development of prompts or cues to help people remember specific words, are sometimes beneficial. Speech-language pathologists also help stroke survivors develop strategies for circumventing language disabilities. These strategies can include the use of symbol boards or sign language. Recent advances in computer technology have spurred the development of new types of equipment to enhance communication.

Speech-language pathologists use special types of imaging techniques to study swallowing patterns of stroke survivors and identify the exact source of their impairment. Difficulties with swallowing have many possible causes, including a delayed swallowing reflex, an inability to manipulate food with the tongue, or an inability to detect food remaining lodged in the cheeks after swallowing. When the cause has been pinpointed, speech-language pathologists work with the individual to devise strategies to overcome or minimize the deficit. Sometimes, simply changing body position and improving posture during eating can bring about improvement. The texture of foods can be modified to make swallowing easier; for example, thin liquids, which often cause choking, can be thickened. Changing eating habits by taking small bites and chewing slowly can also help alleviate dysphagia.

Vocational Therapists

Approximately one-fourth of all strokes occur in people between the ages of 45 and 65. For most people in this age group, returning to work is a major concern. Vocational therapists perform many of the same functions that ordinary career counselors do. They can help people with residual disabilities identify vocational strengths and develop résumés that highlight those strengths. They also can help identify potential employers, assist in specific job searches, and provide referrals to stroke vocational rehabilitation agencies.

Most important, vocational therapists educate disabled individuals about their rights and protections as defined by the Americans with Disabilities Act of 1990. This law requires employers to make "reasonable accommodations" for disabled employees. Vocational therapists frequently act as mediators between employers and employees to negotiate the provision of reasonable accommodations in the workplace.

Chapter 34 | Rehabilitation Facilities

Chapter Contents

Section 34.1 | Care Transition after Hospital Discharge

This section includes text excerpted from "Poststroke Rehabilitation Fact Sheet," National Institute of Neurological Disorders and Stroke (NINDS), March 17, 2020.

At the time of discharge from the hospital, the stroke patient and family coordinate with hospital social workers to locate a suitable living arrangement. Many stroke survivors return home, but some move into some type of medical facility.

INPATIENT REHABILITATION UNITS

Inpatient facilities may be freestanding or part of larger hospital complexes. Patients stay in the facility, usually for two to three weeks, and engage in a coordinated, intensive program of rehabilitation. Such programs often involve at least three hours of active therapy a day, five or six days a week. Inpatient facilities offer a comprehensive range of medical services, including full-time physician supervision and access to the full range of therapists specializing in poststroke rehabilitation.

OUTPATIENT UNITS

Outpatient facilities are often part of a larger hospital complex and provide access to physicians and the full range of therapists specializing in stroke rehabilitation. Patients typically spend several hours, often three days each week, at the facility taking part in coordinated therapy sessions and returning home at night. Comprehensive outpatient facilities frequently offer treatment programs as intense as those of inpatient facilities, but they also can offer less demanding regimens, depending on the patient's physical capacity.

NURSING FACILITIES

Rehabilitative services available at nursing facilities are more variable than are those at inpatient and outpatient units. Skilled nursing facilities usually place a greater emphasis on rehabilitation, whereas traditional nursing homes emphasize residential care. In addition, fewer hours of therapy are offered compared to outpatient and inpatient rehabilitation units.

HOME-BASED REHABILITATION PROGRAMS

Home rehabilitation allows for great flexibility so that patients can tailor their program of rehabilitation and follow individual schedules. Stroke survivors may participate in an intensive level of therapy several hours per week or follow a less demanding regimen. These arrangements are often best suited for people who require treatment by only one type of rehabilitation therapist. Patients dependent on Medicare coverage for their rehabilitation must meet Medicare's "homebound" requirements to qualify for such services; at this time lack of transportation is not a valid reason for home therapy. The major disadvantage of home-based rehabilitation programs is the lack of specialized equipment. However, undergoing treatment at home gives people the advantage of practicing skills and developing compensatory strategies in the context of their own living environment. In the stroke rehabilitation trial, intensive balance and strength rehabilitation in the home was equivalent to treadmill training at a rehabilitation facility in improving walking.

Section 34.2 | Skilled Nursing Facility

This section includes text excerpted from "Nursing Facilities," Centers for Medicare & Medicaid Services (CMS), December 3, 2011. Reviewed May 2020.

Nursing facility services are provided by Medicaid certified nursing homes, which primarily provide three types of services:
- Skilled nursing or medical care and related services
- Rehabilitation needed due to injury, disability, or illness
- Long-term care—health-related care and services (above the level of room and board) not available in the community, needed regularly due to a mental or physical condition

A nursing facility is one of many settings for long-term care, including or other services and supports outside of an institution, provided by Medicaid or other state agencies.

WHERE NURSING FACILITY SERVICES ARE PROVIDED

Medicaid coverage of nursing facility services is available only for services provided in a nursing home licensed and certified by the state survey agency as a Medicaid Nursing Facility (NF). Medicaid NF services are available only when other payment options are unavailable and the individual is eligible for the Medicaid program.

In many cases, it is not necessary to transfer to another nursing home when the payment source changes to Medicaid NF. Many nursing homes are also certified as a Medicare skilled nursing facility (SNF), and most accept long-term care insurance and private payment. For example, commonly an individual will enter a Medicare SNF following a hospitalization that qualifies her or him for a limited period of SNF services. If nursing home services are still required after the period of SNF coverage, the individual may pay privately, and use any long-term care insurance they may have. If the individual exhausts assets and is eligible for Medicaid, and the nursing home is also a Medicaid certified nursing facility, the individual may continue to reside in the nursing home under the Medicaid NF benefit. If the nursing home is not Medicaid certified, she or he would have to transfer to an NF to be covered by the Medicaid NF benefit.

WHO MAY RECEIVE NURSING FACILITY SERVICES

Nursing facility services are required to be provided by state Medicaid programs for individuals 21 years of age or older who need them. States may not limit access to the service, or make it subject to waiting lists, as they may for home and community-based services. Therefore, in some cases, NF services may be more immediately available than other long-term care options. NF residents and their families should investigate other long-term care options in order to transit back to the community as quickly as possible.

The need for nursing facility services is defined by states, all of whom have established the NF level of care criteria. State-level of care requirements must provide access to individuals who meet the coverage criteria defined in federal law and regulation. Individuals with serious mental illness or intellectual disability must also be evaluated by the state's Preadmission Screening and Resident Review program to determine if NF admission is needed and appropriate.

Nursing facility services for individuals under 21 years of age is a separate Medicaid service, optional for states to provide. However, all states provide the service, and in practice, there is no distinction between the services.

In some states, individuals applying for NF residence may be eligible for Medicaid under higher eligibility limits used for residents of an institution.

SERVICES INCLUDED IN THE NURSING FACILITY BENEFIT

A Nursing Facility participating in Medicaid must provide, or arrange for, nursing or related services and specialized rehabilitative services to attain or maintain the highest practicable physical, mental, and psychosocial well-being of each resident.

There is no exhaustive list of services an NF must provide, in that unique resident needs may require particular care or services in order to reach the highest practicable level of well being. The services needed to attain this level of well-being are established in the individual's plan of care.

Specific to each state, the general or usual responsibilities of the NF are shaped by the definition of NF service in the state's Medicaid state plan, which may also specify certain types of limitations to each service. States may also devise levels of service or payment methodologies by acuity or specialization of the nursing facilities.

Federal requirements specify that each NF must provide, (and residents may not be charged for), at least:
- Nursing and related services
- Specialized rehabilitative services (treatment and services required by residents with mental illness or intellectual disability, not provided or arranged for by the state)

Rehabilitation Facilities

- Medically-related social services
- Pharmaceutical services (with the assurance of accurate acquiring, receiving, dispensing, and administering of drugs and biologicals)
- Dietary services individualized to the needs of each resident
- Professionally directed program of activities to meet the interests and needs for well being of each resident
- Emergency dental services (and routine dental services to the extent covered under the state plan)
- Room and bed maintenance services
- Routine personal hygiene items and services

Residents may be charged for:
- Private room, unless medically needed
- Specially prepared food, beyond that, generally prepared by the facility
- Telephone, television, radio
- Personal comfort items including tobacco products and confections
- Cosmetic and grooming items and services in excess of those included in the basic service
- Personal clothing
- Personal reading materials
- Gifts purchased on behalf of a resident
- Flowers and plants
- Social events and activities beyond the activity program
- Special-care services not included in the facility's Medicaid payment

Section 34.3 | Options for Long-Term Care

This section contains text excerpted from the following sources: Text beginning with the heading "Long-Term Care Services" is excerpted from "What Is Long-Term Care?" National Institute on Aging (NIA), National Institutes of Health (NIH), May 1, 2017; Text beginning with the heading "Safety for Patients" is excerpted from "Long-Term Care and Patient Safety," Agency for Healthcare Research and Quality (AHRQ), U.S. Department of Health and Human Services (HHS), September 2019.

LONG-TERM CARE SERVICES

Long-term care involves a variety of services designed to meet a person's health or personal care needs during a short or long period of time. These services help people live as independently and safely as possible when they can no longer perform everyday activities on their own.

Long-term care is provided in different places by different caregivers, depending on a person's needs. Most long-term care is provided at home by unpaid family members and friends. It can also be given in a facility, such as a nursing home or in the community, for example, in an adult day care center.

The most common type of long-term care is personal care—help with everyday activities, also called "activities of daily living." These activities include bathing, dressing, grooming, using the toilet, eating, and moving around—for example, getting out of bed and into a chair.

Long-term care also includes community services such as meals, adult day care, and transportation services. These services may be provided free or for a fee.

People often need long-term care when they have a serious, ongoing health condition or disability. The need for long-term care can arise suddenly, such as after a heart attack or stroke. Most often, however, it develops gradually, as people get older and frailer or as an illness or disability gets worse.

WHO NEEDS LONG-TERM CARE

It is difficult to predict how much or what type of long-term care a person might need. Several things increase the risk of needing long-term care.

- **Age.** The risk generally increases as people get older.
- **Gender.** Women are at higher risk than men, primarily because they often live longer.
- **Marital status.** Single people are more likely than married people to need care from a paid provider.
- **Lifestyle.** Poor diet and exercise habits can increase a person's risk.
- **Health and family history.** These factors also affect risk.

WHAT ARE THE DIFFERENT TYPES OF HOME-BASED LONG-TERM CARE SERVICES?

Home-based long-term care includes health, personal, and support services to help people stay at home and live as independently as possible. Most long-term care is provided either in the home of the person receiving services or at a family member's home. In home services may be short-term—for someone who is recovering from an operation, for example—or long-term, for people who need ongoing help.

Most home-based services involve personal care such as help with bathing, dressing, and taking medications, and supervision to make sure a person is safe. Unpaid family members, partners, friends, and neighbors provide most of this type of care.

Home-based long-term care services can also be provided by paid caregivers, including caregivers found informally, and healthcare professionals such as nurses, home healthcare aides, therapists, and homemakers, who are hired through home healthcare agencies. These services include home healthcare, homemaker services, friendly visitor/companion services, and emergency response systems.

Home Healthcare

Home healthcare involves part-time medical services ordered by a physician for a specific condition. These services may include nursing care to help a person recover from surgery, an accident, or illness. Home healthcare may also include physical, occupational, or speech therapy and temporary home health aide services. These services are provided by home healthcare agencies approved by Medicare, a government insurance program for people over 65 years of age.

Homemaker and Personal Care Services
Home health agencies offer homemaker and personal care services that can be purchased without a physician's order. Homemaker services include help with meal preparation and household chores. Personal care includes help with bathing and dressing. Agencies do not have to be approved by Medicare to provide these kinds of services.

Friendly Visitor and Senior Companion Services
Friendly visitor/companion services are usually staffed by volunteers who regularly pay short visits (less than 2 hours) to someone who is frail or living alone. You can also purchase these services from home health agencies.

Senior Transportation Services
Transportation services help people get to and from medical appointments, shopping centers, and other places in the community. Some senior housing complexes and community groups offer transportation services. Many public transit agencies have services for people with disabilities. Some services are free. Others charge a fee.

Emergency Medical Alert Systems
Emergency response systems automatically respond to medical and other emergencies via electronic monitors. The user wears a necklace or bracelet with a button to push in an emergency. Pushing the button summons emergency help to the home. This type of service is especially useful for people who live alone or are at risk of falling. A monthly fee is charged.

LONG-TERM CARE PLANNING
You can never know for sure if you will need long-term care. Maybe you will never need it. But, an unexpected accident, illness, or

injury can change your needs, sometimes suddenly. The best time to think about long-term care is before you need it.

Planning for the possibility of long-term care gives you time to learn about services in your community and what they cost. It also allows you to make important decisions while you are still able.

People with Alzheimer disease or other cognitive impairment should begin planning for long-term care as soon as possible.

MAKING DECISIONS ABOUT LONG-TERM CARE

Begin by thinking about what would happen if you became seriously ill or disabled. Talk with your family, friends, and lawyer about who would provide care if you needed help for a long time.

You might delay or prevent the need for long-term care by staying healthy and independent. Talk to your doctor about your medical and family history and lifestyle. She or he may suggest actions you can take to improve your health.

Healthy eating, regular physical activity, not smoking, and limited drinking of alcohol can help you stay healthy. So can an active social life, a safe home, and regular healthcare.

MAKING HOUSING DECISIONS: AGING IN PLACE

In thinking about long-term care, it is important to consider where you will live as you age and how your place of residence can best support your needs if you can no longer fully care for yourself.

Most people prefer to stay in their own homes for as long as possible.

MAKING FINANCIAL DECISIONS FOR LONG-TERM CARE

Long-term care can be expensive. Americans spend billions of dollars a year on various services. How people pay for long-term care depends on their financial situation and the kinds of services they use. Often, they rely on a variety of payment sources, including:

- Personal funds including pensions, savings, and income from stocks

- Government health insurance programs, such as Medicaid (Medicare does not cover long-term care, but may cover some costs of short-term care in a nursing home after a hospital stay.)
- Private financing options, such as long-term care insurance
- Veterans' benefits
- Services through the Older Americans Act (OAA)

SAFETY FOR PATIENTS

The patient safety field has primarily focused on improving safety in hospital and ambulatory settings. Yet a large and growing number of Americans who do not require hospital-level care, but are unable to be safely cared for at home reside in settings referred to as "long-term care." These settings include skilled nursing facilities (SNFs), inpatient rehabilitation facilities, and long-term acute-care hospitals. There were more than 1.6 million residents of SNFs in 2011, and long-term acute-care hospital admissions among Medicare beneficiaries have more than doubled over the past 15 years.

LONG-TERM CARE SETTINGS

Patients in long-term care settings may be particularly vulnerable to safety problems in the course of their care. Patients requiring care in long-term care facilities are disproportionately older and chronically ill, and they often enter long-term care after an acute hospitalization. Healthcare utilization after entering long-term care is high—a study by the Office of the Inspector General (OIG) found that nearly 25 percent of Medicare SNF residents require hospitalization each year.

Each type of long-term care setting provides different services and is suitable for different types of patients:

- Long-term acute-care hospitals care for medically complex patients expected to require care for weeks to months. These patients are often chronically critically ill, most commonly recovering from a hospitalization that included an intensive care unit stay. These facilities provide services very similar to acute-care hospitals, including the ability to care for patients requiring mechanical ventilation, complex wound care, or hemodialysis. The facilities may be freestanding or attached to an acute hospital, and they are subject to the same licensing and credentialing requirements as traditional hospitals. Patients at long-term acute-care hospitals generally require daily evaluation by a physician.

- Inpatient rehabilitation facilities care for patients recovering from surgery, trauma, or an acute illness. They provide intensive rehabilitation—patients must be able to tolerate 3 hours of physical or occupational therapy daily—with the goal of restoring patients to their premorbid functional status. Care is overseen by a multidisciplinary team that includes a physician, typically a specialist in rehabilitation medicine.
- Skilled nursing facilities generally care for patients who may be chronically ill, but are considered medically stable. In general, these patients do not require daily evaluation by a physician but do require services, such as physical therapy or wound care.

Patients often enter long-term care after an acute hospitalization. Data from 2011 indicates that nearly 40 percent of Medicare beneficiaries are discharged to some form of long-term care facility—most often an SNF—after hospital discharge. Therefore, the term postacute care is also used to refer to the utilization of long-term care facilities to provide continuing care after hospitalization. Postacute patients represent an increasing proportion of the overall SNF patient population, and these patients—who are often medically complex and frail—may tax the ability of SNFs to provide safe care. As a result of all these factors, the safety field is starting to examine and address safety issues faced by patients in long-term care.

SAFETY CONCERNS IN LONG-TERM CARE

Preventable adverse events are common in long-term care. In 2014 the Office of the Inspector General (OIG) found that 22 percent of Medicare beneficiaries in skilled nursing facilities (SNFs) experienced an adverse event during their stay, half of which were preventable. More than half of the patients who experienced an adverse event at an SNF required hospitalization. A separate OIG found an even higher incidence of adverse events at rehabilitation facilities. Among these are hazards that are well documented in older patients such as medication errors, healthcare-associated infections, delirium, falls, and pressure ulcers. Adverse drug events were the most common type of adverse event in the OIG study as well as in other studies of long-term care populations. While patient complexity explains some of these events, it is also worth noting that computerized provider order entry and other medication safety strategies have not been implemented as widely in SNFs as in hospitals. Healthcare-associated infections (HAIs)—particularly catheter-associated urinary tract infections (CAUTIs)—are also common in long-term care, and efforts are underway to address this problem.

Establishing a robust culture of safety is essential for minimizing patient harm. Unfortunately, safety culture in many long-term care facilities is poorer than that found in hospitals and ambulatory clinics. A 2006 study using the AHRQ Hospital Survey on Patient Safety Culture found that nursing home administrators perceived safety culture in their facilities to be lower than hospital benchmarks across nearly all domains of the survey. AHRQ subsequently developed a safety culture survey instrument for nursing homes and has released biannual benchmarking data since 2008. The most recent (2014) data indicates overall improvement in long-term care safety culture, but respondents still raise concerns about potential patient harm due to inadequate staffing and an overly punitive culture.

HOW TO IMPROVE SAFETY IN LONG-TERM CARE

Improving safety in long-term care facilities will require research into the safety problems faced by patients, education, and training of healthcare providers in long-term care settings, system-level interventions to enhance care coordination, and greater incentives for long-term care facilities to prioritize patient safety.

Rehabilitation Facilities

The federal government is leading many efforts to improve the safety and quality of care at long-term care facilities. The Centers for Medicare & Medicaid Services (CMS) Nursing Home Compare website (www.medicare.gov/nursinghomecompare/search.html) allows patients and providers to compare long-term care facilities on various quality metrics, including measures of patient safety (such as the proportion of patients who experience a healthcare-associated infection). CMS has also proposed revisions to long-term care facilities' conditions of participation in the Medicare and Medicaid programs, which explicitly emphasize a focus on ensuring the quality of care for long-term care facility residents. AHRQ is funding research to examine the epidemiology of adverse events in long-term care settings and identify effective preventive strategies. AHRQ has also developed a number of resources to examine and address safety in long-term care, including training programs for staff, an ongoing collaborative program to prevent catheter-associated urinary tract infections, and a guide to help nursing homes appropriately use antibiotics.

The Joint Commission offers accreditation programs for nursing care centers that provide postacute care services. These include SNFs and most inpatient rehabilitation facilities. The accreditation process emphasizes the importance of patient safety and efforts to prevent hospital admissions among long-term care patients. The Joint Commission National Patient Safety Goals for long-term care facilities were updated in 2016. These require SNFs to have measures in place to prevent specific clinical harms (such as falls, pressure ulcers, and healthcare-associated infections) and to conduct medication reconciliation. Long-term acute-care hospitals and inpatient rehabilitation facilities are accredited in the same fashion as acute-care hospitals, and they are subject to the same National Patient Safety Goals (which were also updated in 2016).

While these efforts are important (and are beginning to bear fruit), fundamental healthcare system issues must be addressed in order to improve safety in long-term care. In the 2015 WebM&M commentary, neither hospitals nor long-term care facilities are incentivized to improve care transitions under the prospective payment system. CMS is developing novel-care models and payment systems to encourage healthcare systems to prioritize safe-care

317

transitions between different types of facilities. Although the data on these new models—which include accountable care organizations, bundled payments for specific diagnoses, and financial penalties for hospitals with high readmission rates—is still preliminary, there are early indications that healthcare systems are shifting their orientation toward caring for patients across the continuum of care rather than in single episodes.

Chapter 35 | Boosting Education for Stroke Survivors and Their Caregivers

Stroke is a leading cause of death in the United States. According to the Centers for Disease Control and Prevention (CDC), someone in the United States has a stroke every 40 seconds, and every four minutes someone dies of a stroke. Although stroke risk increases with age, strokes can and do occur at any age. Nearly a quarter of strokes occur in people under 65 years of age. Approximately 6.2 million people are living with the consequences of stroke.

While many people survive their first stroke, stroke survivors and their caregivers often do not have the information they need to manage their recovery process at home. A competent and knowledgeable caregiver is critical in determining whether a stroke survivor's mental and physical health is improving and whether the survivor or a stroke is institutionalized or can remain at home in her or his community.

Because strokes occur suddenly, survivors and caregivers need extensive education to prevent second strokes and to manage the aftermath of a stroke. In a presentation given at the 2012 Horizons in Rehabilitation Conference, a team of Veteran Affairs nurses evaluated two-stroke education programs developed by VA, one

This chapter includes text excerpted from "Boosting Education for Stroke Survivors and Their Caregivers," U.S. Department of Veterans Affairs (VA), February 11, 2014. Reviewed May 2020.

administered in person and one Web-based—and found that both were important new tools in helping Veterans with stroke and their caregivers to manage the disease.

"Education is a vital aspect of care and management of debilitating illnesses, especially stroke," says Constance R. Uphold, PhD, a researcher with the VA North Florida/South Georgia Veterans Health System and an associate professor at the University of Florida, one of the study's co-presenters.

One of the programs the team evaluated was an in-person educational series developed by the VA Puget Sound Healthcare System, based in Seattle, Wash. The hospital's interdisciplinary stroke team developed an educational series to provide Veterans and caregivers with information on understanding, preventing, and managing stroke.

Participants meet twice a month and listen to lectures on topics including understanding stroke, functional recovery, and communication and cognition. After the lecture, those in attendance hold interactive discussions with the hospital's stroke team and also discuss appropriate support for each individual participant.

Different educational methods are effective in improved stroke-related outcomes, and the in-person education series provides social support and a forum for survivors and caregivers to learn from each other. And the RESCUE website provides a breadth of stroke-related information and reaches a large number of persons.

Part 5 | Life after Stroke

Chapter 36 | Stroke Recovery: A Caregiver Guide

Chapter Contents

Section 36.1 | Changes in Body Function

This section includes text excerpted from "Changes in Body Function," U.S. Department of Veterans Affairs (VA), January 5, 2011. Reviewed May 2020.

The physical effects of stroke can range from muscle weakness to total paralysis. The physical effects will depend on where and how the stroke injured the brain.

WHAT DO YOU NEED TO KNOW ABOUT PARALYSIS AND WEAKNESS?
Paralysis

Paralysis is when muscles are unable to move on their own. There is often a loss of feeling. Paralysis in the arm or leg is the most common problem. If one side of the body is paralyzed, it is known as "hemiplegia."

Weakness

Weakness means a lack of strength. When muscles are weak, they do not move as easily. Muscles may feel heavy or numb. Weakness affecting one whole side of the body is called "hemiparesis."

Rehabilitation

Rehabilitation (rehab) helps strengthen weak muscles. It helps stroke survivors who have hemiparesis regain some movement. Most importantly, rehab teaches your loved one how to deal with the changes. Rehab will help your loved one achieve the best quality of life (QOL).

Treatments

The treatments are also being developed. One treatment is electrical stimulation. This treatment sends small electrical charges to the muscles. These electrical charges improve muscle strength and function.

Constraint-induced movement therapy (CIMT) is another treatment. CIMT involves restricting movement in the unaffected arm or the arm with normal strength. Then, the stroke survivor is forced to use the weak or affected arm.

HOW CAN STROKE AFFECT PROBLEMS WITH BALANCE?

Your loved one may have trouble with balance after stroke. She or he may feel dizzy or unsteady. This can cause your loved one to lose confidence in walking. Falls often happen after a stroke. Almost half of the survivors suffer a serious fall in the first year. It is important that your loved one be evaluated for the risk of falls.

Balance problems can be treated. Have your loved one evaluated by a physical therapist. Exercises, such as yoga and tai chi help to improve balance.

HOW CAN STROKE AFFECT SENSATIONS OR FEELING?

Your loved one may experience a change in sensations. Sensations can be decreased or be felt more strongly. Sensations may also be painful. Unpleasant feelings, like "pins and needles" may occur. These sensations often lessen over time. Some survivors report that sensations are worse when they are tired. Getting plenty of rest will help your loved one.

Safety is a concern for those with decreased sensations. The risk of falls and other injuries is greater. To prevent burns, test water temperature before bathing your loved one. Check affected limbs for bruises, cuts, or sores. Make sure to change positions regularly to prevent pressure sores. Talk to your healthcare team about other safety tips.

WHAT IS SPASTICITY?

Spasticity is a condition where muscles become stiff or rigid. Movement is limited. Over time, the muscle may shorten permanently. When the muscles shorten, the joints can "freeze" into position. This painful condition is known as a "contracture." Contractures prevent normal movement and interfere with doing daily tasks. Proper positioning of spastic limbs can prevent contractures. The physical therapist can teach you proper positioning.

Treatment for spasticity includes other types of physical therapy, such as exercise and stretching. The goals of treatment are to relieve symptoms, reduce pain, and improve movement.

WHAT IS FOOT DROP?
Stroke can weaken the muscles that help lift the foot. This will cause the toes to drag when walking. Some survivors try to help this by bending the knee to lift the foot higher. This uses more energy and makes walking harder.

Your loved one can be fitted with a brace or shoe insert. This will make walking more comfortable. Talk to the physical therapist about gait training exercises. These exercises help your loved one relearn how to walk safely. In some cases, surgery may be needed.

WHAT IS FATIGUE?
Many stroke survivors feel very tired or have fatigue. Simple tasks, such as sitting or standing up may be exhausting. Fatigue can slow down your loved one's recovery. The good news is that there are treatments and ways to decrease fatigue. Physical and occupational therapy can help.

HOW CAN ASSISTIVE DEVICES HELP YOUR LOVED ONE?
Ask your healthcare team about assistive devices. These include wheelchairs, canes, and walkers. Agency supportive services can be arranged if needed.

Assistive Devices
- Help your loved one move around easier
- Provide support and balance
- Help prevent falls
- Helps your loved one be more independent

Some survivors may not want to use assistive devices. They may be embarrassed or afraid. Talk to your loved one about her or his feelings.

HELPFUL TIPS
- **Watch for things that can cause falls when walking—** Uneven sidewalks, doorsteps, liquid spills, ice, and pets can cause falls.
- **Help your loved one stay active—**Work with your healthcare team to develop an exercise plan.
- **Attend rehab sessions as often as possible with your loved one—**This will keep you informed of their progress. Ask questions and talk to the rehab team about your concerns.
- **Listen and be supportive—**The physical effects of stroke can be mentally and physically stressful. Allow your loved one to express their feelings.

REMEMBER
- Has your loved one been evaluated for the risk of falls. Falls are common after stroke.
- Think about finding rehabilitation (rehab) services for your loved one. Rehab can help stroke survivors achieve the best quality of life.
- Encourage your loved one to exercise. Exercise builds strength and improves movement. Contact a physical therapist to set up an exercise program for your loved one.
- Think about getting assistive devices, such as walkers or canes for your loved one. Assistive devices can help your loved one be more independent.

Section 36.2 | Spasticity

This section includes text excerpted from "Spasticity," U.S. Department of Veterans Affairs (VA), January 5, 2011. Reviewed May 2020.

Spasticity is a condition in which muscles become stiff or rigid. The muscles resist being stretched, which limits movement. Spasticity can develop in any muscle in the body. It is most common in the arms, fingers, and legs.

WHY IS IT IMPORTANT TO GET HELP FOR SPASTICITY?

Spasticity develops slowly over weeks or months. It ranges from slight muscle stiffness to muscle shortening. When the muscles shorten, the joints can "freeze" into position. This painful condition is known as a "contracture." Contractures prevent normal movement and interfere with doing daily tasks. Properly positioning spastic limbs helps prevent contractures.

Symptoms of spasticity include:
- Stiffness or tightness of muscles and joints
- Painful muscle spasms or cramping of muscles
- Involuntary (uncontrollable) jerking motions
- Exaggerated deep tendon reflexes (knee-jerk reflex)
- Abnormal position of the arm; tight fist, bent elbow, and arm pressed against the chest
- Abnormal position of the legs; crossing the legs as the tips of scissors would close (scissoring)

WHAT DO YOU NEED TO KNOW?

Spasticity is out of your loved one's control. Things that trigger spasticity or make it worse are:
- Pain (pressure sores)
- Infections (bladder, toenail, ear)
- Cold temperatures
- Constipation
- Fatigue or stress

WHAT TREATMENTS SHOULD YOU DISCUSS WITH YOUR HEALTHCARE TEAM?

Your loved one needs to determine the type of treatment. Often, treatment involves a mix of therapy and medicine. The goals are to relieve symptoms, reduce pain, and improve movement.

Physical exercise and stretching—This will help loosen stiff muscles. A physical therapist works with your loved one. Often, this includes a full range of motion exercises several times a week. Gentle stretching of tight muscles may be needed. The physical therapist may suggest constraint-induced movement therapy (CIMT). CIMT involves restricting movement in the unaffected arm to force the use of the affected arm.

Braces and splints—These assistive devices hold the muscles in a more normal position. This helps to prevent contractures and improve comfort.

Oral medicines—There are medicines to treat the effects of spasticity. Some work to temporarily block nerve impulses. Others work to relax the muscles. Talk to your healthcare team about medicines for your loved one.

Injections of a medicine—Medicines, such as Botox®** help to block nerve activity. This loosens the muscles. Intrathecal baclofen therapy (ITB) is used to treat severe spasticity. A surgically placed pump delivers baclofen** into the spinal fluid. Baclofen is a medicine that relaxes the muscles.

Surgery—This is often the last choice for treating severe, chronic spasticity. It involves operating on the bones, muscles, or nerves. Surgery works to block pain and restore some movement.

**Brand Name and Medicine Disclaimer: *Brand names and types of medicines are provided as examples only. Their inclusion does not mean that these products are endorsed by the U.S. Department of Veterans Affairs (VA) or any other government agency. Also, if a particular brand name is not mentioned, this does not mean or imply that the product is unsatisfactory.*

HELPFUL TIPS

- **Encourage your loved one to remain active**—Exercise and stretching can help ease symptoms and maintain

movement. Reinforce using the affected arm as much as possible for daily tasks.
- **Properly position spastic limbs to prevent contractures**—Proper positioning can keep affected limbs from becoming fixed into a set position. The physical therapist can teach you proper positioning.
- **Watch for skin breakdown**—Spasticity in the fingers can cause the nails to tear into the skin. Spastic limbs may rub against each other. Check the skin regularly for any redness or sores. A good time to do this is during bath time. Talk to your healthcare team about any concerns.
- **Listen and be supportive**—Spasticity can be mentally and physically stressful. Allow your loved one to express her or his feelings.

REMEMBER
- Spasticity develops slowly over weeks or months. Tell your healthcare team if your loved one shows signs of spasticity.
- Check the skin regularly for skin breakdown. Talk to your healthcare team about any concerns.
- Talk to the physical therapist about how to properly position spastic limbs to prevent contractures.

Section 36.3 | Loss of Bladder Control

This section includes text excerpted from "Loss of Bladder Control," U.S. Department of Veterans Affairs (VA), January 5, 2011. Reviewed May 2020.

Urinary incontinence is the loss of ability to hold in urine.

WHAT ARE THE CAUSES OF URINARY INCONTINENCE?

Below are some common reasons why stroke survivors may have trouble controlling their bladder:

- Injury to the part of the brain that controls the urge to pass urine
- Memory problems and forgetting to urinate
- Trouble getting to the bathroom. It may be hard for survivors to walk to the toilet. They may also have a problem talking to people and asking for help.
- Illnesses, such as bladder infections
- Side effects of some medicines

WHAT DO YOU NEED TO KNOW?

Almost all stroke survivors will have some degree of incontinence. Some survivors have accidents once in a while. Others cannot hold their urine at all. The good news is that incontinence can be managed, treated, and sometimes cured.

WHY IS IT IMPORTANT TO GET HELP?

Some problems with controlling the loss of urine are due to illnesses or other easily treated problems. It is important that your loved one be looked at by a healthcare provider. Your healthcare team can work with you and your loved one to help manage the problem.

WHAT TREATMENTS SHOULD YOU DISCUSS WITH YOUR HEALTHCARE TEAM?

Regular or fixed toilet times—Visiting the toilet at fixed times may help to retrain the bladder and prevent accidents.

Bladder retraining with urge suppression—This may help survivors get control over the times they use the toilet. First, establish fixed toilet times. Slowly increase the time between trips to the toilet. Teach survivors to wait at least ten minutes after they feel the need to urinate. Suggest ways to relax and postpone the urge to urinate. For example, have them think about pleasant events.

Exercises—There are exercises that can make the muscles that hold the bladder stronger. These exercises are called "pelvic floor muscle exercises" (Kegel exercises).

A urinary foley catheter—This is a small tube that is sometimes used to pass urine soon after a stroke. The catheter is removed when the survivor no longer needs it. Foley catheters are used only when necessary. MedlinePlus has more information about how to care for catheters.

A condom catheter—This is a pouch-like device that is placed around a human's penis and then connects to a tube. The tube empties urine into a storage bag. MedlinePlus has information on how to care for condom catheters.

Other devices and medicines—For women, medical devices that support the bladder, such as pessaries, are sometimes used. Some medicines can prevent accidents and calm the bladder.

HELPFUL TIPS
Talk about the Problem
- First, talk with your healthcare team. Stroke survivors are often embarrassed and have trouble talking about incontinence. Directly discuss their concerns.
- Use sensitivity and tact. Remember that accidents happen and are not your loved one's fault.

Ways to Manage Bladder Control Problems
- Allow your loved one privacy and plenty of time to sit on the toilet.
- Make sure the survivor drinks four to six glasses of water during the day. Avoid fluids two to three hours before bedtime.

- Help the patient limit foods and beverages that irritate the bladder. Limit caffeine (such as coffee, tea, cola), artificial sweeteners, alcohol, chocolate, acidic foods (such as tomatoes, oranges), and very spicy foods.

Consider the Purchase of Products and Equipment

- A bedside commode or a urinal near the bed is often helpful. Put the commode and urinal in the closet during the day to avoid embarrassing your loved one.
- A raised toilet seat or grab bars in the bathroom may prevent falling.
- Disposable or washable bed pads are available in drug stores or medical supply houses. Place these pads underneath the sheets so they are less noticeable.
- On long trips, disposable undergarments may be used for protection. Designs to choose from include diapers, pads, underwear liners, and undergarments that are worn just like regular underwear. Use these undergarments only when necessary. Your loved one may rely on them and avoid trying other options.

If Your Loved One Has Memory or Communication Problems

- Watch for signs that your loved one needs to use the toilet. Common signs are changes in facial expressions, restlessness, or aimless pulling at clothes.
- Help your loved one to the bathroom every two to three hours.
- Encourage and praise your loved one after toilet use.

If an Accident Occurs, Try the Following to Remove Stains

- Mix together: one cup of hot (not boiling) tap water, one tablespoon of powdered laundry detergent, and one tablespoon of white vinegar.
- With a sponge, apply to the stained area until very wet.
- Place folded towels over the area to absorb the fluid.
- Leave towels in place overnight.

RED FLAG: CHANGES IN URINATION

Call your healthcare provider right away if any of these changes occur:

- Changes in the usual amount, color, and number of times urine is passed
- Pain or great difficulty when urinating
- Blood in urine

REMEMBER

- The first step is to discuss incontinence problems with your healthcare team.
- Be sensitive and remember that accidents are not the fault of your loved one.
- The good news is that incontinence can be managed, treated, and often cured.

Section 36.4 | Pain after Stroke

This section includes text excerpted from "Pain after Stroke," U.S. Department of Veterans Affairs (VA), January 5, 2011. Reviewed May 2020.

Pain is common after a stroke. Pain means that the body is hurt or something is wrong. Every stroke survivor's pain is different. The pain may be mild or severe. It may last for a short time or be constant.

WHAT DO YOU NEED TO KNOW?

Pain after a stroke is caused by many things. Your loved one can have one or more types of pain. The key is to find the cause of the pain so it can be treated.

Local Pain

Local pain results from physical problems. After a part of the body is paralyzed (unable to move) or weakened, the muscles may become tight and stiff. These changes in the muscles can cause pain. This pain is often felt in the joints, most often in the shoulders. Your loved one may also have sore muscles from learning new ways to walk or move. Pain may be caused by lying or sitting in one place for too long. Other common causes are pressure sores or painful leg cramps at night.

Central Pain

Central pain is a direct result of damage to the brain from the stroke. Sensations like light touch are felt as pain when they should not be painful. This pain is described as "burning or aching." The pain is usually on the side of the body affected by the stroke. It is often constant and may get worse over time. Changes in cold and hot temperatures may increase the pain. Movement or touching may increase the pain.

WHY IS IT IMPORTANT TO GET HELP?

Talk to the healthcare team about your loved one's pain. Pain often leads to other problems. For instance, pain can cause depression and loss of sleep. Your loved one may stop moving a painful part of the body. Over time, the joint of this body part may "lockup" and your loved one will lose movement.

WHAT TREATMENTS SHOULD YOU DISCUSS WITH YOUR HEALTHCARE TEAM?

The pain usually lessens with treatment. There are many treatments to ask about.

Pain Medicines

Pain medicines are one of the most important treatments. Use pain medicines that your healthcare team suggests. Follow the directions on the label of the medicine. Give pain medicines on a regular basis. Do not wait until the pain gets bad to give pain medicines. Do not stop using medicines for fear of addiction. When pain medicines are used correctly, they do not cause addiction.

Over-the-counter (OTC) pain medicines, such as Tylenol®** or Advil®** relieve mild pain. These OTC medicines may interact with other medicines your loved one takes. Check with your healthcare team before taking any OTC medicines. For more severe pain, stronger prescription pain medicines, such as narcotics are often needed.

Medicines used to treat depression, spasticity (tightness and stiffness of muscles), or seizures may relieve central pain. Shots or injections of cortisone (steroids) into joints like the shoulder may help.

Brand Name and Medicine Disclaimer: *Brand names and types of medicines are provided as examples only. Their inclusion does not mean that these products are endorsed by the U.S. Department of Veterans Affairs (VA) or any other government agency. Also, if a particular brand name is not mentioned, this does not mean or imply that the product is unsatisfactory.*

Exercises
Exercises to strengthen muscles can help your loved one move better. For example, stretching exercises decrease the tightness and soreness of the muscles. Talk with a physical therapist about the best exercise plan.

Heat Therapy
Heat therapy, such as heating pads and warm baths may soothe sore muscles and stiff joints.

Electrical Nerve Stimulation
Electrical nerve stimulation (often called "TENS" or "TNS") improves the strength of the muscles and often reduces pain. Patches or electrodes are placed on the skin. A mild electrical current runs through these patches. This is not painful.

Complementary or Alternative Therapies
Complementary or alternative therapies such as acupuncture, massage therapy, and yoga often relieve pain.

WHAT IF THE PAIN CONTINUES

Everyone has the right to good pain control. Ask your healthcare team to try different treatments to relieve the pain. If the pain continues, ask about other types of care.

- Pain clinics are helpful for people whose pain is difficult to treat. Ask about pain clinics in your area.
- Psychologists help stroke survivors find ways to live with pain that cannot be completely relieved. Psychologists also help survivors who are sad or depressed due to living with pain.

HOW CAN YOU HELP YOUR LOVED ONE DESCRIBE THE PAIN?

Your healthcare team needs to know how your loved one feels. Ask your loved one to rate the pain. Use a pain scale of "0–10," with "0" being no pain and "10" being the worst pain your loved one has ever felt.

Take note of where your loved one hurts. What things bring on the pain? What makes it worse? When does the pain occur? How does it feel? Report these symptoms to your healthcare team.

Remember that some stroke survivors have trouble speaking. Watch for signs of pain, such as moaning or changes in behaviors. Some stroke survivors may not feel pain. They may not know when they are cut or burned by hot water. Watch for sores and other injuries.

Talk with Your Loved One about the Pain

- The pain almost always is a real problem. Believe your loved one's complaints.
- Allow time for your loved one to talk about the pain.
- Talk about feelings of sadness related to the pain. Watch for signs of depression. Report problems to your healthcare team.

HELPFUL TIPS

- Help your loved one remain active to keep muscles strong and reduce pain.

338

- Talk with your healthcare team about the correct ways to exercise. Also, ask about how best to position paralyzed or weak arms and legs. Splints or other devices may be helpful.
- Support a weak or paralyzed arm to reduce pain in the shoulder. Ask your healthcare team about using an arm sling. Provide support for the arm on a lapboard or raised armrest. Use pillows while lying in bed.
- Have your loved one wear loose, comfortable clothing.
- Help your loved one relax. Find an activity that your loved one enjoys such as playing with the dog or watching television. Suggest activities, such as listening to music, reading a book, prayer, or meditation.
- Use warm baths, showers, warm washcloths, or heating pads. Be sure to check the temperature so as not to cause burns. Cool clothes and ice may also help. Talk with your healthcare team about the best plan.

REMEMBER
- Pain is almost always a real problem. Believe your loved one. Get help for any signs of problems of pain.
- Pain can cause other problems, such as depression and loss of sleep.
- Treatment is based on what is causing the pain. Ask about the pain. Help your loved one describe the pain to the healthcare team.
- Everyone has the right to good pain control. Ask for different treatments if the pain is not relieved.

Section 36.5 | Swallowing Problems

This section includes text excerpted from "Swallowing Problems," U.S. Department of Veterans Affairs (VA), January 5, 2011. Reviewed May 2020.

Difficulty swallowing, or dysphagia, is common after stroke. Over half of survivors will have some trouble swallowing. If not treated, dysphagia can lead to serious health problems.

WHAT DO YOU NEED TO KNOW?

Strokes can damage the nerves that supply the muscles involved in chewing and swallowing. These include the lips, tongue, and throat. For example, strokes may result in:

- Weakened muscles in the lips, tongue, pharynx (throat)
- Loss or change of sensation in the lips or tongue
- Decreased ability to chew food, keep it in the mouth, and prepare the food to swallow
- Inability to cough or clear food that goes into the lungs (down the "wrong pipe")

WHAT ARE SIGNS THAT YOUR LOVED ONE IS HAVING TROUBLE SWALLOWING?

- Coughing or choking while eating or drinking
- Drooling; food or drink leaking out the side of the mouth
- Food left in the mouth after swallowing; food getting stuck in the throat
- Gurgling or wet sounding voice during or right after eating or drinking
- Unexplained weight loss

WHY IS IT IMPORTANT TO GET HELP?

Dysphagia can make eating and drinking difficult. It can keep your loved one from taking in enough food and fluids. This can lead to malnutrition and dehydration. Malnutrition is when the body does not get enough nutrients. Dehydration is when the body loses more fluid than it takes in. If left untreated, these conditions can lead to serious illness and death.

There is also a risk of food or liquid getting diverted. This is called "aspiration." It happens when food or liquid goes into the windpipe and lungs instead of down the esophagus to the stomach. Normally, it can be coughed back up, but after a stroke, sensations may be decreased. Your loved one may not know that food has been aspirated. This is a very dangerous condition known as "silent aspiration." Food or liquid that has been aspirated can lead to chest infections, pneumonia, and even death.

HOW CAN YOU REDUCE THE RISK OF ASPIRATION?

- Have your loved one sit upright at a 90-degree angle while eating. Your loved one should stay upright for 30 minutes after eating.
- Allow plenty of time for meals. Keep the environment or surroundings free from distractions like television.
- Encourage your loved one to take small bites of food.
- Ask your loved one to take small sips from a cup. Do not use a straw.
- Encourage your loved one to cough if they feel food in their throat.

HOW IS DYSPHAGIA DIAGNOSED?

After the stroke, your loved one's swallowing will be checked. This will be done before they are allowed to eat or drink. The healthcare team will do a simple swallow test. A few teaspoons of water will be given by mouth. Foods of different consistency may also be tried. If no coughing or choking is present, the test is repeated. Next, a small glass of water will be tried. If there are no swallowing problems, normal eating and drinking can usually be resumed. Sometimes there may be a few restrictions in eating and drinking.

If there is difficulty with swallowing, a complete assessment will be done. A speech-language therapist and a dietitian will assess your loved one. Your loved one's swallowing will be checked daily. They will be screened for the risk of aspiration.

Special tests to assess swallowing include:
- **Video-fluoroscopy** involves swallowing a barium fluid along with different foods and liquid consistencies while x-rays are taken. The barium will show up on the x-ray. This will help find the location of the swallowing problems.
- **Endoscopy** involves inserting a lighted scope inside the digestive tract. X-rays are taken to watch for swallowing problems in the throat, esophagus, or stomach.

WHAT TREATMENTS SHOULD YOU DISCUSS WITH YOUR HEALTHCARE TEAM?

Dysphagia is treatable. Most survivors will regain safe swallowing within a few weeks. Others may take longer. A small number of survivors will never regain the ability to swallow. Talk to your healthcare team about the best treatment for your loved one.

A speech-language therapist may recommend:
- Exercises to coordinate and strengthen muscles for swallowing
- Strategies or positions to help your loved one swallow more effectively
- Changes in food consistency (texture) to make swallowing easier

Long-Term Treatment

If dysphagia is severe, a feeding tube may be needed. Nourishment or food will be given through the tube instead of by mouth. The type of feeding tube used will depend on the long-term need.
- A nasogastric (NG) tube is placed for short-term use. This is a narrow tube that is placed through the nose into the stomach. The NG tube will be removed when swallowing is regained.
- A percutaneous endoscopic gastrostomy (PEG) tube is placed for long-term use. This tube is inserted into the stomach through the abdominal wall. It will remain in place and be monitored by the healthcare team.

HELPFUL TIPS

Cut foods into small pieces—Avoid foods that are more likely to cause choking. Some of these include nuts, carrots, hot dogs, whole grapes, marshmallows, and meat.

Change the consistency of foods—Some foods can be puréed (blended) to make them soft. Check with your speech-language pathologist first.

Use thickeners for drinks—Thin liquids are harder to swallow. Thin liquids are more easily aspirated. Try using a product, such as Thick-it®**.

Avoid foods with mixed consistencies—For example, avoid soups that have broth (thin liquid) and beans, vegetables, and/or meat (which needs to be chewed).

**Brand Name and Medicine Disclaimer: *Brand names and types of medicines are provided as examples only. Their inclusion does not mean that these products are endorsed by the U.S. Department of Veterans Affairs (VA) or any other government agency. Also, if a particular brand name is not mentioned, this does not mean or imply that the product is unsatisfactory.*

REMEMBER

- Watch for signs that your loved one is having trouble swallowing. Talk to your healthcare team about any concerns.
- Talk to your speech-language pathologist about the best consistency of food for your loved one.
- Have your loved one sit upright while eating and 30 minutes after eating. This will help prevent aspiration.

Section 36.6 | Fatigue after Stroke

This section includes text excerpted from "Feeling Tired after Stroke," U.S. Department of Veterans Affairs (VA), January 5, 2011. Reviewed May 2020.

Fatigue is defined as loss of energy or strength. Around 30 to 70 percent of stroke survivors feel very tired or have fatigue.

WHAT DO YOU NEED TO KNOW FATIGUE?

It is normal for your loved one to tire easily. After a stroke, simple tasks, such as sitting or standing up, may be exhausting. With time, your loved one should get back strength and energy.

Health issues that decrease energy after a stroke include:
- Muscle weakness
- Paralysis
- Pain
- Poor nutrition and weight loss
- Sadness or depression

WHY IS IT IMPORTANT TO GET HELP FOR FATIGUE?

Fatigue can slow down your loved one's recovery. It is important for your healthcare team to learn the cause of fatigue. Sometimes fatigue is due to medical problems that can be treated. At other times, fatigue is due to side effects of medicines. The good news is there are treatments and ways to decrease fatigue.

WHAT TREATMENTS SHOULD YOU DISCUSS WITH YOUR HEALTHCARE TEAM FOR FATIGUE?

- Medicines often help if fatigue is due to pain or depression.
- A social worker, psychologist, or psychiatrist can help your loved one with depression.
- A physical therapist (PT) can teach exercises to build strength. A PT can show your loved one how to move and save energy.

- An occupational therapist (OT) can teach new ways to do everyday tasks to save energy. An OT can suggest changes to make in your home to help your loved one move around.

HELPFUL TIPS
- Encourage your loved one to eat healthy foods, such as fruits and vegetables.
- Give your loved one plenty of water to drink. Decreased amounts of liquids can cause fatigue.
- Plan frequent rest periods.
- Help your loved one to get a good night's sleep; limit caffeine after lunch; and to get up and go to bed at the same time each day.
- Help your loved one stay active. Too much bed rest can weaken muscles.
- Work with your healthcare team to develop an exercise plan.

REMEMBER
- Fatigue is a common problem after stroke.
- Talk with your healthcare team about your loved one's fatigue.
- Frequent rest periods are important.
- Help your loved one exercise and stay active.

Section 36.7 | Vision Problems after Stroke

"Vision Problems after Stroke" © 2017 Omnigraphics. Reviewed May 2020.

Vision problems are very common after stroke, with up to two-thirds of patients experiencing at least some degree of vision impairment. These issues occur most often in cases in which the

345

right side of the brain is affected, but they can result from other types of stroke damage, as well. Sight involves not just the eyes but also the optic nerves, which travel the entire length of the brain. And although the occipital lobe at the back of the brain is the primary area that processes visual information, almost all areas of the brain receive input from vision, so there are many ways that a stroke can affect the way a patient sees. Like other effects of stroke, vision problems can be permanent, but in most cases they can improve over time, especially with proper treatment.

COMMON VISION PROBLEMS AFTER STROKE

There is a wide variety of visual impairment that can occur following a stroke, but some of the most common problems include:

- **Visual field loss.** The visual field is the portion of a person's surroundings that can be seen at any given time. Visual field loss, called "hemianopia," results in patients only being able to see either the right or left side of what they are looking at.
- **Central field loss.** With this condition, the center part of the vision field is affected. The patient might only be able to see objects at the very edges of the field but not in the middle.
- **Double vision.** Known as "diplopia," double vision is most often the result of stroke damage to the brainstem. Here, the patient might see two of the same object, lose depth perception, and become disoriented.
- **Visual neglect.** Visual neglect, or inattention, usually results from damage to the parietal lobe of the brain, where spatial information is processed. With this condition, patients may not be aware of objects on one side. For example, they might only eat food on half of their plates, being unaware that the other half exists.
- **Eye movement issues.** Vision requires the coordinated movement of both eyes, and stroke can affect the way the brain controls these movements. This could result in problems, such as difficulty focusing on objects or continuous jerky movement of the eyes.

346

- **Visual agnosia.** With this unusual disorder, the patient is able to see objects or people but is unable to identify them because of damage to the visual processing area of the brain. However, the patient may be able to recognize objects by touch or smell.

Other problems caused by vision problems resulting from stroke can include difficulty identifying colors, inability to calculate distance to objects, dizziness, and hallucinations.

TREATMENT FOR VISION PROBLEMS AFTER STROKE

Because there are so many different types of visual impairment following a stroke, treatment can vary considerably. Depending on the condition, an ophthalmologist (eye doctor), optometrist (eye-care professional), orthoptist (eye muscle specialist), and optician (eyeglasses and contact lens dispenser) can all be involved in designing and carrying out a treatment plan. Some possible treatments include:

- **Optical therapy.** Also called "vision field relocation," this treatment uses prisms or mirrors—usually mounted on glasses—to shift images from the impaired side to the side with better vision, sometimes increasing the visual field by 20 percent.
- **Visual restoration therapy.** Here, flashing lights and images on a computer screen are used to stimulate neural cells and improve vision in blind areas of the visual field. By performing a set of vigorous exercises every day for several months, partially blind stroke patients can often improve vision significantly.
- **Eye movement therapy.** This type of treatment helps train a patient's eyes to scan objects within her or his poststroke visual field. Exercises focus on strengthening and retraining eye muscles for improved control and stamina.
- **Surgery.** In some cases, surgical repair of eye muscles can correct double vision and movement disorders.

VISION AIDS

Most patients who experience visual impairment after stroke improve at least to some degree with treatment. But in cases in which the problems persist (or while therapy continues), there are various devices that can help patients cope with vision issues. These include:

- **Eye patches.** While eye patches may not permanently correct conditions like double vision, they can be a simple, inexpensive means of coping with certain perception issues.
- **Magnifiers.** All types of magnifiers are available to help make reading easier. These range from simple pocket-sized magnifying glasses to large, lighted tabletop models.
- **Typoscope.** This is a dark piece of nonreflective black cardboard with a rectangular slot in the center. When placed over reading material, it eliminates glare from the surrounding white spaces and makes it easier to focus on a line of text.
- **Reading stands.** A stand cannot only position reading material closer and hold it steady, it can also prevent stooping to read, reducing neck strain and headaches.
- **Proper lighting.** Adequate lighting is important for individuals experiencing vision problems following a stroke. Adjustable lamps focus light on reading material or objects, keeping it out of the person's eyes. And if vision is better in one eye, an adjustable lamp can be positioned over the shoulder of the unaffected eye.
- **Binoculars or telescopes.** A small telescope or set of binoculars can be helpful for reading street signs or viewing distant objects. Some binoculars can be mounted on eyeglasses for added convenience.
- **Sunglasses.** Tinted glasses cannot only protect the eyes from glare, they can also help in improving distance vision and depth perception.

References

1. "Common Problems after Stroke," Stroke Association (UK), February 2015.
2. Gupta, Mrinali Patel, MD. "Stroke/Hemianopsia," Visionaware.org, n.d.
3. Lazarony, Lucy. "Overcome Poststroke Vision Challenges," Strokesmart.org, June 17, 2014.
4. "Stroke-Related Eye Conditions," Royal National Institute of Blind People (UK), 2016.
5. "Vision," National Stroke Association (NSA), n.d.
6. "Vision Disturbances after Stroke," American Stroke Association, November 15, 2016.

Chapter 37 | Reconstructing Everyday Life

Chapter Contents

Section 37.1 | Activities of Daily Living

This section includes text excerpted from "Everyday Personal Care," U.S. Department of Veterans Affairs (VA), January 5, 2011. Reviewed May 2020.

After a stroke, your loved one may need help with personal-care activities. These include bathing, dressing, toileting, and oral or mouth care.

WHAT DO YOU NEED TO KNOW?

It may be hard for your loved one to accept your help. Feeling embarrassed or ashamed are normal emotions. Listen to your loved one talk about how they feel. Be supportive and understanding. Allow your loved one to do as much as possible. Be close by to help if needed.

HELPFUL TIPS
Bathing

- Plan bathing at the time of day when your loved one has the most energy.
- Gather all supplies ahead of time. Never leave an unsteady loved one alone in the bath or shower.
- Check the temperature of the water before you start. Make sure the water is not "too hot" or "too cold."
- Let your loved one do as much as possible. Allow her or him to wash the parts within reach.
- Use assistive devices to make bathing easier and safer. These can include a shower bench, nonskid bath mats, and grab bars.

WHAT IF YOUR LOVED ONE IS BEDRIDDEN?

If your loved one is bedridden (unable to get out of bed), you can do a bed bath. To make it easier, perform the bed bath in steps.

- First, cover the body with towels.
- Wash in sections, removing only one towel at a time.

- Cover the area again after drying. This will provide privacy and keep your loved one warm.

Dressing

- Assistive devices, such as zipper pulls, can help your loved one dress themselves. Velcro® closures can be used to replace buttons, zippers, and shoe laces.
- Loose-fitting clothes are best. It is harder to put on tight-fitting clothes. Pants or skirts with elastic waistbands are easy to pull on and off.
- Clothes should fasten in the front. Avoid clothing that needs to be pulled over the head.
- Have your loved one sit down to dress. Put the affected arm/leg into clothes first. When undressing, take the affected arm/leg out of the clothes last.
- Shoes should have a nonskid tread and not slip off easily. Use shoes with Velcro®** fasteners.

Grooming

- Shaving can be made safer by using an electric razor. This will reduce the risk of cuts and nicks.
- Long handle hair brushes or combs will be easier for your loved one to use.

Toileting

- Make sure the walkway to the bathroom is well-lit.
- If needed, place a bedside commode or a urinal near the bed at night. Put the commode and urinal in the closet during the day to avoid embarrassing your loved one.
- Only use adult diapers as a last resort.

Oral or Mouth Care

- Help your loved one brush their or his teeth twice a day.
- Remember to brush the tongue. The tongue is covered with bacteria that can lead to dental problems.

- Take note of the color of gums and condition of teeth. Notify the dentist if you have concerns.

Skin Care

- Avoid using soaps and bubble baths with fragrances. Chemicals in these items often irritate the skin. Itching and rashes may occur. Make sure to completely rinse the skin with clean water after washing.
- Avoid using laundry detergents or fabric softeners with fragrances. They also can irritate the skin. Use dye-free products instead.
- Use a lotion after bathing to keep the skin moist. Avoid using lotions with perfumes or alcohol. Use a lotion high in petroleum, such as Aquaphor™** to prevent dry skin.
- Check the skin regularly for any rashes or sores. A good time to do this is during bath time. Talk to your healthcare team about any concerns.

Brand Name and Medicine Disclaimer: *Brand names and types of medicines are provided as examples only. Their inclusion does not mean that these products are endorsed by the U.S. Department of Veterans Affairs (VA) or any other government agency. Also, if a particular brand name is not mentioned, this does not mean or imply that the product is unsatisfactory.*

IS YOUR LOVED ONE AT RISK FOR PRESSURE SORES?

Being confined to a bed or a wheelchair raises the risk of pressure sores. Pressure sores happen when "pressure" to parts of the body decreases the blood flow. This can occur from laying or sitting too long. The most common areas for pressure sores are boney areas. These include heels, elbows, hips, and tailbone.

To prevent pressure sores:
- Change position at least every two hours. Use a lifting sheet to move your loved one. This will keep the skin from being dragged across the bedsheets.

- Change bed sheets daily or more often to keep your loved one clean and dry. Skin that sits in urine or sweat is more likely to develop a sore.
- Keep bed sheets pulled flat. Wrinkles in sheets can rub skin and cause pressure sores.
- Place pillows or pads between the knees and under elbows and ankles.
- If possible, get your loved one up and moving. This will increase blood flow and lower the chance of pressure sores.

REMEMBER
- Be supportive and listen. Your loved one may be ashamed to accept help.
- Let your loved one do as much as possible.
- Use assistive devices to make personal care easier and safer.

Section 37.2 | Recommendations for Nutrition and Exercise during Stroke Recovery

This section includes text excerpted from "Healthy Eating," U.S. Department of Veterans Affairs (VA), January 5, 2012. Reviewed May 2020.

Good nutrition or healthy eating is a key to stroke recovery. Healthy eating can help to keep your loved one's blood pressure, blood sugar, and weight under control. Healthy eating may even help prevent another stroke.

WHAT DO YOU NEED TO KNOW?
Grains
Include grains in your loved one's diet every day. Grains have fiber, vitamins, and minerals. Fiber lowers the chance of having another stroke. Wheat, rice, oats, and barley are common grains. Whole

grains are best. Whole grain cereals, brown rice, whole-wheat pasta, and whole wheat breads are good choices. Make at least half of your grains "whole" grains.

Vegetables

Vegetables are another good source of fiber, vitamins, and minerals. Choose dark green, leafy vegetables such as spinach, broccoli, and collard greens. The darker the leaves, the more healthy the vegetable. Orange vegetables, such as sweet potatoes and carrots are good choices too. Vary your vegetables. Make half of your plate fruits and vegetables.

Fruits

Fruits are also good sources of fiber, vitamins, and minerals. Choose different fresh, dried, canned, or frozen fruits. It is best to choose whole fruits rather than juices. Juices have more sugar and less fiber than whole fruits.

Milk, Yogurt, and Cheese

Dairy products contain calcium and vitamin D. They help keep bones strong. Switch to low-fat (1%) or fat-free milk (skim) products. If your loved one cannot have milk products, there are other choices. For instance, some cereals and juices are fortified or have extra calcium and vitamin D. Mackerel, salmon, and sardines are high in calcium and vitamin D. Lactose-free products or calcium supplements can also be taken in place of milk products.

Meats, Beans, and Other Protein Sources

Proteins are found in meat, fish, beans, eggs, and nuts. Proteins help with muscle, bone, and skin health. Pinto beans, kidney beans, chickpeas, and split peas are also high in protein. It is important to limit red meat, which is high in saturated fat. Fish and poultry are better choices. Eat at least eight ounces of cooked seafood per week. Avoid processed foods, as they have a lot of salt. Too much salt can raise blood pressure. Stay away from frying. Instead, boil, bake, or grill meats. Be sure to remove the skin and extra fat before cooking.

Fats, Oils, and Sweets

A healthy diet includes some fats. The key is to choose healthy fats. Vegetable fats such as olive, corn, and soybean oils are better for the heart than animal fats, such as butter and lard. Trans fats are human-made fats. Trans fats are unhealthy and increase the chances of heart attacks and strokes. Trans fats are found in baked goods and some restaurant food. Soft, low-fat tub margarine is better to use than stick margarine. Snacking on nuts is a healthy choice. Encourage your loved one to decrease sweets and high-fat foods. For example, limit added fats to the size of the top of a thumb.

WHY SHOULD YOUR LOVED ONE DRINK PLENTY OF LIQUIDS?

Drinking liquids helps prevent constipation (trouble having a bowel movement). Drinking water is one of the best ways to get the right amount of liquids. To improve flavor, add a lemon or lime slice. Drink water instead of sugary drinks. Unsweetened tea, low-fat or fat-free milk, and 100 percent fruit juice are good choices, too. Liquids are also found in foods, such as fruits and vegetables.

WHAT ABOUT SALT?

Too much salt can raise your loved one's blood pressure. Cut back on salty snacks and processed food. Remember that your loved one should have only 2/3 of a teaspoon of table salt each day. This includes everything your loved one eats or drinks, not just what is added when cooking or eating. Remember that canned foods and many canned soups have added salt. Compare the sodium content and choose the foods with lower numbers.

Helpful Tips

- Cook several extra meals at one time. Date and freeze the extra meals to eat later.

- Read the food labels or "nutrition facts" on packaged or processed foods. Many of these products are high in fat and salt.
- Add more salads, vegetables, and fruits to your loved one's diet.
- Season foods with lemon juice, herbs, and spices instead of salt or butter.

DOES YOUR LOVED ONE HAVE PROBLEMS EATING?
Dysphagia

After a stroke, some survivors have dysphagia or trouble swallowing. This makes eating difficult. The healthcare team will perform tests to find the cause of the problem. Most people recover from dysphagia in a short time. Sometimes surgery or medicine is needed. Speech pathologists are helpful in improving eating problems from dysphagia. Exercises to strengthen the muscles used for eating are often helpful. Your loved one may be taught to eat in a special way. For example, sometimes turning the head to the side while eating helps. Adding special thickening to drinks is helpful for some people who have problems swallowing liquid. Other tips are to sit up straight and to slowly eat and drink. Suggest that your loved one take small sips of liquids and small bites of food. If it is unsafe for your loved one to swallow anything by mouth, a tube for feeding may be needed.

Decreased Appetite

Your loved one may feel less hungry after a stroke. Speak to your healthcare team to see if medicines are to blame. Try giving your loved one smaller meals throughout the day. If possible, have someone eat with your loved one. Talk with a dietitian (nutritionist) about other tips to improve your loved one's appetite.

Change in Taste

The stroke may have changed your loved one's sense of taste. This can also be caused by some medicines. To help, serve foods with strong flavors. Use spices and herbs to add flavor.

Remember

- Plan meals to include poultry (chicken), fish, beans, fruits, vegetables, and whole grains. Drink low-fat or fat-free milk.
- Bake, grill, or broil foods, rather than frying foods.
- Use only 2/3 of a teaspoon of salt each day in all foods and drinks.
- Encourage your loved one to drink plenty of liquids.

Section 37.3 | Recommendations for Exercise during Stroke Recovery

This section includes text excerpted from "Exercise after Stroke," U.S. Department of Veterans Affairs (VA), January 5, 2011. Reviewed May 2020.

PHYSICAL ACTIVITY

Physical activity or exercise can be any activity that gets the body moving. This includes things, such as walking and dancing. It can even include household chores, such as sweeping.

Why Is It Important?

Exercise is good for both the mind and body. It can help your loved one get back strength that was lost due to stroke. It can make muscles more flexible. This will help improve how your loved one moves.

Physical exercise is important in reducing the risk of your loved one having another stroke. Stroke guidelines suggest that the survivor gets 20 to 60 minutes of aerobic exercise three to seven days per week. To make it easier, the exercise can be broken into smaller times. Walking for 10 to 15 minutes several times a day is a good way to get aerobic exercise.

Physical Benefits of Exercise

- Improves energy level

- Makes bones and muscles stronger
- Lowers blood pressure
- Helps improve sleep
- Improves flexibility
- Reduces risk of falls
- Lowers chance of another stroke

Mental Benefits of Exercise
- Reduces stress
- Lowers feelings of depression and anxiety
- Improves self-worth
- Promotes independence

WHAT DO YOU NEED TO KNOW?
Stroke can reduce your loved one's ability to exercise. If they are depressed, the motivation to exercise may be lowered. With decreased physical activity, muscles become weaker. The chances of another stroke or other health problem will increase.

It is important for your loved one to get regular exercise. Most survivors are able to do some form of exercise after their stroke. The type of exercise your loved one can do depends on the disability. The key is to stay as physically active as possible. Talk to your healthcare team before your loved one starts an exercise program.

WHAT ARE THE DIFFERENT TYPES OF EXERCISE?
Aerobic Exercise
- Includes walking, dancing, or riding a bike
- Helps to lower blood pressure and maintain a healthy body weight
- Low-impact exercises, such as swimming help protect the joints

Do 30 minutes of moderate exercise 5 days a week or 20 minutes of intense exercise three days a week.

Strengthening Exercise
- Includes conditioning exercises, such as sit-ups and push-ups
- Includes using balance balls and weights
- Helps to make muscles stronger

Do muscle strengthening exercises at least two times a week.

Flexibility Exercise
- Includes stretching and yoga
- Helps to keep joints flexible
- Lowers chance of injury

Do exercises that increase flexibility at least two times a week.
RED FLAG: Signs to Stop Exercising
Stop exercising right away and contact your healthcare team if your loved one:
- Feels dizzy
- Has trouble breathing
- Has pain (especially chest pain)

HOW DO YOU GET YOUR LOVED ONE TO EXERCISE?
- Help your loved one choose activities they enjoy doing. Walking the dog or gardening can be a fun way to get exercise.
- Join in on the exercise. You can improve your health together.
- Be a cheerleader for your loved one. Even small progress deserves praise.
- Keep an activity journal. Seeing the progress made can help motivate your loved one to continue.
- Look into adaptive recreation if your loved one has a disability. Adaptive recreation allows people with disabilities to get involved in sports or other fitness activities. The Adaptive Resource Information Center can help you find activities in your area.

Helpful Tips
- Have your loved one start slowly. Do not overdo it.
- Remember to have them warm-up and cool down when exercising.
- Make sure your loved one drinks plenty of water before, during, and after exercise.

Remember
- Exercise is important in reducing the risk of your loved one having another stroke. It is good for both the mind and body.
- Talk to your healthcare team before your loved one starts exercising.
- Exercise with your loved one and improve your health too.

Section 37.4 | Return to Work

This section includes text excerpted from "VA/DoD Clinical Practice Guideline for the Management of Stroke Rehabilitation," U.S. Department of Veterans Affairs (VA), July 2019.

INTERVENTIONS REGARDING RETURN TO WORK

Work has long been thought to be beneficial to the overall psychological well-being of individuals who have experienced a stroke and return to work is a frequent goal. The best approach to achieving that goal, however, has been the focus of limited research. It is thought that there may be long-term improved cognitive status after stroke by returning to work.

Lack of vocational rehabilitation within existing stroke rehabilitation services highlights the urgent need for research to facilitate return to work for individuals who have experienced stroke. In general, there is a lack of evidence examining effectiveness of interventions, including vocational rehabilitation services, in improving the likelihood of returning to work. In addition, there are multiple barriers to the provision of services.

Vocational rehabilitation is not often a part of the inpatient or discharge process, and involvement by vocational rehabilitation in the interdisciplinary team is infrequent. Patients are rarely referred for assistance post discharge.

Section 37.5 | Driving: How to Get behind the Wheels Safely

This section includes text excerpted from "Drivewell Driving after You Have a Stroke," National Highway Traffic Safety Administration (NHTSA), February 23, 2015. Reviewed May 2020.

You have been a safe driver for years. For you, driving means freedom and control. As you get older, changes in your physical and mental health can affect how safely you drive.

Driving is a major concern after you have a stroke. A stroke is a "brain attack" that occurs when the blood flow to the brain is interrupted. A stroke makes brain cells die and damages the brain. Brain injury may change the way you do things, especially your ability to drive safely.

HOW CAN A STROKE AFFECT THE WAY YOU DRIVE?

At first, you may not realize all the effects of the stroke. So it is crucial that you talk with your family and work closely with your healthcare provider before you start driving again after you have a stroke. Below are some ways a stroke may affect the way you drive:

- You may not be able to speak, to think or see clearly, or to control your body.
- You may have temporary or permanent weakness, or paralysis on one side of your body.
- You may be forgetful, careless, or irritable.
- You may get frustrated easily and be confused while driving.
- You may drift across lane markings, into other lanes.

CAN YOU STILL DRIVE AFTER A STROKE?

You may be able to drive after a stroke. It depends on where the stroke took place in your brain and how much damage it caused. Many people recover after a stroke and are able to drive safely. But, many others will have some type of disability afterward. Your healthcare provider will tell you how the stroke affected you, and when and if you can drive. It is important to note that in many areas, it is dangerous and even illegal to drive after a stroke without your doctor's consent.

WHAT CAN YOU DO WHEN A STROKE AFFECTS YOUR DRIVING SAFETY?

You may not realize how a stroke has changed your ability to drive safely. After initial treatment, your healthcare provider can tell you about warning signs and symptoms of stroke. Warning signs tend to come on suddenly and may include:

- Numbness or weakness of the face, arm, or leg, especially on one side of the body
- Confusion, trouble speaking, or understanding
- Trouble seeing in one or both eyes
- Trouble walking, dizziness, loss of balance, or coordination
- Severe headache with no known cause

Your healthcare provider can give you information about rehabilitation after the stroke. She or he also may suggest that you see a driver rehabilitation specialist to help you adjust to any changes caused by the stroke. A driver rehabilitation specialist can test how well you drive on and off the road. This specialist also may help you improve your driving skills by training you to use special equipment that can be fitted on your car to make it easier for you to drive safely.

To find a driver rehabilitation specialist, go to (www.aota.org/olderdriver.) Under "Driving and Community Mobility," click the button in the center of the page marked "Search for a Driver Rehabilitation Specialist." This will link you to a national database.

There you can search for names and addresses of local driver rehabilitation specialists.

WHAT CAN YOU DO IF YOU HAVE TO LIMIT OR STOP DRIVING?

With proper treatment and support, you may be able to drive safely after a stroke. Even if you have to limit or give up driving, you can stay active and do the things you like to do.

First, plan ahead. Talk with family and friends about how you can shift from driver to passenger. Below are some ways to get where you want to go and see the people you want to see:

- Rides with family and friends
- Taxis
- Shuttle buses or vans
- Public buses, trains, and subways
- Walking
- Paratransit services (special transportation services for people with disabilities; some offer door-to-door service)

Take someone with you. You may want to have a family member or friend go with you when you use public transportation or when you walk. Having someone with you can help you get where you want to go without confusion.

Find out about transportation services in your area. Many community-based volunteer programs offer free or low-cost transportation.

Section 37.6 | **Sex and Intimacy after Stroke**

This section includes text excerpted from "Sex after Stroke," U.S. Department of Veterans Affairs (VA), January 5, 2011. Reviewed May 2020.

A stroke can change how someone walks, talks, thinks, and feels. If that person is your spouse or partner, a stroke can also affect your sexual relationship.

After a stroke, sex may be difficult. It can be hard to talk about, but it is important. Talk to each other about your feelings. Seek help from your healthcare team, if needed.

WHAT ARE PHYSICAL REASONS WHY SEX MAY BE DIFFICULT?
Erectile Dysfunction
The male survivor may have trouble getting or keeping an erection. This may be a direct result of stroke. It may also be a result of poor health, stress, or depression. Erectile dysfunction (ED) can be treated in different ways. Lifestyle changes like stopping smoking and eating healthier may help. Medicines like Viagra®** can be prescribed. Talk to your healthcare team about treatment.

Vaginal Dryness
The female survivor may have vaginal dryness. She may take longer to become sexually excited. A vaginal lubricant like KY Jelly®** may help to make sex more comfortable. Be patient and take your time.

Immobility
Stroke may cause decreased movement in the arms and/or legs. The survivor may suffer from paralysis (lack of movement). There may also be weakness or spasticity (rigid muscles). To help, support the affected side with pillows during sex.

Incontinence
The survivor may be unable to hold urine or bowel movements after stroke. They may be afraid of having an accident during sex. Have your loved one use the bathroom before sexual activity.

Fatigue

Lack of energy and motivation can limit many activities, including sex. Rest and a healthy diet may help. Have your loved one conserve energy when possible. You may need to take on the more active role during sex.

Side Effects of Medicines

Some medicines may lessen sexual desire or activity. Medicines that treat high blood pressure and depression often cause sexual problems. Talk to your healthcare team about your concerns.

Brand Name and Medicine Disclaimer: *Brand names and types of medicines are provided as examples only. Their inclusion does not mean that these products are endorsed by the U.S. Department of Veterans Affairs (VA) or any other government agency. Also, if a particular brand name is not mentioned, this does not mean or imply that the product is unsatisfactory.*

HOW CAN CHANGES IN EMOTIONS AFFECT SEX?

Fear of another stroke—The survivor may worry that sex could cause another stroke. This is a common concern after a stroke. Sexual activity can begin again when the survivor is ready. Talk to your healthcare team about your concerns.

Decreased libido (desire for sex)—This is common after stroke. Changes in body image may cause low self-esteem. This can affect your loved one's desire for sex. It may take time for the survivor to feel attractive and desirable again. Be patient and supportive. Seek professional counseling if needed.

Depression (feeling blue)—Brain injury and changes after a stroke often lead to depression. Your loved one may feel sad or guilty about needing your help. Encourage your loved one to talk about their feelings. Talk with your healthcare team.

ARE YOU HAVING A HARD TIME ADJUSTING?

Depression can be treated. If you find you are having a hard time adjusting, it may be because of some of these changes:

Altered Appearance

Your partner's physical appearance may have changed. You may not feel the same sexual attraction. Give yourself time to adjust. Focus on the emotional connection you share.

Role Change

You may have difficulty shifting from giving physical care to being a lover. Make time to spend with your loved one to reconnect.

Depression

Caregiving can make you feel sad. It can decrease your desire for sex. Depression can be treated. Talk to your healthcare team.

WHAT TREATMENTS SHOULD YOU DISCUSS WITH YOUR HEALTHCARE TEAM?

If you are worried about your sexual relationship, you are not alone. Talk to your healthcare team about your concerns. Do not be afraid to seek couples counseling. Most stroke survivors are able to resume sexual activity with time. If sexual intercourse is not possible, remember that there are other sexual activities that you can enjoy.

HELPFUL TIPS

- Plan for sexual activity in advance. Allow for privacy and adequate time.
- Explore different positions to see what is most comfortable for both of you. Be creative and have fun.
- Take your time and enjoy each other's company.

REMEMBER

- Share your feelings with each other.
- Talk to your healthcare team. There are treatments and ways to improve your sexual relationship.
- Be patient and offer support.

Chapter 38 | Living at Home after Stroke

Chapter Contents

Section 38.1 | Independent Living with Assistive Technology

This section includes text excerpted from "Assistive Devices," U.S. Department of Veterans Affairs (VA), January 5, 2011. Reviewed May 2020.

After a stroke, a person may have trouble walking, talking, or moving around. Tasks, such as dressing oneself may be difficult. Assistive devices can help.

WHAT ARE ASSISTIVE DEVICES?

Assistive devices can help a person function better and be more independent. Assistive devices can make daily tasks easier. These devices may help ease the burden on you as a caregiver.

WHAT DO YOU NEED TO KNOW?

There are many different assistive devices to choose from. They can range from simple to complex. Focus on your loved one's needs to guide you. Schedule an appointment with a physical or occupational therapist to assess your loved one. Ask questions about what devices would be best. Be sure to include your loved one in the decisions.

WHAT ARE THE DIFFERENT TYPES OF INDEPENDENT LIVING AIDS?

Many devices are available to help with activities of daily living (ADLs). ADLs are the normal everyday tasks that people do. These include cooking, eating, and house cleaning. ADLs also include personal care tasks like bathing and using the bathroom. Examples of helpful devices are listed below.

Kitchen Aids Help with Cooking and Feeding Oneself
- Rocker knives for one-handed cutting
- Easy to grip silverware
- Jar openers
- Reaching tools

Bedroom Aids Make Moving around at Night Safer
- Bedside commodes
- Transfer boards
- Night light

Bathroom Aids Help with Bathing and Toileting
- Hand-held shower head
- Transfer bench for tub
- Shower chair
- Grab bars for toilet

Dressing Aids Make Dressing Oneself Easier
- Zipper pulls and Velcro®** tabs
- Elastic or nontie shoelaces
- Easy-to-pull sock and pantyhose aids

Grooming Aids Help with Personal Hygiene Needs
- Long-handled combs and brushes
- Electric toothbrushes
- No-rinse shampoo and body wash

Brand Name and Medicine Disclaimer: *Brand names and types of medicines are provided as examples only. Their inclusion does not mean that these products are endorsed by the U.S. Department of Veterans Affairs (VA) or any other government agency. Also, if a particular brand name is not mentioned, this does not mean or imply that the product is unsatisfactory.*

WHAT ARE THE DIFFERENT TYPES OF MOBILITY AIDS?
Mobility aids help with walking or moving from place to place. They can help prevent falls and improve independence.

Gait Belts and Lift Vests
- Make lifts and transfers safer
- Provide secure handhold for caregivers when walking is unstable

- Help caregiver balance survivor

Canes
- Decrease stress on the weak or affected leg
- Simple, but effective walking tools
- Widen the base of support
- Various types of canes are available

Crutches
- Provide support under the arm to take stress off the leg
- More stable than canes
- Various types of crutches are available

Walkers
- Offer additional support to make up for lost strength
- Provide maximum stability
- Should be sized to fit user
- Various types of walkers are available

WHAT ARE THE DIFFERENT TYPES OF WHEELCHAIRS?
Wheelchairs are designed to help those who can no longer walk safely. They come in many shapes, sizes, and varieties.

Manual Wheelchairs
- Depend on physical strength of the user or attendant
- Require arm or leg strength to move—unless there is someone to push
- Lightweight; easy to push and maneuver (dependent on weight of user)
- Less costly than motorized wheelchairs

Motorized or Electric Wheelchairs
- Powered by battery or electricity
- Less physical exertion is required

- No one needs to assist user
- Your loved one must be able to make decisions and maneuver safely

Scooters
- Work well for people who can get in and out of a chair
- Often less expensive than powered wheelchairs
- Easier to maneuver than a standard wheelchair

WHAT KINDS OF FINANCIAL HELP ARE AVAILABLE?
No one insurance or public program covers all the costs of assistive devices. Some coverage will depend on the state you live in. Some assistive devices can be replaced free of charge every three to five years. Check with your social worker. See below for where you can find help paying for devices.

Medicare—Benefits may include assistive devices, such as wheelchairs and scooters. Certain medical criteria must be met.

Medicaid—A program providing health coverage for lower income and disabled people. Benefits will vary by state.

Private insurance—Insurance policies vary. Most policies cover at least some of the cost of assistive devices. Check with your insurance company to find out what is covered.

Associations and foundations—Some associations and foundations will help pay for assistive devices.

WHERE CAN YOU BUY ASSISTIVE DEVICES?
Check your phone book for medical equipment and supply stores. Ask your physical or occupational therapist. There are also online healthcare product stores.

HELPFUL TIPS TO DECIDE WHICH ASSISTIVE DEVICES TO USE
- Think about what tasks your loved one needs and wants to do. Look for devices that would help with these tasks.

- Pick the simplest device to meet your loved one's needs. Complex devices are often harder to use.
- Ask your healthcare team for advice. An occupational therapist (OT) or physical therapist (PT) can guide your decisions.

REMEMBER
- Assistive devices can help your stroke survivor be more independent.
- Have your loved one evaluated by a physical or occupational therapist.

Section 38.2 | Preventing Falls

This section includes text excerpted from "Preventing Falls," U.S. Department of Veterans Affairs (VA), January 5, 2011. Reviewed May 2020.

Falls are common after a stroke. The good news is that you can help! There are ways to protect your loved one from falls.

WHAT ARE RISK FACTORS FOR FALLS?
- Past falls
- Trouble walking or getting up
- Balance problems
- Feeling weak and dizzy
- Problems with vision and hearing
- Side effects of medicines

WHY IS IT IMPORTANT TO GET HELP?
Falls can cause broken bones, head injuries, and even death. Ask your healthcare team for help. Your healthcare team can identify your loved one's risks for falling. Ask about a falls assessment. Occupational therapists can come to your home and help make

your house safer. Physical therapists can teach exercises to prevent falls.

RED FLAG: Signs of Trouble

If your loved one falls, get help if they:
- Pass out or lose consciousness
- Feel dizzy
- Have pain
- Have trouble walking
- Have a fever
- Have trouble breathing
- Are taking warfarin

HOW CAN YOU MAKE THE HOME SAFER TO PREVENT FALLS?
Keep Floors Clear

- Remove throw rugs or tape them down.
- Pick up shoes and other items from the floor.
- Push furniture far apart to create space to walk safely.
- Move cords out of the way to avoid tripping.

Make Stairs and Hallways Safer

- Install handrails on indoor and outdoor stairs.
- Fix broken steps.
- Make sure carpet is securely attached.
- Keep lighting bright, especially in stairways and doorways.

Keep the Bathroom Safe

- Put nonslip mats and grab bars in bathtubs and showers.
- Install a raised toilet seat.
- Use a plastic seat in the shower or tub.

Prevent Falls in the Bedroom

- Use nightlights in the bedroom to make walking at night safer.
- Place a commode beside the bed. Your loved one would not need to walk to the bathroom at night.

HOW CAN YOUR LOVED ONE CALL FOR HELP IN AN EMERGENCY?

It is important for your loved one to be able to call for help when they need it. Buy a medical alert system that your loved one can wear or carry. Ask your healthcare team about where to buy alert systems. Have your loved one carry a cell or portable phone at all times to call for help. Keep emergency phone numbers in large print beside every phone.

WHAT ARE OTHER WAYS TO PREVENT FALLS?
Exercise with Your Loved One

- Regular exercise lowers the chances of falling.
- Exercises that improve balance, such as tai chi, are helpful.
- Your local health or senior center may have exercise and walking programs.
- The Senior Planning Services has a fact sheet that shows you how to do exercises from home.

Keep an Eye on Medicines

- Ask a pharmacist, doctor, or nurse to review your loved one's medicines.
- Some medicines make people dizzy or sleepy and cause falls.
- Learn the side effects of over-the-counter and prescription medicines. warfarin (Coumadin®**) increases the risk of bleeding. This makes bruises and cuts more serious. Call your healthcare team if your loved one falls while taking warfarin**.
- Watch for side effects. Call your healthcare team with your concerns.

Have Your Loved One's Vision and Hearing Checked

- Good vision and hearing lower the chances of falling.
- Have your loved one's vision checked at least once a year.
- Change hearing aid batteries often.

379

Wear the Right Shoes
- Your loved one's shoes should have rubber soles and heels.
- Buy shoes with short laces or Velcro®** fasteners.
- Avoid slippers or wear nonskid slippers.

Use the Right Devices to Keep Steady
- A cane or walker can provide support.
- Ask your healthcare team about walking aids and how to use them.
- Lehigh Valley Hospital and Health Network has information on fitting yourself for a cane or walker. It also provides tips on how to use one safely.

Brand Name and Medicine Disclaimer: *Brand names and types of medicines are provided as examples only. Their inclusion does not mean that these products are endorsed by the U.S. Department of Veterans Affairs (VA) or any other government agency. Also, if a particular brand name is not mentioned, this does not mean or imply that the product is unsatisfactory.*

HELPFUL TIPS
- Teach your loved one to stand up slowly after sitting.
- After lying down, your loved one should sit on the side of the bed for a few minutes before standing.
- Watch for things that can cause falls when walking. Uneven sidewalks, door steps, liquid spills, ice, and pets can cause falls.

REMEMBER
- Make your home safer to prevent falls.
- Do balance exercises, such as tai chi. These types of exercises can lower the chances of falling.
- Have your loved one's vision and hearing checked regularly.
- Talk with your healthcare team about ways to prevent falls. Ask the team to review your loved one's medicines.

Section 38.3 | Ways to Make the Home Safer (Home Modification)

This section includes text excerpted from "Ways to Make the Home Safer," U.S. Department of Veterans Affairs (VA), January 5, 2011. Reviewed May 2020.

After a stroke, your loved one may fall or have trouble moving around. You can make changes to improve home safety. These types of changes are called "home modification."

WHAT DO YOU NEED TO KNOW?

Some changes are easy and you can do them yourself. For bigger changes, you may need professional help. The changes you make depend on the needs of your loved one.

WHAT CAN YOU DO?

Look around and find ways to make your home safe. Watch your loved one walk in the home to find areas that are unsafe.

Bathroom

- Buy nonslip bath mats, tub or shower benches, and toilet chairs.
- Install handrails beside the toilet and in the tub or shower.
- Install a hand-held shower head so your loved one can sit during a shower.

Kitchen

- Buy a stove with controls in the front. Your loved one will be able to reach the controls when cooking.
- Lower counters to make them easier to reach while sitting.
- Keep oven mitts and heat-proof mats close to the stove. Leave areas near the stove clear to place hot dishes.
- Place a fire extinguisher in easy reach.

Bedroom
- Put bed rails on the bed for safety.
- Place a commode beside the bed so your loved one would not need to walk to the bathroom. This can prevent falls at night.

WHAT CHANGES CAN BE MADE FOR STROKE SURVIVORS WHO USE WHEELCHAIRS?

Remove the cabinet under the stove or sink so your loved one can roll under. Use heat-proof covering (insulation) on pipes in roll-under sinks and stoves to prevent burns.

Stroke survivors may have trouble moving wheelchairs on heavy carpet. Use nonslip flooring if you remove the carpet. Widen doorways to help stroke survivors get in and out of the home. Outdoor and indoor ramps can also be built.

WHAT ARE SOME GENERAL HOME CHANGES?

Place pads on soft furniture to help with toileting accidents— Cover the pads so that other people will not notice.

Remove throw rugs—Use double-sided tape to hold down carpets.

Keep floors clear—Place large furniture far apart to help your loved one move around. Make sure furniture does not move if leaned on. Cover sharp corners of furniture.

Place handrails on both sides of stairs for safety—Elevators or lifts for the home can help stroke survivors who cannot climb stairs.

Replace door knobs and faucet knobs with lever handles— This will help stroke survivors who have trouble using their hands and arms.

WHAT ARE SOME OTHER SAFETY CHANGES?
- Place a phone in each room or give your loved one a cell phone to call for help. Large-button phones are helpful for people who have trouble seeing.
- A medical alert system that the stroke survivor can carry may help.

- Lighting should be bright (use high wattage light bulbs) to prevent falls. Install overhead lights or nightlights in doorways, hallways, and bathrooms.
- Install and regularly check smoke detectors and carbon monoxide detectors.
- Move all cords out of the way. Make sure cords are in good repair to prevent shock or fires.

HELPFUL TIPS
- If possible, have your loved one visit the home before the last day in the hospital. Some hospitals and rehabilitation centers will let patients take weekend trips to visit family. This will help you learn how to make the house safe before your loved one comes home.
- Occupational therapists, visiting nurses, and physical therapists can come to your house and help you make changes.
- Purchase items for home safety at medical equipment stores and through catalogs.

HOW CAN YOU PAY FOR HOME MODIFICATION?
Insurance and Medicaid
Some changes to the home may be covered by insurance. Talk to private insurance companies to see what can be covered. Medicaid may pay for some needed medical items.

Government Funding
Contact other government resources, such as the U.S. Department of Housing and Urban Development (HUD) and the Social Security Administration (SSA) to help with funding. You may also get information from the Eldercare Locator. Talk to the social worker at your hospital to find out more about all of these programs.

Private Funding
Nonprofit and volunteer groups may pay for some home changes. Contact groups like Rebuilding Together and NeighborWorks Network.

REMEMBER
- The needs of your loved one should determine the changes you make. The healthcare team can help you make the right changes.
- Home changes are often easy to make and you do not need a lot of money. Talk to a social worker if money is a problem. There are ways to obtain help in paying for home changes.
- Look around and keep checking your home for ways to make it safe.

Chapter 39 | Self-Care for Family Caregivers

Chapter Contents

Section 39.1 | How Can Caregivers Maintain Their Relationships

This section includes text excerpted from "Changes in Relationships," U.S. Department of Veterans Affairs (VA), January 5, 2011. Reviewed May 2020.

A stroke is a life-changing event. Your loved one may not be the same person as before. This could affect relationships with family and friends.

WHAT DO YOU NEED TO KNOW?

The changes in your loved one will affect the entire family. Tasks they once did may no longer be possible. You and other family members may be faced with new responsibilities. These could include housework, yard work, or managing money.

Some family members may not be able or willing to help. This is often difficult to accept. Some people have a harder time than others dealing with illness. Some may be overwhelmed with taking on new tasks. Try to forgive those who cannot help. With time, they may come around. Seek help from other family members and friends. Talk to your healthcare team about other resources in your area.

HOW DO ROLES CHANGE AFTER STROKE?

A person's "role" or place in the family helps define who they are. For example, a person's role could be that of parent or spouse. When a stroke happens, roles may no longer fit.

Spouse

Being the spouse or partner of a stroke survivor brings special hardships. The person who once was an equal partner may now rely heavily on you. You may begin to feel more like a parent than a husband or wife. Feelings of loneliness are common. Problems with sexual intimacy and financial concerns can also strain the relationship.

Parent and Child

An adult child caring for a parent brings its own challenges. It may seem that you are caring for or "parenting" your parents. The role reversal can be hard for both you and your loved one. Helping with personal care needs, such as bathing can cause anxiety and embarrassment. Another challenge can be learning how to balance caregiving with your own family responsibilities. However, keep in mind that caring for a parent can be one of the best experiences of your life. You will have the chance to grow closer and learn about one another.

- **Remember that your loved one is facing a lot of changes**—Try to understand how hard it is for her or him to accept your care.
- **Realize that your loved one will always be your parent**—It is important to treat your loved one as an adult. Be respectful.
- **Let your loved one make as many choices as possible**—Ask for your loved one's advice. Treat your loved one as an equal.
- **Be direct and firm if your loved one's health or safety is an issue**—Accept that you will make mistakes. Remember that the most important thing is to give love.

WHAT IS YOUR LOVED ONE'S NEW ROLE IN THE FAMILY?

Your loved one may be different physically, mentally, and emotionally. A lot may have changed. What has not changed is that your loved one is still part of the family. Even if your loved one cannot fulfill past roles, she or he can still contribute.

- **Find new roles and things that your loved one can do**—This will boost confidence.
- **Encourage your loved one to do as much as possible**—Help when you need to. But, avoid being too protective.
- **Be patient**—The stroke can make it hard to do simple tasks.
- **Help your loved one relearn skills in small steps**—Start with easy tasks. Slowly, add new skills.

- **Have a daily routine**—Allow short, frequent times in the day to practice skills.

HOW CAN STROKE CHANGE PERSONALITY?

Your loved one's personality may be different after a stroke. Strokes sometimes damage the area of the brain that affects thoughts and emotions. Stroke survivors are often demanding and self-centered. They may be sad and withdrawn. They may have bursts of crying. At other times, they may laugh for no reason.

Remember that the changes in your loved one are due to the stroke. Your loved one has no control over these behaviors. Keep in mind that these difficult behaviors often disappear over time. Accept that these personality changes affect how you feel towards your loved one. Talking to others or your healthcare team may help.

HOW CAN STROKE CHANGE COMMUNICATION?

Your loved one may have trouble listening, speaking, and understanding words. These communication problems affect relationships with family and friends. Get help from a speech therapist. Continue to talk with your loved one. Make your loved one feel part of the family.

WHAT IS THE EFFECT ON FAMILY RELATIONSHIPS?

The stress of caregiving can strain family relationships. Family members may need to sacrifice time and money to help with care. This can lead to feelings of anger and resentment. Arguments over care and money can cause misunderstandings and hurt feelings.

HELPFUL TIPS TO IMPROVE FAMILY RELATIONSHIPS

Hold family meetings—Come together to discuss concerns. Be open and honest about your feelings. Allow others to do the same.

Show appreciation—Caregiving can be a thankless job at times. Be sure to tell each other thank you. Everyone deserves to feel appreciated.

Work together—Include family members in decision making. They will be more likely to want to be involved in care.

WHAT IS THE EFFECT ON RELATIONSHIPS WITH FRIENDS?

Stroke recovery is a long and often slow process. After the crisis stage is over, people return to their own lives. Friends may not call or come by as often. Some may assume that you do not need to be bothered. Others may be afraid of how to interact with the stroke survivor.

Caregiving can be a lonely job. It is hard for anyone who is not going through it to understand. Friends may want to help but may not know how. Reach out to your friends. Tell your friends specific ways they can help. If your friends shy away, find others who can support you. Start by finding a support group for caregivers in your area.

REMEMBER

- Hold family meetings to discuss concerns. Be open and honest about your feelings. Allow others to do the same.
- Find new roles and tasks for your loved one. This will boost confidence and help her or him regain some independence.
- Reach out to family, friends, and others in the community. Talk to them about your specific needs.

Section 39.2 | Balancing Work and Caregiving

This section includes text excerpted from "Working Caregivers Finding a Balance," Administration for Community Living (ACL), August 16, 2019.

Two-thirds of caregivers in the United States work outside of the home. This creates a unique challenge for both working caregivers and their employers. Juggling caregiving and work-related responsibilities is not easy and some caregivers find it necessary to turn down job opportunities, quit their jobs, or take early retirement. Employers face the costs of replacing valuable employees. By working together, employees and employers can create a workplace environment that is productive and meets everyone's needs.

Below you will find information on how to cope with the stress and emotions related to caregiving and suggestions on how you can better balance caregiving and work responsibilities.

CAREGIVER STRESS

By developing some coping strategies, you may be able to avoid reaching the point of exhaustion and burnout. You are experiencing burnout if you become numb to your loved one's needs and feelings and you just don't care. Do not let it go that far; it may be difficult or impossible to recover.

- Remember you are not alone.
- Seek out resources that can assist you during this emotionally stressful time (books, organizations, web pages, and support groups).
- Find an Eldercare Specialist, a trained expert, who can help you find the services and support you need. Set a positive tone.

EDUCATE YOURSELF ABOUT THE DISEASE OR MEDICAL CONDITION

Whether you care for someone with heart disease, stroke, or dementia or whether care takes place in your own home or at a distance, many of the daily challenges are similar.

- Learn new information and skills and learn how to adapt to the challenges you encounter.
- Get up-to-date and accurate information through books, fact sheets, and brochures regarding your relative's condition.
- Contact the appropriate disease-related organization, that can guide you to other resources, such as hospital-based education programs and support groups.

CAREGIVER EMOTIONS

Providing care for someone you love who is no longer able to take care of herself or himself produces a wide range of emotions. It is natural to feel sadness and grief for your loved one's losses and for the loss of your own previous life. Over time, more emotions may surface.

You May Have Days When You Feel
- Angry and resentful
- Guilty and impatient
- Ashamed and lonely
- Sorry for yourself
- Fearful of the future

Some of these may shock you or seem "bad." These feelings are not self-centered or wicked. It is a normal response to the extreme changes that providing care can bring to your life.

As a caregiver, you donate a great deal of your time and energy to someone else's needs, and often ignore your own. When difficult emotions surface, remember that you have your own needs. Let your feelings prompt you to do something for yourself. Take a break: watch the birds, read a magazine, listen to a favorite song, or just meditate.

REACTION TO LOSS AND CHANGE

There are many losses as one deals with change. Recognizing these will help one address them.
- Guilt
- Sadness
- Anxiety
- Withdrawal
- Irritability
- Feeling overwhelmed
- Anger/frustration
- Feeling helpless
- Change in appetite

STEPS FOR COPING WITH LOSS

- **Talk about your feelings.** Reach out to others (friends, family, spiritual leaders)—this will help reduce feelings of isolation.
- **Join a support group.** Support groups provide caregivers with the opportunity to share with other caregivers and learn from one another.
- **Write your feelings down.** For people who enjoy writing, this can be a wonderful way to express feelings.
- **Read a book on coping with grief.** There are several books available on the issues of caregiving, grieving, and loss.
- **Get help when needed.** Professionals are available and a third party analyzing the situation can be a reliable ally. The Internet is another resource for finding help nationally and in your community. The U.S. Administration on Aging's (AoA) Eldercare Locator (800-677-1116) can connect you to services in your community.

WORKING AND CAREGIVING: FINDING THE BALANCE

- **Prioritize your time at home and at work.** Keeping a calendar of activities helps to identify priorities.
- **Learn to delegate.** Share your responsibilities with others. Do not be afraid to ask for help. It is not a sign of weakness.
- **Help your company** recognize your needs and the needs of other employed caregivers.
- **Keep communication channels open** with your supervisor or your Human Resource department.
- **Utilize your company's available resources.** Remember that businesses want and need to keep good workers. They want to provide support for their employees.
- **Use your vacation time** and make sure the time is spent nurturing you.
- **Make time for you.** Do what works for you. Spend time with friends, family members, or participate in a group.

Spend time alone. Plant a garden, go for long walks, read, take a hot aromatherapy bath. Do whatever it takes to nurture yourself. Always include doing things that are important to you.

Section 39.3 | Fulfilling Your Role as a Long-Distance Caregiver

This section contains text excerpted from the following sources: Text beginning with the heading "Who Is a Long-Distance Caregiver?" is excerpted from "Getting Started with Long-Distance Caregiving," National Institute on Aging (NIA), National Institutes of Health (NIH), May 2, 2017; Text beginning with heading "What Are the Special Challenges for the Long-Distance Caregiver?" is excerpted from "Rescue Fact Sheet—Long-Distance Caregiving," U.S. Department of Veterans Affairs (VA), January 5, 2011. Reviewed May 2020.

WHO IS A LONG-DISTANCE CAREGIVER?

Anyone, anywhere, can be a long-distance caregiver, no matter your gender, income, age, social status, or employment. If you are living an hour or more away from a person who needs your help, you are probably a long-distance caregiver. Anyone who is caring for an aging friend, relative, or parent from afar can be considered a long-distance caregiver.

WHAT CAN A CAREGIVER REALLY DO FROM AFAR?

Long-distance caregivers take on different roles. You may:
- Help with finances, money management, or bill paying
- Arrange for in-home care—hire professional caregivers or home health or nursing aides and help get needed durable medical equipment
- Locate care in an assisted living facility or nursing home (also known as a "skilled nursing facility")
- Provide emotional support and occasional respite care for a primary caregiver, the person who takes on most of the everyday caregiving responsibilities
- Serve as an information coordinator—research health problems or medicines, help navigate through a maze of new needs, and clarify insurance benefits and claims

- Keep family and friends updated and informed
- Create a plan and get paperwork in order in case of an emergency
- Evaluate the house and make sure it is safe for the older person's needs

Over time, as your family member's needs change, so will your role as long-distance caregiver.

First Steps for New Long-Distance Caregivers
To get started:
- Ask the primary caregiver, if there is one, and the care recipient how you can be most helpful.
- Talk to friends who are caregivers to see if they have suggestions about ways to help.
- Find out more about local resources that might be useful.
- Develop a good understanding of the person's health issues and other needs.
- Visit as often as you can; not only might you notice something that needs to be done and can be taken care of from a distance, but you can also relieve a primary caregiver for a short time.

Many of us do not automatically have a lot of caregiver skills. Information about training opportunities is available. Some local chapters of the American Red Cross might offer courses, as do some nonprofit organizations focused on caregiving. Medicare and Medicaid will sometimes pay for this training.

WHAT DO CAREGIVERS NEED TO KNOW ABOUT THEIR FAMILY MEMBER'S HEALTH?
Learn as much as you can about your family member's condition and any treatment. This can help you understand what is going on, anticipate the course of an illness, prevent crises, and assist in healthcare management. It can also make talking with the doctor easier.

Get written permission, as needed under the Health Insurance Portability and Accountability (HIPAA) Act Privacy Rule, to receive medical and financial information. To the extent possible, the family member with permission should be the one to talk with all healthcare providers. Try putting together a notebook, on paper or online, that includes all the vital information about medical care, social services, contact numbers, financial issues, and so on. Make copies for other caregivers, and keep it up-to-date.

MAKING THE MOST OUT OF VISITS WITH AGING PARENTS OR RELATIVES

Talk to the care recipient ahead of time and find out what she or he would like to do during your visit. Also check with the primary caregiver, if appropriate, to learn what she or he needs, such as handling some caregiving responsibilities while you are in town. This may help you set clear-cut and realistic goals for the visit. Decide on the priorities and leave other tasks to another visit.

Remember to actually spend time visiting with your family member. Try to make time to do things unrelated to being a caregiver such as watching a movie, playing a game, or taking a drive. Finding time to do something simple and relaxing can help everyone—it can be fun and build family memories. And, try to let outside distractions wait until you are home again.

HOW CAN YOU STAY CONNECTED WITH AN AGING PARENT OR RELATIVE FROM FAR AWAY?

Try to find people who live near your loved one and can provide a realistic view of what is going on. This may be your other parent. A social worker may be able to provide updates and help with making decisions. Many families schedule conference calls with doctors, the assisted living facility team, or nursing home staff so that several relatives can be in one conversation and get the same up-to-date information about health and progress.

Do not underestimate the value of a phone and e-mail contact list. It is a simple way to keep everyone updated on your parents' needs.

You may also want to give the person you care for a cell phone (and make sure she or he knows how to use it). Or, if your family member lives in a nursing home, consider having a private phone line installed in her or his room. Program telephone numbers of doctors, friends, family members, and yourself into the phone, and perhaps provide a list of the speed-dial numbers to keep with the phone. Such simple strategies can be a lifeline. But try to be prepared should you find yourself inundated with calls from your parents.

WHAT ARE THE SPECIAL CHALLENGES FOR THE LONG-DISTANCE CAREGIVER?

Living far away presents extra challenges in caregiving. Traveling to your loved one can be costly. It may be hard to take time off of work.

If you are not the primary caregiver, you face other challenges. Working with another caregiver involves good communication and understanding. You may not always see eye to eye. Remember that you both are trying to provide the best care. Listen to each other and be supportive.

WHAT ARE THE FIRST THINGS YOU SHOULD DO AS A LONG-DISTANCE CAREGIVER?

- Plan a visit to your loved one to assess the situation.
- Talk to your loved one about what she or he needs.
- Work closely with the local caregiver, if there is one. The local caregiver is the best judge of what is needed.

WHAT QUESTIONS SHOULD YOU ASK TO PLAN YOUR LOVED ONE'S CARE?

- What can your loved one (and the local caregiver) do without help from others?
- What specific help does your loved one need and want?
- How will services be paid for?
- How can you help?

HOW CAN YOU FIND SERVICES IN THE LOCAL AREA?

- **Use the telephone and Internet to find local services**—It can be difficult to find services when you are not familiar with the local area.
- **Contact the local Area Agency on Aging (AAA)**— They can assess your loved one's needs and eligibility for services. They can help you find local services. These include housekeeping, personal care, and other services.
- **Use a phone book from your loved one's area**—You can find one online. The Blue Pages list state and local services.
- **Find help in your community**—Check with the local church, Veterans' association, or community groups for support.
- **Talk to a geriatric care manager or care coordinator**—A geriatric care manager or care coordinator is a specialist in planning care for older people. The local AAA can help you find one. The National Association of Professional Geriatric Care Managers can also help.

WHAT CAN YOU DO LIVING FAR AWAY?

You cannot provide daily care. But, you can help in other ways.
- Arrange services and hire healthcare workers.
- Help with finances; you can pay bills online or through direct deposits or the mail service.
- Obtain information about insurance benefits.
- Learn all you can about your loved one's medical problems and treatments.
- Show your love by telephoning, and sending gifts and letters.

WHY IS IT IMPORTANT TO TALK WITH YOUR LOVED ONE AND LOCAL CAREGIVER OFTEN?

Your loved one's needs will change over time. Plan conference calls with your family, professionals, and other workers. A geriatric care manager can also keep tabs on how things are going.

WHAT IS THE FAMILY AND MEDICAL LEAVE ACT?

You can take leave for some family reasons. Check with your employer. The Family and Medical Leave Act (FMLA) requires some employers to allow up to 12 weeks of unpaid leave. Some states have laws that expand leave.

HELPFUL TIPS

- It is normal to feel guilty that you are not doing enough—Remind yourself that you are doing the best you can.
- Coordinate care from a distance—Keep a list of friends, local people, and agencies that can help.

REMEMBER

- Work as a team with your loved one and local caregiver to plan care.
- You can do many things as a long-distance caregiver. You can pay bills, find information, and offer support.
- Contact a social worker, a geriatric care manager, or look online to find help.

Section 39.4 | Caregiver Stress and Depression

This section includes text excerpted from "Caregiver Stress and Depression," U.S. Department of Veterans Affairs (VA), January 5, 2011. Reviewed May 2020.

Taking care of someone else can be stressful. Caregivers often sacrifice their own well-being to provide care for their loved ones. The stress of caregiving can cause headaches and chronic neck and back pain. It can affect thoughts and feelings, leading to depression. Caregiving stress can cause serious health problems.

Zarit Scale	Never (0)	Rarely (1)	Sometimes (2)	Quite Frequently (3)	Nearly Always (4)
1) Do you feel that because of the time you spend with the stroke survivor that you don't have enough time for yourself?					
2) Do you feel stressed between caring for the stroke survivor and trying to meet other responsibilities (work/family)?					
3) Do you feel strained when you are around the stroke survivor?					
4) Do you feel uncertain about what to do about the stroke survivor?					
Total Score:					

Figure 39.1. Applied Psychological Measurement

WHAT DO YOU NEED TO KNOW ABOUT CAREGIVER STRESS AND DEPRESSION?

You may have feelings of anger, guilt, and sadness. You may worry that you are not doing the right things. You may feel lonely and resent your new role. These are feelings that most caregivers have from time to time. Pay attention to how caregiving is affecting you. Talk to your healthcare team about your negative feelings.

DO YOU FEEL STRESSED?

Answer the questions on the Zarit scale to find out your stress level. A score of eight or above shows a high level of stress. Talk to your healthcare team about ways to reduce stress.

WHY IS IT IMPORTANT TO GET HELP?

The stress of caregiving may be overwhelming and affect the care you give. Taking care of yourself will make you a better caregiver. Get help from your healthcare team. Proper treatments help most people.

DEPRESSION AND CAREGIVING

Caregivers suffer from depression twice as often as noncaregivers. Depression is not a sign of personal weakness. Depression cannot be wished away.

HOW DO YOU KNOW IF YOU ARE DEPRESSED?

The signs and symptoms of depression vary from person-to-person. Without treatment, symptoms of depression can last for weeks, months, or years. Here is a list of the signs and symptoms of depression. If you have any of these signs for more than two weeks, talk to your healthcare team.

- Sadness or an "empty" mood
- Feeling guilty, worthless, or helpless
- Problems concentrating, remembering, or making decisions
- Change in eating habits and/or weight changes
- Feeling hopeless
- Lack of energy or feeling tired and "slowed down"
- Problems with sleep such as trouble getting to sleep, staying asleep, or sleeping too much
- Easily angered or irritable
- Wanting to be alone or spending much time alone
- Loss of interest or pleasure in hobbies and activities, including sex, that were once enjoyed

WHAT TREATMENTS SHOULD YOU DISCUSS WITH YOUR HEALTHCARE TEAM?

Ignoring the stress of caregiving is the number one cause of caregiver burn-out. Be honest with yourself about what you are feeling. Do not pretend that everything is okay. Proper treatment helps most people with depression. Ask your healthcare team about the best treatment for you.

- Medicines, such as anti-depressants are almost always helpful.
- Psychotherapy (talk therapy) is used along with medicines. Talk therapy gives you a safe place to talk about your feelings.
- Support groups provide a place to share your feelings with other caregivers.
- Other caregivers understand what you are going through. They can help you find solutions to your problems.

HOW CAN YOU TAKE BETTER CARE OF YOURSELF?
Taking care of yourself will make you a better caregiver.
- **Put taking care of yourself at the top of your list**—Have regular medical checkups. Eat right and exercise.
- **Ask for help**—Take on only what you can manage. Do not try to do everything by yourself. Be prepared with a mental list of ways other people can help.
- **Find time for yourself**—You need breaks from caregiving. Do things you enjoy. Go for walks or visit your friends. Take yoga or relaxation classes. Get a massage. Treat yourself to special outings on a regular basis.
- **Laugh and have fun**—Joke with your loved one. Laugh out loud. Read a funny book. Watch a funny movie or a comedy on TV.

HELPFUL TIPS
- **Accept your feelings**—Feelings of anger and sadness are normal from time to time. Be patient with yourself.
- **Remember that caregiving has rewards**—About half of all caregivers report positive feelings about caregiving. Caregiving often leads to stronger relationships with loved ones. Many stroke survivors do not show their true feelings. But, know that your loved one needs and appreciates your care.
- **Do not take things personally**—Your loved one may say or do hurtful things. Remember that these behaviors are due to their illness.
- **Practice getting rid of negative thoughts**—Replace negative thoughts with positive thinking or memories. Practice this every day. Focus on the things you can do. Relax about those things that you cannot. Forget and forgive your mistakes. We all make them.
- **Get information**—Learn about strokes. Learn about resources and ways to provide good care. This will help you plan for the future.

REMEMBER
- Take care of your health. You will be a better caregiver.
- Ask for help. Prepare a list of ways others can help.
- Depression cannot be wished away. It is not a sign of weakness.
- Proper treatment helps most people with stress and depression. Talk with your healthcare team.

Section 39.5 | Spirituality in Caregiving

This section contains text excerpted from the following sources: Text beginning with the heading "What You Need to Know about Caregiver Spirituality and Health?" is excerpted from "Caregiver Spirituality and Health," U.S. Department of Veterans Affairs (VA), January 17, 2012. Reviewed May 2020; Text beginning with the heading "Caregivers" is excerpted from "Caregivers Who Work Outside of the Home," U.S. Department of Veterans Affairs (VA), January 5, 2011. Reviewed May 2020.

WHAT YOU NEED TO KNOW ABOUT CAREGIVER SPIRITUALITY AND HEALTH?
Caregivers often sacrifice their own well-being to provide care for others. This sacrifice can disrupt your beliefs and cause spiritual distress. Symptoms of spiritual distress include:
- Loss of purpose or meaning
- Questioning your faith, values, and beliefs
- Feeling abandoned or punished by God
- Feeling worthless, hopeless, and alone in the world
- Withdrawal from family and friends

WHY IS SPIRITUALITY IMPORTANT TO YOUR HEALTH?
There seems to be a connection between the mind, body, and spirit. When you have spiritual distress, your entire being is affected. While physical health is easy to measure, spiritual health is not. Being healthy spiritually means showing love to yourself and others. You have a sense of inner peace and contentment. You value life and are thankful for what you have. Being spiritually healthy can help you cope with the stress of being a caregiver.

WHAT TO DISCUSS WITH HEALTHCARE TEAM

Talk to your healthcare provider if you are feeling spiritual distress. Your provider can refer you to a local clergyman or spiritual advisor. If you attend a house of worship, speak to your pastor or priest. Ask your healthcare provider about support groups in your area.

Helpful Tips

Think about what nourishes your spirit and makes you feel at peace. Set aside time each day to practice these things. This may include:

- **Practicing prayer or meditation.** Some people find prayer or meditation to be helpful. Benefits include lower stress and better overall health.
- **Volunteering in the community.** Helping others can put your problems into perspective. It can also provide you with a sense of purpose and pride.
- **Read the Bible or other inspirational books.** Some people find comfort in God's word. Reading about other's triumphs over adversity can inspire you.
- **Attend a house of worship.** Some people find a sense of community when surrounded by others who share their beliefs.
- **Go on a nature walk.** Connecting with nature can bring spiritual peace.
- **Keep a journal to express your thoughts and feelings.** Writing down your problems can help you sort them out.

Remember

- Strengthening your spiritual side can help you cope with the stress of caregiving.
- There seems to be a connection between the mind, body, and spirit. When you have spiritual distress, other areas of your body and mind are affected.
- Think about what nourishes your spirit and makes you feel at peace. Set aside time every day to practice these things.

CAREGIVERS

Most working caregivers have little time to relax. They often give up hobbies and social activities to care for their loved one. There are ways to balance the demands of home life and work. Caregivers work for many reasons. You may work out of need to support your family. You may work for enjoyment or to build a career. No matter why you work, there are ways to lessen your stress.

WHAT DO YOU NEED TO KNOW?

- Talk with your boss about your caregiving responsibilities. Explain that you want to do a good job at work.
- Ask if the Family and Medical Leave Act applies to your workplace. Some workers may take unpaid leave to care for loved ones.
- Ask if your employer offers insurance benefits and other benefits to help you care for your loved one.
- Talk to your boss about flexible work schedules. Tasks in some jobs can be done from home. Consider working fewer hours. Think about sharing a job with another employee.

HOW CAN YOU FIND HELP?

- Ask your employer or local Area Agency on Aging (AAA) about the National Family Caregiver Support Program's (NFCSP) benefits and services in your state.
- Use respite care and adult day services.

Helpful Tips

- **Make time for yourself**—You will be a better caregiver if you do things you enjoy.
- **Set priorities**—Decide what things are most important. Say "no" to those of less importance.
- **Accept that you cannot do everything**—Do not feel guilty about working. Get help from others. Make a schedule for family, friends, and community helpers.

- **Have a "back up" plan**—Be prepared for other persons to provide care in emergencies.
- **Find ways to make your life easier**—Hire someone to do chores if you can afford it. Use organizing tools. A dry erase calendar can help track tasks and care.

Remember

- Be open with your boss. Ask about insurance benefits, leave time, and flexible work hours.
- Find ways to make your life easier. Ask for help from family and friends. Get services from volunteer and community agencies.
- Take care of yourself. Find time to relax and enjoy with your family and friends.

Chapter 40 | Respite Care and Stroke Support

Chapter Contents

Section 40.1 | Community Services

This section includes text excerpted from "Community Services," U.S. Department of Veterans Affairs (VA), January 5, 2011. Reviewed May 2020.

Caring for your stroke survivor can be a big task. Sometimes you need more help. There are many types of community agencies that provide services. These agencies may be for-profit or not-for-profit.

WHY ARE COMMUNITY SERVICES IMPORTANT?

Community services can help you provide better care. The services may help your loved one feel less dependent on you. They may allow your loved one to remain at home for a longer period of time.

WHAT DO YOU NEED TO KNOW?

Decide what services best meet you and your stroke survivor's needs. Talk with your loved one and family members. Plan for the services you will need in the future. Learn about the services in your community.

HOW CAN YOU FIND COMMUNITY SERVICES?

- Ask a social worker. Social workers at other hospitals and home health agencies can help.
- Look in your local telephone book for a "Guide to Human Services" or a similar title. Most have a section that lists community agencies.
- Call your local Area Agency on Aging (AAA).
- Contact other agencies, such as the United Way or Catholic Charities.
- Talk with other people, such as clergy or staff at your local senior center. The phone book will have the number for your local senior center.
- Contact a case manager or a geriatric care manager.

WHO ARE CASE MANAGERS AND GERIATRIC CARE MANAGERS?
Case Manager

A case manager can help you find the right services. A case manager visits your home and determines you and your loved one's needs. They will assess your loved one's eligibility for services. The case manager will link you to local services. The case manager will help find resources to pay for services. They will make sure the services you receive are good.

Your local Area Agency on Aging (AAA) can also help you find a case manager. Services from a case manager through the AAA may be free or at a reduced cost.

Geriatric Care Manager

Professional geriatric care managers provide case management services. These professionals are experts in finding services for older adults. They are paid for by the family or the stroke survivor.

WHAT SERVICES CAN YOU GET FOR YOUR LOVED ONE AT HOME?
Home Health Services

Home health services are provided by different types of healthcare workers. Nurses provide services, such as changing wound dressings and checking vital signs. Nursing care may include cleaning urinary catheters and giving tube feedings. Nurses may teach your loved one how to correctly take medicines. Nursing assistants may give baths or help with other personal care. Physical, occupational, and speech therapists may also provide home health services.

Your stroke survivor must have a medical need to receive these services. Medicare or other insurance may pay for services if they are ordered by a healthcare provider. Otherwise, the family or stroke survivor pays for the services.

Home Care Services

Home care services are nonmedical services. They include help with chores and personal care. Personal care is helped with bathing, eating, and other personal activities. Services may also include housekeeping, errands, and home repairs. Home helpers may prepare light meals. They also provide company for your loved one.

Meal Delivery Programs

Meal delivery programs are usually known as "meals-on-wheels." Workers, mainly volunteers, deliver meals to the home. A healthy, hot lunch is delivered with a cold meal for later in the day. Usually, the program delivers meals five days a week. There are special diets, such as diabetic and low salt diets. Your loved one may benefit from the personal contact of the person who delivers the meals. Also, some grocery stores deliver meals to the home.

Respite Care

Respite care can be provided at home. Workers come and stay with the stroke survivor. This gives the caregiver time to do activities outside the home. Some places, such as nursing homes, also have respite care.

WHAT SERVICES ARE AVAILABLE IN SETTINGS OUTSIDE OF THE HOME?
Adult Day Care

Adult day care is for people with health or memory problems. The services vary. Adult day care centers may offer personal care. Personal care can be helped with eating and personal hygiene. Day care centers may provide nursing care, such as taking blood pressures. These centers often provide meals, exercise, and social activities. Some centers offer occupational, speech, and physical therapies. Others have recreation activities such as arts, crafts, and music.

Day care can help you and your loved one. Your loved one can do fun activities. They can enjoy the company of other people. Day care can give you a break. It can help you keep working outside the home.

411

Senior Centers

Senior centers are places that often provide meals, and health and wellness programs. They may have recreation, arts, and social activities. They often have information about other community services.

Congregate Meal Programs

Congregate meal programs are offered in places, such as senior centers. Older people are served healthy meals. Your loved one can go there and meet other people.

WHAT ARE OTHER TYPES OF SERVICES?
Medical Alarm Systems

Medical alarm systems help seniors call for emergency help from their homes. With a simple push of a button, help is available 24 hours a day. These systems will give you peace of mind that your loved one is safe. Buy these systems at your pharmacy or check on the Internet.

Transportation Services

Transportation services take your loved one to medical appointments and other places. Local service clubs sometimes have transportation programs. They also may have volunteer drivers.

HELPFUL TIPS

- Begin planning services before your stroke survivor comes home. There may be waiting lists for services.
- Get references if using a home helper who is not employed by an agency.
- Contact a social worker or case manager about how to pay for services. Some services may be free. You may be able to pay a reduced cost for some services.

REMEMBER

- Community services can help both your loved one and you.

- You can choose from many different kinds of community services.
- Your local Area Agency on Aging is a good source of information for community services.

Section 40.2 | Getting Help from Family, Friends, and Community

This section includes text excerpted from "Getting Help from Family, Friends, and Community," U.S. Department of Veterans Affairs (VA), January 5, 2011. Reviewed May 2020.

Caregiving is a lot of work. Help is available. You are not alone in caring for your loved one. Your loved one is important and so are you. Family, friends, and community volunteers may want to help. You just need to ask.

WHAT DO YOU NEED TO KNOW?

Caregiving can be a full-time job. Make a list of what tasks you need and who you can ask. Here are ways others can help:
- Household chores such as cooking meals, washing the laundry, house-cleaning, house repair, and lawn care
- Other help such as transportation to medical visits, shopping and gathering information on services, and financial assistance
- Social visits. Remind others that your loved one enjoys friendly visits. During these visits, you can get a short break. Think about going shopping or having lunch with a friend.

WHY IS IT IMPORTANT TO GET HELP FROM FAMILY AND FRIENDS?

Family, friends, and community volunteers can help you give better care. This is important because:
- Sharing the work will help you keep your loved one at home.
- Getting support will help you take care of yourself.

- Everyone feels part of the family when they can help. Give them a chance.

Ask for the Help You Need

Ask your loved one how they feel about getting help from others. Your loved one has the right to be involved. Be sure your loved one is comfortable with the people who help. Be clear and ask for what you need. Tell each person who helps how the stroke affected your loved one.

HOW DO YOU FIND VOLUNTEERS IN THE COMMUNITY?

Contact your church, local community or senior center, or local Veterans organization. Also, contact these agencies and ask for local volunteers.
- A social worker in the local hospital
- Local Area Agency on Aging (AAA)
- The Family Care Navigator

HOW DO YOU PLAN FOR EMERGENCIES BEFORE YOU NEED HELP?

- Keep a list of phone numbers of people who can help.
- Plan who can help with different emergency needs. Who can take your loved one to the hospital? Who can pick up medicines late at night? Who could stay with your loved one during an illness?
- Prepare an emergency kit that has medicines, clothes, and special foods. Also, include a list of care instructions about your loved one.

HELPFUL TIPS

- Have a meeting with your family, friends, and volunteers. Work together to get the best help for your loved one.
- Realize that asking for help may be hard for you.
- Say "thank you" to each person who helps—it is the best reward.

- Screen people before hiring them. Check at least two references before hiring anyone who does not work for an agency.

REMEMBER
- Sharing the work will help you keep your loved one at home.
- Your well being is important, too. Ask for help. You will find that family, friends, and others want to help.

Section 40.3 | Stroke Support Groups

This section includes text excerpted from "Stroke Support Groups," U.S. Department of Veterans Affairs (VA), January 5, 2011. Reviewed May 2020.

Stroke support groups help survivors and families cope with life after stroke. Support group members share experiences and encourage one another.

WHY ARE THEY IMPORTANT?
Life after a stroke is often difficult. Talking to others who have been through stroke and recovery may help. Support groups focus on their strengths and successes. Some support groups invite guest speakers who are healthcare providers. Support groups are a good place to make friends.

They Can Help You and Your Loved One
- Solve problems and get tips on caregiving
- Find local resources
- Get information on ways to improve health
- Learn about strokes and recovery
- Try new things, such as bowling or taking a dance class

WHAT DO YOU NEED TO KNOW?

Stroke support groups are often run by hospitals, the stroke-related volunteer groups. Many groups include members trained to answer your questions. There are different types of stroke support groups. Some groups include people with other medical conditions. To some, this makes the group more interesting. There are also support groups for caregivers only. Groups meet at days and times convenient for members.

HOW DO YOU FIND A STROKE SUPPORT GROUP?

If you are looking for a stroke support group in your area, consider the following resources.

Other healthcare professionals such as nurses, psychologists, and physical therapists can help.

- Search the National Stroke Association's Stroke Group Registry.
- Call the American Stroke Association's "Warmline." It connects families with other stroke support groups.
- Check your local newspaper for announcements about stroke support groups.

HOW DO YOU FIND STROKE SUPPORT GROUPS ONLINE?

You may prefer an online support group. Online support groups are often helpful if you lack the time or cannot leave the house.

You can find online support groups through these websites:

- The Stroke Network (www.strokenetwork.org)
- The American Stroke Association (www.stroke.org)

HELPFUL TIPS

- You may have to visit several support groups to find the right one.
- Support groups do not take the place of medical care. Your healthcare provider knows what is best for you and your loved one.
- You can even start a stroke support group.

REMEMBER
- It is hard to adjust to the changes after stroke. Stroke support groups offer help and encouragement. They can help people get back into social activities.
- Different kinds of stroke support groups are available. Your loved one and you may go to a local group. You also may use an online group.
- Stroke support groups do not take the place of medical care.

Section 40.4 | Taking a Break from Caregiving (Respite Care)

This section includes text excerpted from "Taking a Break from Caregiving," U.S. Department of Veterans Affairs (VA), January 5, 2011. Reviewed May 2020.

Respite care lets you take a break from caregiving. It may be for a few hours or several days or weeks. Respite care may be provided in the home. Adult day care centers, assisted living centers and nursing homes may also provide respite care.

WHY IS RESPITE CARE IMPORTANT?
Respite care gives you a chance to take care of yourself. It allows you time to take a vacation, shop, or visit friends. Taking care of your own needs will help you be a better caregiver. It can help keep your loved one at home after a stroke.

WHAT DO YOU NEED TO KNOW?
First, include your loved one in planning for respite care— Decide together what help you need. Ask your loved one about having help from others. Would your loved one be comfortable for a short time staying in a care facility?

Include other family members in the planning—Give them information. Let everyone express their concerns. Give everyone a chance to help.

Make a plan for your loved one's future—Plan for emergencies before you need help.

Create a care team to help with your loved one's needs—The team may include professionals hired to help. Use volunteers, family, friends, neighbors, and church members.

WHERE CAN YOU GET HELP?

- Talk with the social worker at your local medical center. Each center has different types of respite care.
- Think about taking help from a geriatric care manager. Geriatric care managers are specialists who plan and manage care for older people. They can assess your loved one's needs. They can arrange for services. Some charge a fee. Contact the National Association of Professional Geriatric Care Managers.
- Clergy, staff in senior centers, and local organizations can help.
- Your local Area Agency on Aging can also help. Find your Area Agency on Aging through the Eldercare Locator.

HOW CAN YOU PAY FOR RESPITE CARE?

- Some private insurance companies pay for respite care.
- Medicare or Medicaid may pay for respite care.
- You may find other ways to pay for respite care where you live. Check with your local Area Agency on Aging.

HELPFUL TIPS

- Ask for and accept help. Accepting help can improve everyone's quality of life.
- Screen people before hiring them. Check at least two references before hiring anyone not from an agency.

REMEMBER

- Respite care can give you a much-needed break from caregiving.

Respite Care and Stroke Support

- Check with the social worker at your local medical center. A number of local and community resources are available.
- Plan for respite care before you need it.

Chapter 41 | Managing Financial and Legal Issues

Chapter Contents

Section 41.1 | Managing Finances

This section includes text excerpted from "Managing Your Loved One's Finances," U.S. Department of Veterans Affairs (VA), January 5, 2011. Reviewed May 2020.

After a stroke, your loved one may need help with managing finances. Handling money issues is often a difficult task for caregivers. Involve your loved one in financial decisions as much as possible. If your loved one cannot make decisions, you may need to take over.

HOW CAN YOU PLAN AHEAD?

Talk to your loved one about finances while they still can. Make sure you know your loved one's wishes. Here are steps for getting your loved one's financial affairs in order:

- Gather everything about income, expenses, property, investments, insurance, and savings.
- Keep your loved one's financial papers in one place. For example, you could set up a home file cabinet. If papers are in a safe deposit box, keep copies in the home file.
- Tell a person you trust where you put important papers. If you do not have someone you trust, ask a lawyer for help.

WHAT ARE THE WARNING SIGNS YOUR LOVED ONE IS HAVING TROUBLE WITH FINANCES?

- Unopened mail piling up and unpaid bills
- Mishandling money
- Calls from creditors
- Costly new purchases and hobbies
- Complaining about not having enough money
- Physically not able to go to the bank or pay bills

HOW DO YOU AVOID FRAUD AND SCAMS?

Help your loved one from becoming a victim of scams and fraud. These can include telemarketing, home repair, and get-rich-quick schemes. Check junk mail and telephone logs. Each state should have an agency that handles elder fraud cases. The Eldercare Locator can help you find your local Area Agency on Aging.

HOW DO YOU DECIDE ON WHICH FINANCIAL TASKS YOUR LOVED ONE NEEDS HELP?

It may be hard for your loved one to give up financial tasks. You can start slowly by helping to write checks for bills. You can deposit checks. Later you can set up automatic bill payments. For other tasks, you may need a professional. For example, a lawyer or accountant can help with the following:

- Budget planning
- Talking with creditors or lenders
- Filing taxes
- Managing investments

WHAT FINANCIAL ADVANCE PLANNING DO YOU NEED?

Below are ways to make sure your loved one's wishes are followed. It is best to contact an attorney to help set up these arrangements.

Durable Power of Attorney

A durable power of attorney (POA) gives someone the right to act for another person. This could include making financial or legal decisions. It could include writing checks to pay your loved one's bills. It stays in place if your loved one becomes unable to make decisions.

Living Trust

A living trust gives instructions about a person's estate. An estate includes a person's property and funds. The trust appoints someone to handle the estate when the person becomes unable. Trust instructions state how assets should be distributed at death. A trust can avoid the expense and delay of probate. Probate is when the courts say that a will is valid.

Will
A will states how a person wants assets distributed at death. A will lists who is in charge of a person's assets. A will can include other things, such as gifts or funeral wishes.

Guardianship
In a guardianship, the court appoints someone to make decisions when a person no longer can. The court also decides when a person cannot make decisions. The family may need this if other advance planning documents are not in place. This process can take some time.

Estate Planning
Estate planning is developing a plan for others to manage assets if a person dies or becomes incapable. Estate planning can include writing wills and naming beneficiaries. It can also include creating trusts and making funeral arrangements.

Joint Accounts
Joint accounts allow another person to handle someone's affairs. These can be checking, investment, or other accounts. Contact an attorney before setting up a joint account.

WHAT KINDS OF HELP ARE AVAILABLE?
Below are experts who may be helpful.

Financial Caregivers
Financial caregivers help with daily financial tasks. Tasks include paying bills or keeping records. Fees are reasonable, usually from $25 to $60 an hour. Contact the National Association of Professional Geriatric Care Managers (NAPGCM) or the American Association of Daily Money Managers (AADMM). You may also call your local Area Agency on Aging for a referral.

Elder Law Attorneys

Elder law attorneys help families interpret individual state laws. They help plan how wishes will be carried out. They help families understand financial choices. They provide advice about ways to keep financial assets secure. Look in your local phone book for elder law attorneys.

Bank Representatives

Bank representatives provide advice on ways to access your loved one's accounts to pay bills. They can help set up a joint checking account.

Accountants

Accountants prepare tax forms. They can help you organize your loved one's records.

Financial Advisors

Financial advisors provide advice about resources to pay for your loved one's care. Financial advisors know if you are eligible for caregiver tax benefits. Learn about paying for community services.

Fiduciaries

The fiduciaries are people who are given a position of trust to handle the funds of another person who is incapable.

HELPFUL TIPS

- Ask someone at your local VA medical center about forms and financial planning resources.
- Find out if your loved one's insurance offers finance management help.
- Get references before hiring someone to help with finances. From time to time, check hired assistants' work. Make sure they do an honest and responsible job.
- Review plans regularly and update documents when needed.

426

REMEMBER

- Plan ahead for managing your loved one's finances. Take care of financial matters while your loved one can think clearly.
- It is difficult to talk to your loved one about managing finances. Include them as much as possible in financial decisions and tasks.
- Gather and organize your loved one's financial information.
- Qualified experts can help you manage your loved one's finances.

Section 41.2 | Getting Help with Legal Matters

This section includes text excerpted from "Getting Help with Legal Matters," U.S. Department of Veterans Affairs (VA), January 5, 2011. Reviewed May 2020.

Everyone should have their legal matters in order. Your stroke survivor could lose the ability to make decisions. Careful planning will make sure your loved one's wishes are followed.

WHAT DO YOU NEED TO KNOW ABOUT LEGAL MATTERS?

Plan ahead. Talk to your stroke survivor about legal matters early. Your loved one must have mental capacity to sign legal documents. Mental capacity means they can understand and make decisions.

You may need legal advice on the following:
- Advance planning, such as a living will
- Public benefits
- Long-term care and other housing
- Abuse and neglect

WHERE CAN YOU FIND HELP WITH LEGAL MATTERS?

If possible, use an elder law attorney or attorney familiar with disability. Contact the National Academy of Elder Law Attorneys. Your local Area Agency on Aging (AAA) can refer you to an attorney. Some AAAs provide legal services for seniors. Find your local AAA on the Eldercare Locator.

Community legal aid agencies offer help at low or no cost. The bar association in your area can refer you to an attorney. First visits often include a small fee. Look in your local phone book to find these agencies.

WHAT LEGAL DOCUMENTS DO YOU NEED?

The documents below will protect your loved one's rights.

Durable Power of Attorney

The durable power of attorney (POA) gives someone the right to act for another person. This could include making financial or legal decisions. It could include writing checks to pay for bills. It stays in place if your loved one becomes unable to make decisions.

Durable Power of Attorney for Healthcare

The durable power of attorney for healthcare names a person to make healthcare decisions for someone who cannot. For example, the person could decide to continue or stop a feeding tube. The person is usually a family member or close friend. They may be called a "healthcare surrogate" or "healthcare proxy."

Health Insurance Portability and Accountability Act

The Health Insurance Portability and Accountability (HIPAA) Act provides privacy for a person's medical records. Your loved one should sign a HIPAA release. The release says who can see your loved one's medical records.

Living Will

A living will states in advance a person's wishes about medical care. Your loved one can say what medical treatments should be done. This may include a feeding tube or breathing machine.

The document often allows naming someone to make healthcare decisions.

Do Not Resuscitate Order
A do not resuscitate order (DNR) states not to revive a person who stops breathing.

Will
A will states how a person wants assets (property and belongings) distributed at death. A will lists who is in charge of a person's assets. A will can include other things, such as gifts or funeral wishes.

WHAT ARE SOME OTHER LEGAL MATTERS YOU SHOULD KNOW ABOUT?
Guardianship
In a guardianship, the court appoints someone to make decisions when a person no longer can. The court also decides when a person cannot make decisions. The family may need this if other advance planning documents are not in place. This process can take a long time.

Living Trust
A living trust gives instructions about a person's estate. An estate includes a person's property and funds. The trust appoints someone to handle the estate when the person becomes unable. Trust instructions state how assets should be distributed at death. A trust can avoid the expense and delay of probate. Probate is when the courts say that a will is valid.

Estate Planning
Estate planning is developing a plan for others to manage assets if a person dies or becomes unable. Estate planning can include writing wills and naming beneficiaries. A beneficiary is someone

429

who receives benefits or assets. Estate planning can include creating trusts and making funeral plans.

Joint Accounts

Joint accounts allow another person to handle someone's affairs. These can be checking, investment, or other accounts. Contact an attorney before setting up a joint account.

HELPFUL TIPS

- Educate yourself on legal matters.
- Keep important legal documents up-to-date. Review them often to make needed changes.
- Store your loved one's legal documents in a safe place. Tell someone you trust where you put these documents.

REMEMBER

- Take care of legal matters early. Discuss legal matters while your loved one is able to think clearly. Your loved one must be mentally capable to sign legal documents.
- Talk to an attorney. If possible, find an elder law attorney or attorney familiar with disability.

Section 41.3 | Paying for Community Services

This section includes text excerpted from "Paying for Community Services," U.S. Department of Veterans Affairs (VA), January 5, 2011. Reviewed May 2020.

Your loved one may need community services after a stroke. Examples are home health, household chores, or meals-on-wheels. It is common to need help paying for services.

COMMUNITY SERVICES

Some community services are free or have reduced rates. The government may pay for services. Getting financial help may relieve your stress.

430

WHAT KINDS OF FINANCIAL HELP ARE AVAILABLE?

Requirements for getting financial help vary for different programs. Some are based on age, disability, or income. Most Veterans' programs are based on service-related disabilities.

The Area Agency on Aging (AAA) has information on local, state, and federal programs. To find your local AAA, use the online Eldercare Locator.

- Some hospitals have home healthcare services programs. The patient usually qualifies for these services if the disability is service-related. If not service-related, other benefits may be available for Veterans with low incomes. Some states have special programs for Veterans.
- Other agencies may help you pay for services. For example, the United Way, your local Council on Aging, or Catholic Charities may help. Most phone books have sections listing community agencies. Look in the front for the "Guide to Human Services" or a similar title.

WHICH INSURANCE PROGRAMS HELP PAY FOR COMMUNITY SERVICES?

- Medicare may pay for nursing care or therapy at home. You will need a prescription from a healthcare provider. Medicare may pay for nonmedical services for patients getting home care. These services could include making meals and household chores.
- Medicaid helps low-income people who have few assets. It may pay for services, such as personal or home healthcare. Personal care is helped with tasks, such as bathing and dressing. Programs vary by state.
- Other kinds of insurance may pay for community services. For example, some long-term care and private insurance may pay for services. Check with your insurance company.

HELPFUL TIPS

- Plan ahead—Seek financial help before you need it. First talk to your loved one about her or his financial needs.

431

Ask questions about retirement, savings, insurance, and social security.
- Shop around—Interview several agencies before choosing one to provide services. Check out references.
- Ask for help—Ask for help from family, friends, community groups, or churches.

REMEMBER
- The Area Agency on Aging has information.
- Some insurance plans, such as Medicare and Medicaid, may pay for services.

Section 41.4 | Health Insurance Information for Stroke Patients

This section includes text excerpted from "Stroke Recovery—Medicare Can Help," Centers for Medicare & Medicaid Services (CMS), May 7, 2018.

Did you know that more than half a million people over 65 years of age suffer a stroke each year? If you are recovering from a stroke and suffering major side effects such as problems with hearing or vision, paralysis, balance problems, or difficulty walking or moving around in daily life, Medicare covers rehabilitation services to help you regain your normal functions.

Medicare covers medical and rehabilitation services while you are in a hospital or skilled nursing facility (SNF). It also helps pay for medically-necessary outpatient physical therapy and occupational therapy. If you need rehabilitation after a stroke, visit Inpatient Rehabilitation Facility Compare to find and compare rehabilitation facilities in your ZIP code. You can compare facilities based on quality of care, such as how often patients get infections or pressure ulcers.

There are certain risk factors that can increase your chances of having a recurring stroke such as smoking and drinking, high blood pressure, high cholesterol, diabetes, and bad eating habits.

Knowing your risk factors can help prevent a stroke from happening again. You can also prevent 80 percent of recurring strokes through lifestyle changes and medical interventions. Medicare covers these preventive services that can help you, and in most cases, you will pay nothing for these services:

- Cardiovascular disease screening (includes blood test screening for cholesterol)
- Cardiovascular disease (behavioral therapy)
- Alcohol misuse screening and counseling
- Diabetes screenings and self-management training
- Nutrition therapy services and obesity screening and counseling
- Smoking and tobacco use cessation counseling (to stop smoking or using tobacco products)
- Suffering a stroke can be scary, and for some, the recovery can be life changing. Having the resources you need to take control of your health can help you with your recovery and perhaps prevent another stroke.

Chapter 42 | End-of-Life Care after Stroke

Chapter Contents

Section 42.1 | Understanding End-of-Life Decisions

This section includes text excerpted from "Understanding Healthcare Decisions at the End of Life," National Institute on Aging (NIA), National Institutes of Health (NIH), May 17, 2017.

It can be overwhelming to be asked to make healthcare decisions for someone who is dying and is no longer able to make her or his own decisions. It is even more difficult if you do not have written or verbal guidance. How do you decide what type of care is right for someone? Even when you have written documents, some decisions still might not be clear since the documents may not address every situation you could face.

Two approaches might be useful. One is to put yourself in the place of the person who is dying and try to choose as she or he would. This is called "substituted judgment." Some experts believe that decisions should be based on substituted judgment whenever possible.

Another approach, known as "best interests," is to decide what would be best for the dying person. This is sometimes combined with substituted judgment.

If you are making decisions for someone at the end of life and are trying to use one of these approaches, it may be helpful to think about the following questions:

Has the dying person ever talked about what she or he would want at the end of life?

Has she or he expressed an opinion about how someone else was being treated?

What were her or his values in life? What gave meaning to life? Maybe it was being close to family—watching them grow and making memories together. Perhaps just being alive was the most important thing.

As a decision-maker without specific guidance from the dying person, you need as much information as possible on which to base your actions. You might ask the doctor:

- What you might expect to happen in the next few hours, days, or weeks if you continue your current course of treatment?

437

- Why is this new test being suggested?
- Will it change the current treatment plan?
- Will a new treatment help your relative get better?
- How would the new treatment change her or his quality of life (QOL)?
- Will it give more quality time with family and friends?
- How long will this treatment take to make a difference?
- If you choose to try this treatment, can you stop it at any time? For any reason?
- What are the side effects of the approach you are suggesting?
- If you try this new treatment and it does not work, what then?
- If you do not try this treatment, what will happen?
- Is the improvement you saw today an overall positive sign or just something temporary?

It is a good idea to have someone with you when discussing these issues with medical staff. Having someone take notes or remember details can be very helpful. If you are unclear about something you are told, do not be afraid to ask the doctor or nurse to repeat it or to say it another way that does make sense to you. Keep asking questions until you have all the information you need to make decisions. Make sure you know how to contact a member of the medical team if you have a question or if the dying person needs something.

Sometimes, the whole family wants to be involved in every decision. Maybe that is the family's cultural tradition. Or, maybe the person dying did not pick one person to make healthcare choices before becoming unable to do so. That is not unusual, but it makes sense to choose one person to be the contact when dealing with medical staff. The doctors and nurses will appreciate having to phone only one person.

Even if one family member is named as the decision-maker, it is a good idea, as much as possible, to have family agreement about the care plan. If you cannot agree on a care plan, a decision-maker, or even a spokesperson, the family might consider a mediator, someone trained to bring people with different opinions to a common decision.

In any case, as soon as it is clear that the patient is nearing the end of life, the family should try to discuss with the medical team which end-of-life care approach they want for their family member. That way, decision making for crucial situations can be planned and may feel less rushed.

COMMON END-OF-LIFE CONCERNS

Maybe you are now faced with making end-of-life choices for someone close to you. You have thought about that person's values and opinions, and you have asked the healthcare team to explain the treatment plan and what you can expect to happen.

But, there are other issues that are important to understand in case they arise. What if the dying person starts to have trouble breathing and a doctor says a ventilator might be needed? Maybe one family member wants the healthcare team to do everything possible to keep this relative alive. What does that involve? Or, what if family members cannot agree on end-of-life care or they disagree with the doctor? What happens then?

Here are some other common end-of-life issues. They will give you a general understanding and may help your conversations with the doctors.

If Someone Says "Do Everything Possible" When Someone Is Dying, What Does That Mean?

This means that if someone is dying, all measures that might keep vital organs working will be tried—for example, using a ventilator to support breathing or starting dialysis for failing kidneys. Such life support can sometimes be a temporary measure that allows the body to heal itself and begin to work normally again. It is not intended to be used indefinitely in someone who is dying.

What Can Be Done If Someone's Heart Stops Beating (Cardiac Arrest)?

Cardiopulmonary resuscitation (CPR) can sometimes restart a stopped heart. It is most effective in people who were generally healthy before their heart stopped. During CPR, the doctor

439

repeatedly pushes on the chest with great force and periodically puts air into the lungs. Electric shocks (called "defibrillation") may also be used to correct an abnormal heart rhythm, and some medicines might also be given. Although not usually shown on television, the force required for CPR can cause broken ribs or a collapsed lung. Often, CPR does not succeed in older adults who have multiple chronic illnesses or who are already frail.

What If Someone Needs Help Breathing or Has Completely Stopped Breathing (Respiratory Arrest)?

If a patient has very severe breathing problems or has stopped breathing, a ventilator may be needed. A ventilator forces the lungs to work. Initially, this involves intubation, putting a tube attached to a ventilator down the throat into the trachea or windpipe. Because this tube can be quite uncomfortable, people are often sedated with very strong intravenous medicines. Restraints may be used to prevent them from pulling out the tube. If the person needs ventilator support for more than a few days, the doctor might suggest a tracheotomy, sometimes called a "trach" (rhymes with "make"). This tube is then attached to the ventilator. This is more comfortable than a tube down the throat and may not require sedation. Inserting the tube into the trachea is a bedside surgery. A tracheotomy can carry risks, including a collapsed lung, a plugged tracheostomy tube, or bleeding.

How Can You Be Sure the Medical Staff Knows That the Patient Has a DNR (Do Not Resuscitate) Order?

Tell the doctor in charge as soon as the patient or person making healthcare decisions decides that CPR or other life-support procedures should not be performed. The doctor will then write this on the patient's chart using terms such as Do Not Resuscitate (DNR), Do Not Attempt to Resuscitate (DNAR), Allow Natural Death (AND), or Do Not Intubate (DNI). DNR forms vary by state and are usually available online.

If end-of-life care is given at home, a special nonhospital DNR, signed by a doctor, is needed. This ensures that if emergency medical technicians (EMTs) are called to the house, they will respect your wishes. Make sure it is kept in a prominent place so EMTs can see it. Without a nonhospital DNR, in many states EMTs are required to perform CPR and similar techniques. Hospice staff can help determine whether a medical condition is part of the normal dying process or something that needs the attention of EMTs.

DNR orders do not stop all treatment. They only mean that CPR and a ventilator will not be used. These orders are not permanent—they can be changed if the situation changes.

Should Pacemakers (or Similar Devices) Be Turned Off When Someone Is Dying?

A pacemaker is a device implanted under the skin on the chest that keeps a heartbeat regular. It will not keep a dying person alive. Some people have an implantable cardioverter-defibrillator (ICD) under the skin. An ICD shocks the heart back into regular rhythm when needed. The ICD should be turned off at the point when life support is no longer wanted. This can be done at the bedside without surgery.

What Does It Mean If the Doctor Suggests a Feeding Tube?

If a patient cannot or would not eat or drink, the doctor might suggest a feeding tube. While a patient recovers from an illness, getting nutrition temporarily through a feeding tube can be helpful. But, at the end of life, a feeding tube might cause more discomfort than not eating. For people with dementia, tube feeding does not prolong life or prevent aspiration.

As death approaches, loss of appetite is common. Body systems start shutting down, and fluids and food are not needed as before. Some experts believe that at this point few nutrients are absorbed from any type of nutrition, including those received through a feeding tube. Further, after a feeding tube is inserted, the family might need to make a difficult decision about when, or if, to remove it.

If tube feeding will be tried, there are two methods that could be used. In the first, a feeding tube, known as a "nasogastric" or "NG tube," is threaded through the nose down to the stomach to give nutrition for a short time. Sometimes, the tube is uncomfortable. Someone with an NG tube might try to remove it. This usually means the person has to be restrained, which could mean binding her or his hands to the bed.

If tube feeding is required for an extended time, then a gastric or G tube is put directly into the stomach through an opening made in the side or abdomen. This second method is sometimes called a "percutaneous endoscopic gastrostomy (PEG) tube." It carries risks of infection, pneumonia, and nausea.

Hand feeding (sometimes called "assisted oral feeding") is an alternative to tube feeding. This approach may have fewer risks, especially for people with dementia.

Should Someone Who Is Dying Be Sedated?

Sometimes, for patients very near the end of life, the doctor might suggest sedation to manage symptoms that are not responding to other treatments and are still making the patient uncomfortable. This means using medicines to put the patient in a sleep-like state. Many doctors suggest continuing to use comfort care measures like pain medicine even if the dying person is sedated. Sedatives can be stopped at any time. A person who is sedated may still be able to hear what you are saying—so try to keep speaking directly to, not about, her or him. Do not say things you would not want the patient to hear.

Are Antibiotics Helpful When Someone Is Dying?

Antibiotics are medicines that fight infections caused by bacteria. Lower respiratory infections (such as pneumonia) and urinary tract infections (UTIs) are often caused by bacteria and are common in older people who are dying. Many antibiotics have side effects, so the value of trying to treat an infection in a dying person should be weighed against any unpleasant side effects. If someone is already dying when the infection begins, giving antibiotics is probably not going to prevent death, but might make the person feel more comfortable.

Do Patients Have the Right to Refuse Treatment?

Choosing to stop treatment that is not curing or controlling an illness, or deciding not to start a new treatment, is completely legal—whether the choice is made by the person who is dying or by the person making healthcare decisions. Some people think this is like allowing death to happen. The law does not consider refusing such treatment to be either suicide or euthanasia, sometimes called "mercy killing."

What Happens If the Doctor and You Have Different Opinions about Care for Someone Who Is Dying

Sometimes medical staff, the patient, and family members disagree about a medical care decision. This can be especially problematic when the dying person cannot tell the doctors what kind of end-of-life care she or he wants. For example, the family might want more active treatment, such as chemotherapy, than the doctors think will be helpful. If there is an advance directive explaining the patient's preferences, those guidelines should determine care.

Without the guidance of an advance directive, if there is a disagreement about medical care, it may be necessary to get a second opinion from a different doctor or to consult the ethics committee or patient representative, also known as an "ombudsman," of the hospital or facility. Palliative care consultation may also be helpful. An arbitrator (mediator) can sometimes assist people with different views to agree on a plan.

The Doctor Does Not Seem Familiar with Your Family's Views about Dying. What Should You Do?

America is a rich melting pot of religions, races, and cultures. Ingrained in each tradition are expectations about what should happen as a life nears its end. It is important for everyone involved in a patient's care to understand how each family background may influence expectations, needs, and choices.

Your background may be different from that of the doctor with whom you are working. Or, you might be used to a different approach to making healthcare decisions at the end of life than

443

your medical team. For example, many healthcare providers look to a single person—the dying person or her or his chosen representative—for important healthcare decisions at the end of life. But, in some cultures, the entire immediate family takes on that role.

It is helpful to discuss your personal and family traditions with your doctors and nurses. If there are religious or cultural customs surrounding death that are important to you, make sure to tell your healthcare providers.

Knowing that these practices will be honored could comfort the dying person. Telling the medical staff ahead of time may also help avoid confusion and misunderstanding when death occurs. Make sure you understand how the available medical options presented by the healthcare team fit into your family's desires for end-of-life care.

COMMUNICATING WITH YOUR HEALTHCARE TEAM

Make sure the healthcare team knows what is important to your family surrounding the end of life. You might say:

In your religion, you . . . (then describe your religious traditions regarding death).

Where you come from . . . (tell what customs are important to you at the time of death).

In your family when someone is dying, you prefer . . . (describe what you hope to have happened).

Section 42.2 | Providing Care and Comfort at the End of Life

This section includes text excerpted from "Providing Care and Comfort at the End of Life," National Institute on Aging (NIA), National Institutes of Health (NIH), May 17, 2017.

Comfort care is an essential part of medical care at the end of life. It is care that helps or soothes a person who is dying. The goals are to prevent or relieve suffering as much as possible and to improve QOL while respecting the dying person's wishes.

You are probably reading this because someone close to you is dying. You wonder what will happen. You want to know how to give comfort, what to say, what to do. You might like to know how to make dying easier—how to help ensure a peaceful death, with treatment consistent with the dying person's wishes.

A peaceful death might mean something different to you than to someone else. Your sister might want to know when death is near so she can have a few last words with the people she loves and take care of personal matters. Your husband might want to die quickly and not linger. Perhaps your mother has said she would like to be at home when she dies, while your father wants to be in a hospital where he can receive treatment for his illness until the very end.

Some people want to be surrounded by family and friends; others want to be alone. Of course, often one does not get to choose. But, avoiding suffering, having your end-of-life wishes followed, and being treated with respect while dying are common hopes.

Generally speaking, people who are dying need care in four areas—physical comfort, mental and emotional needs, spiritual issues, and practical tasks. Their families need support as well. In this section, you will find a number of ways you can help someone who is dying. Always remember to check with the healthcare team to make sure these suggestions are appropriate for your situation.

WHAT IS END-OF-LIFE CARE?

At the end of life, each story is different. Death comes suddenly, or a person lingers, gradually fading. For some older people, the body weakens while the mind stays alert. Others remain physically strong, but cognitive losses take a huge toll. Although everyone dies, each loss is personally felt by those close to the one who has died.

End-of-life care is the term used to describe the support and medical care given during the time surrounding death. Such care does not happen only in the moments before breathing ceases and the heart stops beating. Older people often live with one or more chronic illnesses and need a lot of care for days, weeks, and even months before death.

445

When a doctor says something like, "I'm afraid the news is not good. There are no other treatments for you to try. I'm sorry," it may close the door to the possibility of a cure, but it does not end the need for medical support. Nor does it end the involvement of family and friends.

There are many ways to provide care for an older person who is dying. Such care often involves a team. If you are reading this, then you might be part of such a team.

Being a caregiver for someone at the end of life can be physically and emotionally exhausting. In the end, accept that there may be no perfect death, just the best you can do for the one you love. And, the pain of losing someone close to you may be softened a little because, when you were needed, you did what you could.

END OF LIFE: PROVIDING PHYSICAL COMFORT

There are ways to make a person who is dying more comfortable. Discomfort can come from a variety of problems. For each, there are things you or a healthcare provider can do, depending on the cause. For example, a dying person can be uncomfortable because of:

- Pain
- Breathing problems
- Skin irritation
- Digestive problems
- Temperature sensitivity
- Fatigue

Pain. Watching someone you love die is hard enough, but thinking that person is also in pain makes it worse. Not everyone who is dying experiences pain, but there are things you can do to help someone who does. Experts believe that care for someone who is dying should focus on relieving pain without worrying about possible long-term problems of drug dependence or abuse.

Do not be afraid of giving as much pain medicine as is prescribed by the doctor. Pain is easier to prevent than to relieve, and severe pain is hard to manage. Try to make sure that the level of pain does not get ahead of pain-relieving medicines. Tell the doctor or nurse if the pain is not controlled. Medicines can be increased or changed. If this does not help, then ask for consultation with a palliative medical specialist who has experience in pain management for seriously ill patients

Struggling with severe pain can be draining. It can make it hard for families to be together in a meaningful way. Pain can affect mood—being in pain can make someone seem angry or short-tempered. Although understandable, irritability resulting from pain might make it hard to talk, hard to share thoughts and feelings.

Breathing problems. Shortness of breath or the feeling that breathing is difficult is a common experience at the end of life. The doctor might call this dyspnea. Worrying about the next breath can make it hard for important conversations or connections. Try raising the head of the bed, opening a window, using a humidifier, or having a fan circulating air in the room. Sometimes, morphine or other pain medications can help relieve the sense of breathlessness.

People very near death might have noisy breathing, sometimes called a "death rattle." This is caused by fluids collecting in the throat or by the throat muscles relaxing. It might help to try turning the person to rest on one side. There is also medicine that can be prescribed that may help clear this up. Not all noisy breathing is a death rattle. It may help to know that this noisy breathing is usually not upsetting to the dying person, even if it is to family and friends.

Skin irritation. Skin problems can be very uncomfortable. With age, skin naturally becomes drier and more fragile, so it is important to take extra care with an older person's skin. Gently applying alcohol-free lotion can relieve dry skin and be soothing.

Dryness on parts of the face, such as the lips and eyes, can be a common cause of discomfort near death. A lip balm could keep this from getting worse. A damp cloth placed over closed eyes might relieve dryness. If the inside of the mouth seems dry, giving ice chips (if the person is conscious) or wiping the inside of the mouth with a damp cloth, cotton ball, or specially treated swab might help.

Sitting or lying in one position puts constant pressure on sensitive skin, which can lead to painful bed sores (sometimes called

447

"pressure ulcers"). When a bed sore first forms, the skin gets discolored or darker. Watch carefully for these discolored spots, especially on the heels, hips, lower back, and back of the head.

Turning the person from side to back and to the other side every few hours may help prevent bed sores. Try putting a foam pad under an area, such as a heel or elbow to raise it off the bed and reduce pressure. Ask if a special mattress or chair cushion might also help. Keeping the skin clean and moisturized is always important.

Digestive problems. Nausea, vomiting, constipation, and loss of appetite are common issues at the end of life. The causes and treatments for these symptoms are varied, so talk to a doctor or nurse right away. There are medicines that can control nausea or vomiting or relieve constipation, a common side effect of strong pain medications.

If someone near death wants to eat, but is too tired or weak, you can help with feeding. To address loss of appetite, try gently offering favorite foods in small amounts. Or, try serving frequent, smaller meals rather than three big ones.

You do not have to force a person to eat. Going without food and/or water is generally not painful, and eating can add to discomfort. Losing one's appetite is a common and normal part of dying. Swallowing may also be a problem, especially for people with dementia. A conscious decision to give up food can be part of a person's acceptance that death is near.

Temperature sensitivity. People who are dying may not be able to tell you that they are too hot or too cold, so watch for clues. For example, someone who is too warm might repeatedly try to remove a blanket. You can take off the blanket and try a cool cloth on her or his head.

If a person is hunching her or his shoulders, pulling the covers up, or even shivering—those could be signs of cold. Make sure there is no draft, raise the heat, and add another blanket. Avoid electric blankets because they can get too hot.

Fatigue. It is common for people nearing the end of life to feel tired and have little or no energy. Keep activities simple. For example, a bedside commode can be used instead of walking to the bathroom. A shower stool can save a person's energy, as can switching to sponging off in bed.

END OF LIFE: MANAGING MENTAL AND EMOTIONAL NEEDS

Complete end-of-life care also includes helping the dying person manage mental and emotional distress. Someone who is alert near the end of life might understandably feel depressed or anxious. It is important to treat emotional pain and suffering. Encouraging conversations about feelings might help. You might want to contact a counselor, possibly one familiar with end-of-life issues. If the depression or anxiety is severe, medicine may help.

A dying person may also have some specific fears and concerns. She or he may fear the unknown or worry about those left behind. Some people are afraid of being alone at the very end. This feeling can be made worse by the understandable reactions of family, friends, and even the medical team. For example, when family and friends do not know how to help or what to say, sometimes they stop visiting. Or, someone who is already beginning to grieve may withdraw.

Doctors may feel helpless because they cannot cure their patient. Some seem to avoid a dying patient. This can add to a dying person's sense of isolation. If this is happening, discuss your concerns with the family, friends, or the doctor.

The simple act of physical contact—holding hands, a touch, or a gentle massage—can make a person feel connected to those she or he loves. It can be very soothing. Warm your hands by rubbing them together or running them under warm water.

Try to set a comforting mood. Remember that listening and being present can make a difference. For example, Gordon loved a party, so it was natural for him to want to be around family and friends when he was dying. Ellen always liked spending quiet moments with one or two people at a time, so she was most comfortable with just a few visitors.

Some experts suggest that when death is very near, music at a low volume and soft lighting are soothing. In fact, near the end of life, music therapy might improve mood, help with relaxation, and lessen pain. Listening to music might also evoke memories those present can share. For some people, keeping distracting noises such as televisions and radios to a minimum is important.

Often, just being present with a dying person is enough. It may not be necessary to fill the time with talking or activity. Your quiet presence can be a simple and profound gift for a dying family member or friend.

SPIRITUAL NEEDS AT THE END OF LIFE

People nearing the end of life may have spiritual needs as important as their physical concerns. Spiritual needs include finding meaning in one's life and ending disagreements with others, if possible. The dying person might find peace by resolving unsettled issues with friends or family. Visits from a social worker or a counselor may also help.

Many people find solace in their faith. Others may struggle with their faith or spiritual beliefs. Praying, talking with someone from one's religious community (such as a minister, priest, rabbi, or imam), reading religious texts, or listening to religious music may bring comfort.

Family and friends can talk to the dying person about the importance of their relationship. For example, adult children can share how their father has influenced the course of their lives. Grandchildren can let their grandfather know how much he has meant to them. Friends can relate how they value years of support and companionship. Family and friends who cannot be present could send a recording of what they would like to say or a letter to be read out loud.

Sharing memories of good times is another way some people find peace near death. This can be comforting for everyone. Some doctors think it is possible that even if a patient is unconscious, she or he might still be able to hear. It is probably never too late to say how you feel or to talk about fond memories.

Always talk to, not about, the person who is dying. When you come into the room, it is a good idea to identify yourself, saying something in good words. Another good idea is to have someone write down some of the things said at this time—both by and to the person who is dying. In time, these words might serve as a source of comfort to family and friends. People who are looking for ways to help may welcome the chance to aid the family by writing down what is said.

There may come a time when a dying person who has been confused suddenly seems clear-thinking. Take advantage of these moments, but understand that they might be only temporary, not necessarily a sign she or he is getting better. Sometimes, a dying person may appear to see or talk to someone who is not there. Try to resist the temptation to interrupt or say they are imagining things. Give the dying person the space to experience their own reality.

END OF LIFE: PLANNING AHEAD

Many practical jobs need to be done at the end of life—both to relieve the person who is dying and to support the caregiver. Everyday tasks can be a source of worry for someone who is dying, and they can overwhelm a caregiver. Taking over small daily chores around the house—such as picking up the mail or newspaper, writing down phone messages, doing a load of laundry, feeding the family pet, taking children to soccer practice, or picking up medicine from the pharmacy—can provide a much-needed break for caregivers.

A person who is dying might be worried about who will take care of things when she or he is gone. Offering reassurance is a good thing and also might provide a measure of peace. Reminding the dying person that her or his personal affairs are in good hands can also bring comfort.

Everyone may be asking the family, "What can I do for you?" It helps to make a specific offer. Say to the family, "Let me help with . . . " and suggest something like bringing meals for the caregivers, paying bills, walking the dog, or babysitting. If you are not sure what to offer, talk to someone who has been through a similar situation. Find out what kind of help was useful.

If you want to help, but cannot get away from your own home, you could schedule other friends or family to help with small jobs or to bring in meals. This can allow the immediate family to give their full attention to the person who is dying.

If you are the primary caregiver, ask for help when you need it and accept help when it is offered. Do not hesitate to suggest a specific task to someone who offers to help. Friends and family are probably anxious to do something for you and/or the person who is dying, but they may be reluctant to repeatedly offer when you are so busy.

Keeping close friends and family informed can feel overwhelming. Setting up an outgoing voicemail message, a blog, an e-mail list, a private Facebook page, or even a phone tree can reduce the number of calls you have to make. Some families create a blog or website to share news, thoughts, and wishes. Or, you can assign a close family member or friend to make the updates for you. These can all help reduce the emotional burden of answering frequent questions.

Section 42.3 | Advance Care Planning: Healthcare Directives

This section includes text excerpted from "Advance Care Planning: Healthcare Directives," National Institute on Aging (NIA), National Institutes of Health (NIH), January 15, 2018.

Advance care planning is not just about old age. At any age, a medical crisis could leave you too ill to make your own healthcare decisions. Even if you are not sick now, planning for healthcare in the future is an important step toward making sure you get the medical care you would want, if you are unable to speak for yourself, and doctors and family members are making the decisions for you.

Many Americans face questions about medical treatment, but may not be capable of making those decisions, for example, in an emergency or at the end of life. This will explain the types of decisions that may need to be made in such cases and questions you can think about now so you are prepared later. It can help you think about who you would want to make decisions for you if you cannot make them yourself. It will also discuss ways you can share your wishes with others. Knowing who you want to make decisions on your behalf and how you would decide might take some of the burden off family and friends.

WHAT IS ADVANCE CARE PLANNING?

Advance care planning involves learning about the types of decisions that might need to be made, considering those decisions ahead of time, and then letting others know—both your family and your healthcare providers—about your preferences. These preferences are often put into an advance directive, a legal document that goes into effect only if you are incapacitated and unable to speak for yourself. This could be the result of disease or severe injury—no matter how old you are. It helps others know what type of medical care you want.

An advance directive also allows you to express your values and desires related to end-of-life care. You might think of it as a living document—one that you can adjust as your situation changes because of new information or a change in your health.

ADVANCE CARE PLANNING DECISIONS

Sometimes decisions must be made about the use of emergency treatments to keep you alive. Doctors can use several artificial or mechanical ways to try to do this. Decisions that might come up at this time relate to:

- Cardiopulmonary resuscitation (CPR)
- Ventilator use
- Artificial nutrition (tube feeding) and artificial hydration (IV, or intravenous, fluids)
- Comfort care

What is CPR? Cardiopulmonary resuscitation might restore your heartbeat if your heart stops or is in a life-threatening abnormal rhythm. It involves repeatedly pushing on the chest with force, while putting air into the lungs. This force has to be quite strong, and sometimes ribs are broken or a lung collapses. Electric shocks, known as "defibrillation," and medicines might also be used as part of the process. The heart of a young, otherwise healthy person might resume beating normally after CPR. Often, CPR does not succeed in older adults who have multiple chronic illnesses or who are already frail.

Using a ventilator as emergency treatment. Ventilators are machines that help you breathe. A tube connected to the ventilator is put through the throat into the trachea (windpipe) so the machine can force air into the lungs. Putting the tube down the throat is called "intubation." Because the tube is uncomfortable, medicines are often used to keep you sedated while on a ventilator. If you are expected to remain on a ventilator for a long time, a doctor may perform a tracheotomy or "trach" (rhymes with "make"). During this bedside surgery, the tube is inserted directly into the trachea through a hole in the neck. For long-term help with breathing, a trach is more comfortable, and sedation is not needed. People using such a breathing tube are not able to speak without special help because exhaled air does not go past their vocal cords.

Using artificial nutrition and hydration near the end of life. If you are not able to eat, you may be fed through a feeding tube that is threaded through the nose down to your stomach. If tube feeding is still needed for an extended period, a feeding tube may be surgically inserted directly into your stomach. Hand feeding (sometimes called "assisted oral feeding") is an alternative to tube feeding. This approach may have fewer risks, especially for people with dementia.

If you are not able to drink, you may be provided with IV fluids. These are delivered through a thin plastic tube inserted into a vein.

Artificial nutrition and hydration can be helpful if you are recovering from an illness. However, studies have shown that artificial nutrition toward the end of life does not meaningfully prolong life. Artificial nutrition and hydration may also be harmful if the dying body cannot use nutrition properly.

What is comfort care at the end of life? Comfort care is anything that can be done to soothe you and relieve suffering while staying in line with your wishes. Comfort care includes managing shortness of breath; limiting medical testing; providing spiritual and emotional counseling; and giving medication for pain, anxiety, nausea, or constipation.

GETTING STARTED WITH ADVANCE CARE PLANNING
Start by thinking about what kind of treatment you do or do not want in a medical emergency. It might help to talk with your doctor about how your current health conditions might influence your

health in the future. For example, what decisions would you or your family face if your high blood pressure leads to a stroke? You can ask your doctor to help you understand and think through your choices before you put them in writing. Discussing advance care planning decisions with your doctor is free through Medicare during your annual wellness visit. Private health insurance may also cover these discussions.

If you do not have any medical issues now, your family medical history might be a clue to help you think about the future. Talk with your doctor about decisions that might come up if you develop health problems similar to those of other family members.

In considering treatment decisions, your personal values are the key. Is your main desire to have the most days of life? Or, would your focus be on QOL, as you see it? What if an illness leaves you paralyzed or in a permanent coma and you need to be on a venti-lator? Would you want that?

What makes life meaningful to you? If your heart stops or you have trouble breathing, would you want to undergo life-saving measures if it meant that, in the future, you could be well enough to spend time with your family? Would you be content if the emergency leaves you simply able to spend your days listening to books on tape or gazing out the window?

But, there are many other scenarios. Here are a few. What would you decide?

- If a stroke leaves you unable to move and then your heart stops, would you want CPR? What if you were also mentally impaired by a stroke—does your decision change?
- What if you are in pain at the end of life? Do you want medication to treat the pain, even if it will make you more drowsy and lethargic?
- What if you are permanently unconscious and then develop pneumonia? Would you want antibiotics and to be placed on a ventilator?

For some people, staying alive as long as medically possible, or long enough to see an important event like a grandchild's wedding, is the most important thing. An advance directive can help to make that possible. Others have a clear idea about when they would no longer want to prolong their life. An advance directive can help with that, too.

Your decisions about how to handle any of these situations could be different at age 40 than at age 85. Or, they could be different if you have an incurable condition as opposed to being generally healthy. An advance directive allows you to provide instructions for these types of situations and then to change the instructions as you get older or if your viewpoint changes.

MAKING YOUR ADVANCE CARE WISHES KNOWN

There are two main elements in an advance directive—a living will and a durable power of attorney for healthcare. There are also other documents that can supplement your advance directive. You can choose which documents to create, depending on how you want decisions to be made. These documents include:

- Living will
- Durable power of attorney for healthcare
- Other advance care planning documents

Living will. A living will is a written document that helps you tell doctors how you want to be treated if you are dying or permanently unconscious and cannot make your own decisions about emergency treatment. In a living will, you can say which of the procedures you would want, which ones you would not want, and under which conditions each of your choices applies.

Durable power of attorney for healthcare. A durable power of attorney for healthcare is a legal document naming a healthcare proxy, someone to make medical decisions for you at times when you are unable to do so. Your proxy, also known as a "representative," "surrogate," or "agent," should be familiar with your values and wishes. This means that she or he will be able to decide as you would when treatment decisions need to be made. A proxy can be chosen in addition to or instead of a living will. Having a healthcare proxy helps you plan for situations that cannot be foreseen, such as a serious auto accident.

Some people are reluctant to put specific health decisions in writing. For them, naming a healthcare agent might be a good approach, especially if there is someone they feel comfortable talking with about their values and preferences. A named proxy can evaluate each situation or treatment option independently.

Other advance care planning documents. You might also want to prepare documents to express your wishes about a single medical issue or something not already covered in your advance directive. A living will usually cover only the specific life-sustaining treatments discussed earlier. You might want to give your healthcare proxy specific instructions about other issues, such as blood transfusion or kidney dialysis. This is especially important if your doctor suggests that, given your health condition, such treatments might be needed in the future.

Medical issues that might arise at the end of life include:
- DNR orders
- Organ and tissue donation
- POLST and MOLST forms

A **DNR (do not resuscitate) order** tells medical staff in a hospital or nursing facility that you do not want them to try to return your heart to a normal rhythm if it stops or is beating unsustainably using CPR or other life-support measures. Sometimes this is referred to as a "do not attempt resuscitation" (DNAR) or an "allow natural death" (AND) order. Even though a living will might say CPR is not wanted, it is helpful to have a DNR order as part of your medical file if you go to a hospital. Posting a DNR next to your bed might avoid confusion in an emergency situation. Without a DNR order, medical staff will make every effort to restore your breathing and the normal rhythm of your heart.

A similar document, called a "do not intubate order" (DNI), tells medical staff in a hospital or nursing facility that you do not want to be put on a breathing machine.

A nonhospital DNR order will alert emergency medical personnel to your wishes regarding measures to restore your heartbeat or breathing if you are not in the hospital.

Organ and tissue donation allow organs or body parts from a generally healthy person who has died to be transplanted into people who need them. Commonly, the heart, lungs, pancreas, kidneys, corneas, liver, and skin are donated. There is no age limit for organ and tissue donation. You can carry a donation card in your wallet. Some states allow you to add this decision to your driver's license. Some people also include organ donation in their advance care planning documents.

At the time of death, family members may be asked about organ donation. If those close to you, especially your proxy, know how you feel about organ donation, they will be ready to respond. There is no cost to the donor's family for this gift of life. If the person has requested a DNR order, but wants to donate organs, she or he might have to indicate that the desire to donate supersedes the DNR. That is because it might be necessary to use machines to keep the heart beating until the medical staff is ready to remove the donated organs.

POLST and MOLST forms provide guidance about your medical care preferences in the form of a doctor's orders. Typically you create a Physician Orders for Life-Sustaining Treatment (POLST) or Medical Orders for Life-Sustaining Treatment (MOLST) when you are near the end of life or critically ill and know the specific decisions that might need to be made on your behalf. These forms serve as a medical order in addition to your advance directive. They make it possible for you to provide guidance that healthcare professionals can act on immediately in an emergency.

A number of states use POLST and MOLST forms, which are filled out by your doctor or sometimes by a nurse practitioner or physician's assistant. The doctor fills out a POLST or MOLST after discussing your wishes with you and your family. Once signed by your doctor, this form has the same authority as any other medical order. Check with your state department of health to find out if these forms are available where you live.

HOW TO CHOOSE YOUR HEALTHCARE PROXY

If you decide to choose a proxy, think about people you know who share your views and values about life and medical decisions. Your proxy might be a family member, a friend, your lawyer, or someone in your social or spiritual community. It is a good idea to also name an alternate proxy. It is especially important to have a detailed living will if you choose not to name a proxy.

You can decide how much authority your proxy has over your medical care—whether she or he is entitled to make a wide range of decisions or only a few specific ones. Try not to include guidelines that make it impossible for the proxy to fulfill her or his duties. For example, it is probably not unusual for someone to say in conversation, "I do not want to go to a nursing home," but think carefully about whether you want a restriction such as that in your advance directive. Sometimes, for financial or medical reasons, that may be the best choice for you.

Of course, check with those you choose as your healthcare proxy and alternate before you name them officially. Make sure they are comfortable with this responsibility.

MAKING YOUR HEALTHCARE DIRECTIVES OFFICIAL

Once you have talked with your doctor and have an idea of the types of decisions that could come up in the future and whom you would like as a proxy, if you want one at all, the next step is to fill out the legal forms detailing your wishes. A lawyer can help, but is not required. If you decide to use a lawyer, do not depend on her or him to help you understand different medical treatments. Start the planning process by talking with your doctor.

Many states have their own advance directive forms. Your local Area Agency on Aging can help you locate the right forms.

Some states require your advance directive to be witnessed; a few require your signature to be notarized. A notary is a person licensed by the state to witness signatures. You might find a notary at your bank, post office, or local library, or call your insurance agent. Some notaries charge a fee.

Some states have registries that can store your advance directive for quick access by healthcare providers, your proxy, and anyone else to whom you have given permission. Private firms also will store your advance directive. There may be a fee for storing your form in a registry. If you store your advance directive in a registry and later make changes, you must replace the original with the updated version in the registry.

Some people spend a lot of time in more than one state—for example, visiting children and grandchildren. If that is your situation, consider preparing an advance directive using forms for each state—and keep a copy in each place, too.

WHAT TO DO AFTER YOU SET UP YOUR ADVANCE DIRECTIVE

Give copies of your advance directive to your healthcare proxy and alternate proxy. Give your doctor a copy for your medical records. Tell close family members and friends where you keep a copy. If you have to go to the hospital, give staff there a copy to include in your records. Because you might change your advance directive in the future, it is a good idea to keep track of who receives a copy.

Review your advance care planning decisions from time to time—for example, every 10 years, if not more often. You might want to revise your preferences for care if your situation or your health changes. Or, you might want to make adjustments if you receive a serious diagnosis; if you get married, separated, or divorced; if your spouse dies; or if something happens to your proxy or alternate. If your preferences change, you will want to make sure your doctor, proxy, and family know about them.

BE PREPARED

What happens if you have no advance directive or have made no plans and you become unable to speak for yourself? In such cases, the state where you live will assign someone to make medical decisions on your behalf. This will probably be your spouse, your parents if they are available, or your children if they are adults. If you have no family members, the state will choose someone to represent your best interests.

Always remember: An advance directive is only used if you are in danger of dying and need certain emergency or special measures to keep you alive, but you are not able to make those decisions on your own. An advance directive allows you to make your wishes about medical treatment known.

It is difficult to predict the future with certainty. You may never face a medical situation where you are unable to speak for yourself and make your wishes known. But, having an advance directive may give you and those close to you some peace of mind.

Section 42.4 | End-of-Life Care Settings

This section includes text excerpted from "Where Can I Find Care for a Dying Relative?" National Institute on Aging (NIA), National Institutes of Health (NIH), May 17, 2017.

Decades ago, most people died at home, but medical advances have changed that. Today, most Americans are in hospitals or nursing homes at the end of their lives. Some people enter the hospital to get treated for an illness. Some may already be living in a nursing home.

There is no right place to die. And, of course, where you die is not always something you get to decide. But, if given the choice, each person and/or her or his family should consider which type of care makes the most sense, where that kind of care can be provided, whether family and friends are available to help, and how they will pay for it. This explains some of the care options available to people at the end of life.

END-OF-LIFE CARE IN HOSPITALS

In a hospital setting, medical professionals are available who know what needs to be done for someone who is dying. This can be very reassuring. In addition to the regular care team, some hospitals may have palliative care teams that can assist with managing uncomfortable symptoms and making medical decisions for patients who may or may not be at the end of life.

END-OF-LIFE CARE IN NURSING HOMES

More and more people are in nursing homes at the end of life. In a nursing home, nursing staff are always present. Unlike a hospital, a doctor is not in the facility all the time, but may be available by phone. Plans for end of life care can be arranged ahead of time, so when the time comes, care can be provided as needed without first consulting a doctor.

If the person has lived in the nursing home for a while, the staff and family probably already have a relationship. This can make the care feel more personalized than in a hospital. Additionally, if the person is enrolled in hospice, the hospice team will be available to assist nursing facility staff with end of life care.

As in a hospital, privacy may be an issue in nursing homes. You can ask if arrangements can be made to give your family more time alone when needed.

END-OF-LIFE CARE AT HOME

Home is likely the most familiar setting for someone who needs end-of-life care. Family and friends can come and go freely. Care at home can be a big job for family and friends—physically, emotionally, and financially. But, there are benefits too, and it is often a job caregivers are willing to take on. Hiring a home nurse is an option for people who need additional help and have the financial resources.

Talk with your healthcare provider about the kind of care needed. Frequently, this care does not require a nurse, but can be provided by nursing assistants or family and friends without medical training.

To make comfort care available at home, you will have to arrange for services (such as visiting nurses) and special equipment (like a hospital bed or bedside commode). Health insurance might only cover these services or equipment if they have been ordered by a doctor; make sure you check with your insurance company before ordering.

Work with the doctor to decide what is needed to support comfort care at home. If the seriously ill person is returning home from the hospital, sometimes a hospital discharge planner, often a social worker, can help with the planning. Your local Area Agency on Aging might be able to recommend other sources of help.

A doctor has to be available to oversee the patient's care at home—she or he will arrange for new services, adjust treatment, and order medicines as needed. It is important to follow the doctor's plan in order to make the dying person as comfortable as possible. Talk with the doctor if you think a treatment is no longer helping. Hospice is frequently used to care for people who are home at the end of life.

Section 42.5 | Palliative Care versus Hospice Care

This section includes text excerpted from "What Are Palliative Care and Hospice Care?" National Institute on Aging (NIA), National Institutes of Health (NIH), May 17, 2017.

Many Americans die in facilities, such as hospitals or nursing homes receiving care that is not consistent with their wishes. To make sure that does not happen, older people need to know what their end-of-life care options are and state their preferences to their caregivers in advance. For example, if an older person wants to die at home, receiving end-of-life care for pain and other symptoms, and makes this known to healthcare providers and family, it is less likely she or he will die in a hospital receiving unwanted treatments.

Caregivers have several factors to consider when choosing end-of-life care, including the older person's desire to pursue life-extending or curative treatments, how long she or he has left to live, and the preferred setting for care.

UNDERSTANDING PALLIATIVE CARE

Doctors can provide treatment to seriously ill patients in the hopes of a cure for as long as possible. These patients may also receive medical care for their symptoms, or palliative care, along with curative treatment.

A palliative care consultation team is a multidisciplinary team that works with the patient, family, and the patient's other doctors to provide medical, social, emotional, and practical support. The

463

team is made of palliative care specialist doctors and nurses, and includes others such as social workers, nutritionists, and chaplains.

Palliative care can be provided in hospitals, nursing homes, outpatient palliative care clinics and certain other specialized clinics, or at home. Medicare, Medicaid, and insurance policies may cover palliative care. Veterans may be eligible for palliative care through the Department of Veterans Affairs. Private health insurance might pay for some services. Health insurance providers can answer questions about what they will cover. Check to see if insurance will cover your particular situation.

In palliative care, you do not have to give up treatment that might cure a serious illness. Palliative care can be provided along with curative treatment and may begin at the time of diagnosis. Over time, if the doctor or the palliative care team believes ongoing treatment is no longer helping, there are two possibilities. Palliative care could transition to hospice care if the doctor believes the person is likely to die within 6 months. Or, the palliative care team could continue to help with increasing emphasis on comfort care.

UNDERSTANDING HOSPICE CARE

Increasingly, people are choosing hospice care at the end of life. Hospice can be provided in any setting—home, nursing home, assisted living facility, or inpatient hospital.

At some point, it may not be possible to cure a serious illness, or a patient may choose not to undergo certain treatments. Hospice is designed for this situation. The patient beginning hospice care understands that her or his illness is not responding to medical attempts to cure it or to slow the disease's progress.

Like palliative care, hospice provides comprehensive comfort care as well as support for the family, but, in hospice, attempts to cure the person's illness are stopped. Hospice is provided for a person with a terminal illness whose doctor believes she or he has six months or less to live if the illness runs its natural course.

Hospice is an approach to care, so it is not tied to a specific place. It can be offered in two types of settings—at home or in a facility such as a nursing home, hospital, or even in a separate hospice center.

Hospice care brings together a team of people with special skills—among them nurses, doctors, social workers, spiritual advisors, and trained volunteers. Everyone works together with the person who is dying, the caregiver, and/or the family to provide the medical, emotional, and spiritual support needed.

A member of the hospice team visits regularly, and someone is always available by phone—24 hours a day, seven days a week. Hospice may be covered by Medicare and other insurance companies; check to see if insurance will cover your particular situation.

It is important to remember that stopping treatment aimed at curing an illness does not mean discontinuing all treatment. A good example is an older person with cancer. If the doctor determines that the cancer is not responding to chemotherapy and the patient chooses to enter into hospice care, then the chemotherapy will stop. Other medical care may continue as long as it is helpful. For example, if the person has high blood pressure, she or he will still get medicine for that.

Part 6 | Clinical Trials and Research on Stroke

Chapter 43 | Clinical Trials on Stroke

Chapter Contents

Section 43.1 | What Are Clinical Trials?

This section includes text excerpted from "Clinical Trials: Benefits, Risks, and Safety," National Institute on Aging (NIA), National Institutes of Health (NIH), May 17, 2017.

You may ask yourself, "Why should I try something that researchers are not sure will work?" That is a good question. Being part of a clinical trial may have risks, but it may also have benefits. Past clinical trial history has led many people to hesitate to sign up for research. However, today there are strict rules in place to keep your health and privacy safe.

WHAT ARE THE BENEFITS OF A CLINICAL TRIAL?

- You may get a new treatment for a disease before it is available to everyone.
- You play a more active role in your own healthcare.
- Researchers may provide you with medical care and more frequent health checkups as part of your treatment.
- You may have the chance to help others get a better treatment for their health problems in the future.
- You may be able to get information about support groups and resources.

WHAT ARE THE POTENTIAL RISKS OF A CLINICAL TRIAL?

- The new treatment may cause serious side effects or be uncomfortable.
- The new treatment may not work, or it may not be better than the standard treatment.
- You may NOT be part of the treatment group (or experimental group) that gets the new treatment—for example, a new drug or device. Instead, you may be part of the control group, which means you get the standard treatment or a no-treatment placebo.
- The clinical trial could cause inconvenience to you. For example, medical appointments could take a lot of time. You might need to travel to the study site several times or stay in the hospital.

HOW IS THE SAFETY OF CLINICAL TRIAL PARTICIPANTS PROTECTED?

This is a very important question. The history of clinical research is not perfect. Based on many years of experience and learning, Congress has passed laws to protect study participants. Today, every clinical investigator is required to monitor and make sure that every participant is safe. These safeguards are an essential part of the research. Research abuses like the Tuskegee Syphilis Experiment, which began in 1932, before safeguards were in place, will NOT happen again.

Researchers are required to follow strict rules to make sure that participants are safe. These rules are enforced by the federal government. Each clinical trial also follows a careful study plan or protocol that describes what the researchers will do. The principal investigator, or head researcher, is responsible for making sure that the protocol is followed.

An Institutional Review Board, or IRB, at each study site, must approve every clinical trial in the United States. The IRB is made up of doctors, scientists, and lay people, like yourself, who are dedicated to making sure that the study participants are not exposed to unnecessary risks. The people on the IRB regularly review the study and its results. They make sure that risks (or potential harm) to participants are as low as possible.

Along with the IRB, many clinical trials are closely supervised by a Data and Safety Monitoring Committee. The Committee is made up of experts in your condition who periodically look at the results of the study as it is in progress. If they find that the experimental treatment is not working or is harming participants, they will stop the trial right away.

The informed consent process also helps protect participants. Before joining a clinical trial, you will be told what to expect as a participant and all the things that might happen. For example, someone from the research team will explain possible side effects or other risks of the treatment. As part of the informed consent process, you will have a chance to ask questions about the trial.

After getting all this information, you can think about whether or not you want to participate. If you decide to join the trial, you will be given an informed consent form to sign. By signing the form, you show that you have been told all the details and want to be part of the study. The informed consent form is NOT a contract. You can leave the trial at any time and for any reason without being judged or put in a difficult position regarding your medical care. Researchers must keep health and personal information private.

Section 43.2 | Featured NICHD Clinical Trials

This section includes text excerpted from "Stroke: Clinical Trials," *Eunice Kennedy Shriver* National Institute of Child Health and Human Development (NICHD), December 1, 2016. Reviewed May 2020.

CONTRALATERALLY CONTROLLED FES OF ARM AND HAND FOR SUBACUTE STROKE REHABILITATION

This study seeks to enhance the effect of contralaterally controlled functional electrical stimulation (CCFES) by applying CCFES to elbow extension as well as hand movement. In CCFES, patients receive electrical stimulation to their weak hand as they move it; the patient controls the amount of stimulation with the other hand.

ENHANCING REHABILITATION AFTER STROKE (ENHANCE)

Enhance is a 12-week, randomized, placebo-controlled study to determine if donepezil (Aricept®) treatment during rehabilitation after stroke improves functional recovery. The researchers also will examine the drug's effect on cognitive domains (attention/working memory, information processing speed, and episodic memory) that are relevant to functional outcomes.

ELECTRICAL STIMULATION FOR RECOVERY OF HAND FUNCTION IN CHRONIC STROKE SURVIVORS

The purpose of this study is to estimate the efficacy of CCFES in reducing upper extremity impairment and activity limitation in chronic upper extremity hemiplegia. CCFES is a rehabilitation intervention in which neuromuscular electrical stimulation is applied to the finger and thumb muscles of the paretic upper limb to open the hand. The stroke survivor controls the stimulation intensity, and consequent degree of hand opening, by modulating the degree of opening of the unimpaired hand, which is detected by an instrumented glove. Thus, opening of the unaffected hand produces stimulated opening of the affected hand. The stimulation process is used to assist the stroke survivor in practicing functional tasks with the affected hand.

ELECTRICAL STIMULATION FOR HEMIPLEGIC SHOULDER PAIN

Poststroke shoulder pain is a major rehabilitation problem that affects moderately to severely impaired stroke survivors. Surface electrical stimulation (ES) of muscles surrounding the hemiparetic shoulder has been demonstrated to be beneficial, but despite the evidence for therapeutic benefit, the clinical implementation of surface ES for poststroke shoulder pain has been difficult. To address the limitations of surface ES, the investigative team pioneered the development of percutaneous intramuscular (IM) ES for the treatment of poststroke shoulder pain. The primary objective is to estimate the relative pain reduction associated with IM ES versus "usual care."

ARM REHABILITATION STUDY AFTER STROKE (ICARE)

ICARE is the study about arm and hand recovery after a stroke. The investigators are testing an experimental arm therapy called "Accelerated Skill Acquisition Program" (ASAP), which combines challenging, intensive, and meaningful practice of tasks of the participant's choice compared to two standard types of therapy (usual and customary arm therapy totaling 30 hours and usual and customary arm therapy for a duration indicated on the therapy prescription). A second objective is to characterize current outpatient arm therapy (dosage and content) following stroke for individuals who are eligible for ICARE.

BRAIN STIMULATION-AIDED STROKE REHABILITATION: NEURAL MECHANISMS OF RECOVERY

The purpose of this study is to investigate whether benefits of training the affected hand in patients with stroke can be improved by combining training with a painless, noninvasive technique called "transcranial direct current stimulation" (TDCS). TDCS will be applied over the part of the brain responsible for movements of the affected hand. The investigators also will study the changes in the brain that favor recovery of hand function following combination of training and TDCS.

POSTSTROKE APHASIA AND REPETITIVE TRANSCRANIAL MAGNETIC STIMULATION (RTMS) TREATMENT STUDY (PART)

In this study, the investigators will examine the efficacy of navigated excitatory repetitive transcranial magnetic stimulation (nerTMS) and a combination of nerTMS and constraint-induced aphasia therapy (CIAT) as poststroke aphasia rehabilitation methods. The investigators expect that these new types of rehabilitation, either nerTMS alone or in combination with CIAT, will help patients with aphasia return to their lives as they were prior to the stroke.

Section 43.3 | NIH Stroke Clinical Trials Research Network (NIH StrokeNet)

This section includes text excerpted from "NIH StrokeNet Small Business Innovation Clinical Trials and Biomarker Studies for Stroke Treatment, Recovery, and Prevention," National Institutes of Health (NIH), May 10, 2017.

To facilitate the cooperation and partnering of public and private funding organizations, universities, academic medical centers, research institutes, contract research organizations, biotechnology companies, and pharmaceutical companies in the advancement of interventions for stroke prevention, treatment, and rehabilitation, the National Institute of Neurological Disorders and Stroke

(NINDS) has formed the National Institutes of Health (NIH) Stroke Clinical Trials Research Network (NIH StrokeNet, www. ninds.nih.gov/research/clinical_research/NINDS_stroke_trials_ network.htm). The NIH StrokeNet comprises of a National Clinical Coordinating Center (NCC), a National Data Management Center (NDMC), and 25 geographically distributed Regional Coordinating Centers (RCC) with over 350 affiliated stroke centers.

The NIH StrokeNet network will consider the breadth of cerebrovascular disease, beginning with patients identified with an acute stroke through stroke rehabilitation, and primary and secondary stroke prevention for pediatric and adult patients.

The network will provide a robust, standardized, and accessible infrastructure to facilitate rapid development and implementation of NINDS-funded stroke trials. The network is designed to increase the efficiency of stroke clinical trials by facilitating patient recruitment and retention, supporting novel methodologies and streamlined approaches to accelerate the development of promising stroke therapies, and enabling comparison between approaches.

Section 43.4 | Acute Ischemic Stroke Therapy

This section includes text excerpted from "New Breakthrough in Acute Stroke Therapy," National Institute of Neurological Disorders and Stroke (NINDS), January 19, 2020.

Acute stroke therapy has finally turned a historic corner. Results from four landmark randomized controlled clinical trials were highlighted among numerous studies reported at the International Stroke Conference in Nashville, Tennessee. This breakthrough in acute stroke therapy echoes the treatment of heart attacks, where catheter-based treatments to open the occluded (or blocked) coronary artery have demonstrated lessened mortality.

In 1983, Zeumer, Hacke, and Ringelstein reported that three in five patients with typically fatal strokes caused by occlusion of the basilar artery improved after streptokinase, an agent known to dissolve blood clots (called "thrombolytic agents"), was injected by a catheter into the artery-clogging clot. A year later, Zeumer and Ringelstein reported two cases successfully treated by injection of another thrombolytic agent, urokinase, into clots blocking the intracranial carotid arteries. The basilar and carotid arteries are the major routes of blood flow to the brain. Like basilar occlusion, blockage at the top of the carotid artery is often fatal, or otherwise results in lifelong disability. This pioneering work in Germany offered hope that successful treatment for the most severe strokes was possible. In 1989 at the Mass. General Hospital, the National Institute of Neurological Disorders and Stroke (NINDS) instituted an acute stroke service for the intra-arterial treatment of severe strokes. The "miracle" recoveries that were occasionally seen after opening these brain arteries in the "angio" suite infused a high level of enthusiasm.

The field has taken a number of twists and turns over the past 30 years, but with the reports at the stroke conference, the proce-dure of using a catheter to physically penetrate and then dissolve or remove large clots in brain arteries can now be widely considered to be beneficial.

Intravenous (IV) administration into the circulatory system of tissue plasminogen activator (tPA), also a thrombolytic agent, became standard of care after publication of the NINDS trial in 1995. IV tPA does not penetrate into the clots but instead works at the interface between the clot and the bloodstream. As a result IV tPA had limited ability to dissolve the large clots that caused the most severe strokes. In 1999, an Abbot pharmaceuticals-funded, randomized controlled trial injecting pro-urokinase, a novel throm-bolytic, via a catheter directly into the center of the clot blocking the major brain arteries showed benefit, but the U.S. Food and Drug Administration (FDA) required a confirmatory study and the company decided not to proceed. Beginning in the mid-1990's the NINDS funded a series of linked studies—Emergency Management of Stroke (EMS) followed by the Interventional Management of Stroke (IMS) trials (IMS, IMS I/II, and IMS III)—to test the abil-ity of intra-arterial therapy to rescue patients with severe strokes despite treatment with IV tPA. In 2013, disappointment in the field was palpable when IMS III showed no benefit of intra-arterial therapy in addition to the benefit of IV tPA.

Two major advances that occurred since IMS III was first designed may have led to recent successes. First, the field moved from injecting thrombolytic agents that dissolved clots over time to deploying stents that could capture the clot and remove it from the artery when the device is removed from the vessel. These stent-retrievers are more effective in removing clots and they are easier and faster to deploy than previous devices. The early EMS and IMS trials used the injection approach, whereas IMS III used the injection approach and also began incorporating the newer approach with clot-retrieval devices as their use began to increase during the course of the trial. The latest trials reported this February utilized the Solitaire stent retrieval device made by Covidien (now Medtronic).

The second advance was the use of imaging techniques to select patients for the study who have both large clots and incomplete brain injury. By injecting a common contrast agent intravenously with the brain computed tomography (CT) scan (CT angiography) or magnetic resonance imaging (MRI) (MR angiography), large artery blockages can easily be identified. In addition, CT or MRI techniques can now also define the degree of irreversible injury that is associated with poor outcome even if the vessel is opened, i.e., when it is too late to save brain tissue.

In addition, IMS III results suggested there might be harm associated with performing the angiographic procedures under general anesthesia, which the recently reported studies also confirmed. IMSIII also impressed upon the field that it was crucial to enroll patients into randomized controlled trials, an idea that was not widely held by the community during IMSIII.

After IMS III, the NINDS met with various stakeholders to consider next steps for a trial utilizing noninvasive angiography and tissue imaging to select patients for intra-arterial therapy with the newest devices. However, multiple parties were already planning independent studies with support from industry partners. Thus the results of these four latest trials have been highly anticipated by the community, since they build on decades of investment and development in this new approach that had yet to realize its full potential to revolutionize treatment of severe acute strokes.

Section 43.5 | Intracerebral Hemorrhage Deferoxamine Trial (iDEF Trial)

This section includes text excerpted from "Intracerebral Hemorrhage Deferoxamine Trial—iDEF Trial," National Institute of Neurological Disorders and Stroke (NINDS), March 27, 2019.

The purpose of this trial is to study the effects of deferoxamine on brain or intracranial hemorrhage (ICH). This trial also will help researchers learn more about the safety of the drug.

The ICH occurs when a blood vessel in the brain bursts open. This causes blood to leak into the brain and may lead to a hemorrhagic stroke. A hemorrhagic stroke occurs when blood flow to a part of the brain stops. The blood in the brain also contains iron, which damages the brain.

The focus of this multicenter, double-blind, placebo-controlled study is to evaluate deferoxamine mesylate, or deferoxamine. Deferoxamine has been approved by the U.S. Food and Drug Administration (FDA) for use in other diseases to remove excess iron from the body. It combines with iron in the bloodstream. The combination of iron and deferoxamine is then removed from the body by the kidneys.

In this study, scientists will test if removal of iron from the brain after ICH will reduce the effects of the hemorrhage. The main purpose of this study is to examine how deferoxamine affects ICH. Scientists will specifically look at a person's ability to function and think well after ICH. Researchers also will learn more about the safety of the study drug.

A total of 294 people will be enrolled in this study at sites in the United States and Canada. Participants will be randomized to receive either deferoxamine mesylate or saline placebo for 3 consecutive days. Treatment will begin within 24 hours after ICH symptom onset. All participants will be followed for 6 months and will receive standard of care therapy while participating in the study. Follow-up will include 2 in-person study visits and 2 study through phone calls.

Study duration for participants is about 6 months.

ELIGIBILITY CRITERIA
Inclusion
- Age $\geq$ 18 and $\leq$ 80 years of age
- Diagnosis of ICH is confirmed by brain computed tomography (CT) scan
- NIHSS score $\geq$6 and GCS >6 upon presentation
- Functional independence prior to ICH

Exclusion
- Previous chelation therapy or known hypersensitivity to deferoxamine (DFO) products
- Known severe iron-deficiency anemia
- Abnormal renal function
- Planned surgical evacuation of ICH prior to administration of study drug
- Suspected secondary ICH related to tumor, ruptured aneurysm or arteriovenous malformation, hemorrhagic transformation of an ischemic infarct, or venous sinus thrombosis
- Infratentorial hemorrhage
- Irreversibly impaired brainstem function (bilateral fixed and dilated pupils and extensor motor posturing)
- Complete unconsciousness, defined as a score of 3 on item 1a of the NIH Stroke Scale (NIHSS)
- Preexisting disability
- Coagulopathy; concurrent use of direct thrombin inhibitors (such as dabigatran), direct factor Xa inhibitors (such as rivaroxaban or apixaban), or low-molecular-weight heparin
- People with confirmed aspiration, pneumonia, or evident bilateral pulmonary infiltrates on chest x-ray or CT scan prior to enrollment
- People with significant respiratory disease such as chronic obstructive pulmonary disease, pulmonary fibrosis, or any use (chronic or intermittent) of inhaled O2 at home
- Fraction of inspired oxygen (FiO_2) >0.35 (>4 L/min) prior to enrollment

- Sepsis; Systemic Inflammatory Response Syndrome; respiratory rate >20 or $PaCo_2$ <32 mmHg; white blood cell (WBC) >12, <4, or bands >10%); or shock [systolic blood pressure (SBP) <90 mmHg] at presentation
- The presence of 4 or more of the following risk modifiers for acute respiratory distress syndrome (ARDS) prior to enrollment: tachypnea (respiratory rate >30); pulse oximetry (SpO_2) <95%; obesity (BMI >30); acidosis (pH <7.35); hypoalbuminemia (albumin <3.5 g/dL); or concurrent use of chemotherapy
- Taking iron supplements containing $\geq$ 325 mg of ferrous iron, or prochlorperazine
- Persons with heart failure taking > 500 mg of vitamin C daily
- Known severe hearing loss
- Pregnancy or breastfeeding
- Positive drug screen, alcoholism, or drug dependency
- Any condition which, in the judgment of the investigator, might increase the risk to the patient
- Life expectancy of less than 90 days due to comorbid conditions
- Concurrent participation in another research protocol for investigation of another experimental therapy
- Indication that a new Do Not Resuscitate (DNR) or Comfort Measures Only (CMO) order will be implemented within the first 72 hours of hospitalization

STUDY DESIGN AND LOCATION
Study Design
Allocation: Randomized, Endpoint Classification: Safety/Efficacy Study, Intervention Model: Parallel Assignment, Masking: Double Blind (Subject, Caregiver, Investigator, Outcomes Assessor), Primary Purpose: Treatment

Study Location
Multiple U.S. locations

Chapter 44 | Research on Stroke

Chapter Contents

Section 44.1 | Immune Cells May Heal Bleeding Brain after Strokes

This section includes text excerpted from "Immune Cells May Heal Bleeding Brain after Strokes," National Institute of Neurological Disorders and Stroke (NINDS), September 20, 2017.

While immune cells called "neutrophils" are known to act as infantry in the body's war on germs, a National Institutes of Health (NIH)-funded study suggests they can act as medics as well. By studying rodents, researchers showed that instead of attacking germs, some neutrophils may help heal the brain after an intracerebral hemorrhage, a form of stroke caused by ruptured blood vessels. The study suggests that two neutrophil-related proteins may play critical roles in protecting the brain from stroke-induced damage and could be used as treatments for intracerebral hemorrhage.

"Intracerebral hemorrhage is a damaging and often fatal form of stroke for which there are no effective medicines," said Jaroslaw Aronowski, M.D., Ph.D., professor, department of neurology, at the University of Texas Health Science Center at Houston, and senior author of the study published in *Nature Communications*. "Our results are a hopeful first step towards developing a treatment for this devastating form of stroke."

Accounting for 10 to 15 percent of all strokes, intracerebral hemorrhages happen when blood vessels rupture and leak blood into the brain, often leading to death or long-term disability. Chronic high blood pressure is the leading risk factor for these types of strokes. The initial phase of damage appears to be caused by the pressure of blood leaking into the brain. Over time, further damage may be caused by the accumulation of toxic levels of blood products, infiltrating immune cells, and swelling.

Decades of research suggest that neutrophils are some of the earliest immune cells to respond to a hemorrhage, and that they may both harm and heal the brain. In this study, the researchers found that interleukin-27 (IL-27), a protein that controls the activity of immune cells, may shift the role of neutrophils from harming the brain to helping with recovery.

Injections of IL-27 after a hemorrhage helped mice recover. Days after the strokes, the treated mice had better mobility, including

485

walking, limb stretching, and navigating holes in a floor. In contrast, injections of an antibody that blocked natural IL-27 activity slowed recovery. The brains of the mice treated with IL-27 also showed less damage. They had less swelling around the hemorrhages and lower levels of iron and the blood protein hemoglobin, both of which are toxic at high levels.

"This study shines a spotlight on the critical role the immune system may play in helping the brain heal after a hemorrhage or stroke and opens new avenues for stroke treatment strategies," said Jim Koenig, Ph.D., program director at the NIH's National Institute of Neurological Disorders and Stroke (NINDS).

Neutrophils are born in bone marrow and carry chemicals in hundreds of densely filled packets called "granules," which look like dark spots under a microscope. Typically, when the body senses bacteria or an injury, neutrophils rush to the invasion site and release germ killing chemicals from the granules. This appears to happen minutes after a hemorrhagic stroke.

In this study, the researchers suggested that after a hemorrhagic stroke the brain secretes high levels of IL-27, which leads to a second wave of neutrophils arriving with granules filled with higher amounts of healing molecules. IL-27 levels were elevated in the brain and blood of the mice an hour after hemorrhages and stayed high for three days, peaking at 24 hours later. Further experiments suggested that brain cells called "microglia" produced the IL-27 in response to the presence of red blood cells.

Once released, IL-27 molecules appeared to travel to the bones of the mice, infiltrated the marrow, and changed the role newborn neutrophils played in response to a stroke. When the researchers extracted newborn neutrophils from the bones of mice and treated them with IL-27, the chemical raised the activity of genes associated with healing, especially lactoferrin, while reducing the activity of genes associated with killing cells. Conversely, treating mice with an IL-27 neutralizing antibody after a hemorrhage lowered lactoferrin gene activity.

"Our results suggested that IL-27 links the brain to the bones," said Dr. Aronowski. "We can use these results as a source for ideas for developing potential treatments for hemorrhagic stroke."

Finally, the researchers showed the iron-binding protein lactoferrin may protect the brain from intracerebral hemorrhagic strokes. Mice and rats injected with lactoferrin 30 minutes after hemorrhages recovered faster and had reduced brain damage as compared to animals given placebos. In one set of experiments, the researchers found that giving mice lactoferrin 24 hours after a stroke was also effective.

"Lactoferrin appears to have a long treatment window," said Dr. Aronowski. "This means lactoferrin might one day be used to help patients recover from intracerebral hemorrhage."

Dr. Aronowski's team is taking the next steps toward testing lactoferrin treatment in patients.

by Christopher G. Thomas, Ph.D.

Section 44.2 | Researchers Get a Handle on How to Control Blood Sugar after Stroke

This section includes text excerpted from "Researchers Get a Handle on How to Control Blood Sugar after Stroke," National Institute of Neurological Disorders and Stroke (NINDS), July 24, 2019.

Hyperglycemia, or high levels of glucose, is common in patients with acute ischemic stroke and is associated with worse outcomes compared to normal blood sugar levels. Animal studies also pointed to an effect of high blood sugar in worsening stroke injury. Stroke experts have debated whether intensive glucose management after acute ischemic stroke leads to better outcomes but a new study in *The Journal of the American Medical Association (JAMA)* finds that aggressive methods are not better than standard approaches. The study was supported by the National Institute of Neurological Disorders and Stroke (NINDS), part of the National Institutes of Health (NIH).

"After decades of uncertainty about how to manage blood sugar in acute stroke patients we finally have strong clinical evidence that aggressive lowering does not improve patient outcome," said Walter Koroshetz, M.D., NINDS director.

The Stroke Hyperglycemia Insulin Network Effort (SHINE) study, a large, multisite clinical study led by Karen C. Johnston, M.D., professor of neurology and Associate Vice President of Clinical & Translational Research at the University of Virginia, Charlottesville, compared two commonly used strategies for glucose control in ischemic stroke patients. More than 1100 patients underwent intensive glucose management, which required the use of intravenous delivery of insulin to bring blood sugar levels down to 80 to 130 mg/dL, or standard glucose control using insulin shots, which aimed to get glucose below 180 mg/dL, for up to 72 hours. After 90 days, the patients were evaluated for outcomes, including disability, neurological function, and quality of life.

The results suggested that the two treatments were equally effective at helping the patients recover from their strokes. After 90 days, about 20 percent of the patients showed favorable outcomes regardless of whether they were given intensive or standard treatment.

Intensive glucose therapy increased the risk of very low blood glucose (hypoglycemia) and required a higher level of care, such as increased supervision from nursing staff, compared to standard treatment.

The study was stopped early when a preplanned interim analysis revealed that intensive glucose control did not improve outcomes compared to standard treatment.

"We found that the extra risks associated with aggressive treatment were not worth it," said Dr. Johnston. "We are so grateful to the patients and research teams from across the country who helped us answer this important question. As a result of their participation, patients around the world will benefit."

Section 44.3 | International Study Suggests Combination Therapy May Prevent Stroke in Certain People

This section includes text excerpted from "International Study Suggests Combination Therapy May Prevent Stroke in Certain People," National Institute of Neurological Disorders and Stroke (NINDS), May 17, 2018.

Results from an international clinical trial of more than 4880 participants, published in the *New England Journal of Medicine* (*NEJM*), show that combining clopidogrel and aspirin following a small stroke or experiencing minor stroke symptoms decreases risk of a new stroke, heart attack or other ischemic event within 90 days. The combination therapy was also associated with an increase in major bleeding, although many of those episodes were nonfatal and did not occur in the brain. The results were presented at the 4th European Stroke Organization Conference in Gothenburg, Sweden. The study was supported by the National Institute of Neurological Disorders and Stroke (NINDS), part of the National Institutes of Health (NIH).

"These findings are likely to have a global effect on clinical practice, as these drugs are easily available in many hospitals and clinics," said Walter Koroshetz, M.D., director of NINDS. "As the benefit of the combination was concentrated in the first two weeks while risk of bleeding was constant over 90 days, it may be especially valuable in acute management of a minor ischemic stroke or transient ischemic attack (TIA)."

The Platelet-Oriented Inhibition in New TIA and minor ischemic stroke (POINT) clinical trial follows an earlier study, which showed benefits of this drug combination in a Chinese population. POINT was conducted to see whether the benefits could be expanded to a more diverse group of patients.

The study, led by S. Claiborne Johnston, M.D., Ph.D., dean and professor of neurology at Dell Medical School at The University of Texas at Austin, included patients who had experienced either a minor stroke or a TIA, in which blood supply to a part of the brain is briefly stopped and can be a risk factor for a larger stroke. Study participants were given clopidogrel and aspirin or aspirin alone to see whether the combination therapy could prevent a larger stroke within three months.

Dr. Johnston's team found that the combination of clopidogrel and aspirin prevented more ischemic events, such as stroke and heart attack, compared to aspirin alone. The results showed that 5 percent of patients in the combination therapy group and 6.5 percent of patients taking only aspirin experienced such an event within 90 days. However, the combination therapy was associated with a greater risk of major bleeding, or hemorrhage, than aspirin alone. In the aspirin-only group, 0.4 percent of patients suffered a major hemorrhage but 0.9 percent of patients taking clopidogrel and aspirin had severe bleeding.

The findings suggest that for 1000 patients, clopidogrel plus aspirin would prevent 15 ischemic attacks but may cause five instances of major hemorrhage. The majority of these hemorrhages occurred outside of the brain and were not fatal.

"We saw a real benefit with the combination therapy, but that treatment does come with a risk," said Dr. Johnston. "Overall, the risk of severe bleeding was very small, but it was not zero."

The study was stopped early because the combination therapy was found to be more effective than aspirin alone in preventing severe strokes but also due to the risk of severe hemorrhage.

Clopidogrel and aspirin prevent platelets from sticking together and forming clots in blood vessels, although they work in different ways. Aspirin blocks molecules that activate the clotting process while clopidogrel prevents a specific chemical from attaching to a receptor.

"Each year, strokes cause millions of disabilities around the world and preventing many of those would lead to not only tremendous health savings, but improved quality of life for many individuals and their families," said Dr. Johnston.

Section 44.4 | Eye Could Provide "Window to the Brain" after Stroke

This section includes text excerpted from "Eye Could Provide 'Window to the Brain' after Stroke," National Institute of Neurological Disorders and Stroke (NINDS), February 7, 2018.

Research into curious bright spots in the eyes on stroke patients' brain images could one day alter the way these individuals are assessed and treated. A team of scientists at the National Institutes of Health (NIH) found that a chemical routinely given to stroke patients undergoing brain scans can leak into their eyes, highlighting those areas and potentially provide insight into their strokes. The study was published in *Neurology*.

"We were kind of astounded by this—it is a very unrecognized phenomenon," said Richard Leigh, M.D., an assistant clinical investigator at the NIH's National Institute of Neurological Disorders and Stroke (NINDS) and the paper's senior author. "It raises the question of whether there is something we can observe in the eye that would help clinicians evaluate the severity of a stroke and guide us on how best to help patients."

The eyes glowed so brightly on those images due to gadolinium, a harmless, transparent chemical often given to patients during magnetic resonance imaging (MRI) scans to highlight abnormalities in the brain. In healthy individuals, gadolinium remains in the bloodstream and is filtered out by the kidneys. However, when someone experiences damage to the blood-brain barrier, which controls whether substances in the blood can enter the brain, gadolinium leaks into the brain, creating bright spots that mark the location of brain damage.

Previous research had shown that certain eye diseases could cause a similar disruption to the blood-ocular barrier, which does for the eye what the blood-brain barrier does for the brain. Dr. Leigh's team discovered that a stroke can also compromise the blood-ocular barrier and that the gadolinium that leaked into a patient's eyes could provide information about her or his stroke.

"It looks like the stroke is influencing the eye, and so the eye is reflective of what is going on in the brain," Dr. Leigh said. "Clearly

491

these results are preliminary, so future studies will have to be attuned to this to fully understand its impact."

The researchers performed MRI scans on 167 stroke patients upon admission to the hospital without administering gadolinium and compared them to scans taken using gadolinium two hours and 24 hours later. Because gadolinium is transparent, it did not affect patients' vision and could only be detected with MRI scans. Roughly three-quarters of the patients experienced gadolinium leakage into their eyes on one of the scans, with 66 percent showing it on the two-hour scan and 75 percent on the 24-hour scan. The phenomenon was present in both untreated patients and patients who received a treatment, called "tPA," to dissolve the blood clot responsible for their strokes.

Gadolinium was typically present in the front part of the eye, called the "aqueous chamber," after two hours, and in a region towards the back, called the "vitreous chamber," after 24 hours. Patients showing gadolinium in the vitreous chamber at the later timepoint tended to be of older age, have a history of hypertension, and have more bright spots on their brain scans, called "white matter hyperintensities," that are associated with brain aging and decreased cognitive function.

In a minority of patients, the two-hour scan showed gadolinium in both eye chambers. The strokes in those patients tended to affect a larger portion of the brain and cause even more damage to the blood-brain barrier than the strokes of patients with a slower pattern of gadolinium leakage or no leakage at all. The findings raise the possibility that, in the future, clinicians could administer a substance to patients that would collect in the eye just like gadolinium and quickly yield important information about their strokes without the need for an MRI.

"It is much easier for us to look inside somebody's eye than to look into somebody's brain," Dr. Leigh said. "So if the eye truly is a window to the brain, we can use one to learn about the other."

Despite the relationship between gadolinium leakage and stroke severity, the phenomenon was not found to be related to the level of disability the patients developed following their strokes. It also remains unclear whether gadolinium can enter the eye in healthy people.

Section 44.5 | Brain-Scan Guided Emergency Stroke Treatment Can Save More Lives

This section includes text excerpted from "Brain-Scan Guided Emergency Stroke Treatment Can Save More Lives," National Institute of Neurological Disorders and Stroke (NINDS), January 24, 2018.

Advances in brain imaging can identify a greater number of stroke patients who can receive therapy later than previously believed, according to a new study. The results of the Endovascular Therapy Following Imaging Evaluation for the Ischemic Stroke (DEFUSE 3) trial, presented at the International Stroke Conference 2018 in Los Angeles and published on Jan. 24 in the *New England Journal of Medicine* (*NEJM*), demonstrated that physically removing brain clots up to 16 hours after symptom onset in selected patients led to improved outcomes compared to standard medical therapy. The study was funded by the National Institute of Neurological Disorders and Stroke (NINDS), part of the National Institutes of Health (NIH).

"These striking results will have an immediate impact and save people from life-long disability or death," said Walter Koroshetz, M.D., director NINDS. "I really cannot overstate the size of this effect. The study shows that one in three stroke patients who present with at-risk brain tissue on their scans improve and some may walk out of the hospital saved from what would otherwise have been a devastating brain injury."

DEFUSE 3 was a large, multisite study supported by the NINDS' StrokeNet, which is a network of hospitals providing research infrastructure for multi-site clinical trials. This study was conducted at 38 centers across the United States and was led by Gregory W. Albers, M.D., professor of neurology and neurological sciences at Stanford University School of Medicine, in California, and director of the Stanford Stroke Center. The study was ended early by the NIH on recommendation of the independent Data and Safety and Monitoring Board because of overwhelming evidence of benefit from the clot removal procedure.

Ischemic stroke occurs when a cerebral blood vessel becomes blocked, cutting off the delivery of oxygen and nutrients to brain

493

tissue. Brain tissue in the immediate area of the blockage, known as the "core," cannot typically be saved from dying, and it can enlarge over time. However, it has long been thought that the area surrounding the core (known as the "ischemic penumbra") has the potential to be saved based on how quickly the blood flow can be restored. Over the past two decades, scientists have been working to develop brain scanning methods, called "perfusion imaging," that could identify patients with brain tissue that can still be salvaged by removing the blockage. In perfusion imaging, a standard dye is injected and scanned for a few minutes as it passes through the brain.

Using an automated software known as "RAPID" to analyze perfusion MRI or CT scans, the DEFUSE 3 researchers identified patients thought to have salvageable tissue up to 16 hours after stroke onset. The participants were randomized to either receive endovascular thrombectomy plus standard medical therapy or medical therapy alone.

Endovascular thrombectomy, or the physical removal of the blockage, is currently approved for use up to six hours following onset of stroke symptoms. Dr. Albers and the DEFUSE 3 researchers discovered that this intervention can be effective up to 16 hours after symptoms began in this select group of patients. The findings showed that patients in the thrombectomy group had substantially better outcomes 90 days after treatment compared to those in the control group. For example, 45 percent of the patients treated with the clot removal procedure achieved functional independence compared to 17 percent in the control group. In addition, thrombectomy was associated with improved survival. According to the results 14 percent of the treated group had died within 90 days of the study, compared to 26 percent in the control group.

"Although stroke is a medical emergency that should be treated as soon as possible, DEFUSE 3 opens the door to treatment even for some patients who wake up with a stroke or arrive at the hospital many hours after their initial symptoms," said Dr. Albers.

DEFUSE 3 builds on results from the two earlier DEFUSE studies as well as the industry-sponsored DAWN trial, which used perfusion imaging technology to identify patients most likely to

494

benefit from interventions, such as thrombectomy. Those studies suggested that the advanced brain imaging could identify which patients could benefit from restoring blood flow in an extended treatment window.

- by Barbara I. McMakin

Section 44.6 | Hibernating Ground Squirrels Provide Clues to New Stroke Treatments

This section includes text excerpted from "Hibernating Ground Squirrels Provide Clues to New Stroke Treatments," National Institute of Neurological Disorders and Stroke (NINDS), November 17, 2017.

In the fight against brain damage caused by stroke, researchers have turned to an unlikely source of inspiration: hibernating ground squirrels.

While the animals' brains experience dramatically reduced blood flow during hibernation, just like human patients after a certain type of stroke, the squirrels emerge from their extended naps suffering no ill effects. Now, a team of National Institutes of Health (NIH)-funded scientists have identified a potential drug that could grant the same resilience to the brains of ischemic stroke patients by mimicking the cellular changes that protect the brains of those animals. The study was published in The FASEB Journal, the official journal of the Foundation of American Societies for Experimental Biology (FASEB).

"For decades scientists have been searching for an effective brain-protecting stroke therapy to no avail. If the compound identified in this study successfully reduces tissue death and improves recovery in further experiments, it could lead to new approaches for preserving brain cells after an ischemic stroke," said Francesca Bosetti, Ph.D., Pharm.D., program director at the NIH's National Institute of Neurological Disorders and Stroke (NINDS).

An ischemic stroke occurs when a clot cuts off blood flow to part of the brain, depriving those cells of oxygen and nutrients like the blood sugar glucose that they need to survive. Nearly

800,000 Americans experience a stroke every year and 87 percent of those are ischemic strokes.

Currently, the only way to minimize stroke-induced cell death is to remove the clot as soon as possible. A treatment to help brain cells survive a stroke-induced lack of oxygen and glucose could dramatically improve patient outcomes, but no such neuroprotective agents for stroke patients exist.

Recently, researchers led by John Hallenbeck, M.D., an NINDS senior investigator and co-senior author of the study, found that a cellular process called "SUMOylation" goes into overdrive in a certain species of ground squirrel during hibernation. Dr. Hallenbeck suspected this was how the animals' brains survived the reduced blood flow caused by hibernation, and subsequent experiments in cells and mice confirmed his suspicions.

"If we could only turn on the process hibernators appear to use to protect their brains, we could help protect the brain during a stroke and ultimately help people recover," said Joshua Bernstock, a graduate student in Dr. Hallenbeck's lab and the study's first author.

SUMOylation occurs when an enzyme attaches a molecular tag called a "Small Ubiquitin-like Modifier" (SUMO) to a protein, altering its activity and location in the cell. Other enzymes called "SUMO-specific proteases" (SENPs) can then detach those tags, thereby decreasing SUMOylation. In the current study, Bernstock and his colleagues teamed up with researchers from the NIH's National Center for Advancing Translational Sciences (NCATS) to examine whether any of over 4,000 molecules from the NCATS small molecule collections could boost SUMOylation by blocking a SENP called "SENP2," which would theoretically protect cells from a shortage of life-sustaining substances.

The researchers first used an automated process to examine whether the compounds prevented SENP2 from severing the connection between a tiny metal bead and an artificial SUMO protein created in the lab of Wei Yang, Ph.D., the study's other senior author and an associate professor at Duke University in Durham, NC. This system, along with computer modeling and further tests performed both in and outside of cells, whittled the thousands of candidate molecules down to eight that could bind to SENP2 in cells and were nontoxic. Two of those—ebselen and 6-thioguanine—were then found to both boost SUMOylation in rat cells and keep them alive in the absence of oxygen and glucose.

A final experiment showed that ebselen boosted SUMOylation in the brains of healthy mice more than a control injection. 6-thioguanine was not tested because it is a chemotherapy drug with side effects that make it unsuitable as a potential stroke treatment. The researchers now plan to test whether ebselen can protect the brains of animal models of stroke.

Because SUMOylation affects a variety of molecules, Bernstock believes his group's approach could inspire similar attempts to treat neurological conditions by targeting pathways with wide-ranging effects. He also hopes it will prompt others to look to natural models, as he and Dr. Hallenbeck did with the ground squirrel.

"As a physician-scientist, I really like to work on projects that have clear relevance for patients," Bernstock said. "I always want outcomes that can lend themselves to new therapeutics for people who are in need."

Part 7 | **Additional Help and Information**

Chapter 45 | Glossary of Terms Related to Stroke

acupuncture: A form of complementary and alternative medicine that involves inserting thin needles through the skin at specific points on the body to control pain and other symptoms.

acute stroke: A stage of stroke starting at the onset of symptoms and lasting for a few hours thereafter.

advance directive(s): Written instructions letting others know the type of care you want if you are seriously ill or dying. These include a living will and durable power of attorney.

agnosia: A cognitive disability characterized by ignorance of or inability to acknowledge one side of the body or one side of the visual field.

Alzheimer disease (AD): A brain disease that cripples the brain's nerve cells over time and destroys memory and learning.

amputation: Removal of part or all of a body part, except for organs in the body.

anemia: When the amount of red blood cells or hemoglobin (the substance in the blood that carries oxygen to organs) becomes reduced, causing fatigue that can be severe.

anesthesia: The use of medicine to prevent the feeling of pain or another sensation during surgery or other procedures that might be painful.

aneurysm: A weak or thin spot on an artery wall that has stretched or ballooned out from the wall and filled with blood, or damage to an artery leading to pooling of blood between the layers of the blood vessel walls.

angina: A recurring pain or discomfort in the chest that happens when some part of the heart does not receive enough blood. It is a common symptom of

This glossary contains terms excerpted from documents produced by several sources deemed reliable.

coronary heart disease, which occurs when vessels that carry blood to the heart become narrowed and blocked due to atherosclerosis. Angina feels like a pressing or squeezing pain, usually in the chest under the breast bone, but sometimes in the shoulders, arms, neck, jaws, or back. Angina is usually brought on by exertion, and relieved within a few minutes by resting or by taking prescribed angina medicine.

antibiotics: Drugs used to fight many infections caused by bacteria. Some antibiotics are effective against only certain types of bacteria; others can effectively fight a wide range of bacteria. Antibiotics do not work against viral infections.

anticoagulants: A drug therapy used to prevent the formation of blood clots that can become lodged in cerebral arteries and cause strokes.

antidepressants: A name for a category of medications used to treat depression.

aphasia: Total or partial loss of the ability to use or understand language; usually caused by stroke, brain disease, or injury.

apraxia: A movement disorder characterized by the inability to perform skilled or purposeful voluntary movements, generally caused by damage to the areas of the brain responsible for voluntary movement.

arteries: Blood vessels that carry oxygen and blood to the heart, brain, and other parts of the body.

arteriography: An x-ray of the carotid artery taken when a special dye is injected into the artery.

arteriovenous malformation (AVM): A congenital disorder characterized by a complex tangled web of arteries and veins.

atherosclerosis: A blood vessel disease characterized by deposits of lipid material on the inside of the walls of large to medium-sized arteries which make the artery walls thick, hard, brittle, and prone to breaking.

atrial fibrillation: Irregular beating of the left atrium, or left upper chamber, of the heart.

bacteria: Microorganisms that can cause infections.

beta-blockers: A type of medication that reduces nerve impulses to the heart and blood vessels. This makes the heart beat slower and with less force. Blood pressure drops and the heart works less hard.

biological: Having to do with, or related to, living things.

Glossary of Terms Related to Stroke

biopsy: Removal of a small piece of tissue for testing or examination under a microscope.

bladder: The organ in the human body that stores urine. It is found in the lower part of the abdomen.

blood: Fluid in the body made up of plasma, red and white blood cells, and platelets. Blood carries oxygen and nutrients to and waste materials away from all body tissues. In the breast, blood nourishes the breast tissue and provides nutrients needed for milk production.

blood glucose level: Also called "blood sugar level," it is the amount of glucose, or sugar, in the blood. Too much glucose in the blood for a long time can cause diabetes and damage many parts of the body such as the heart, blood vessels, eyes, and kidneys.

blood pressure: The force of blood against the walls of arteries. Blood pressure is noted as two numbers—the systolic pressure (as the heart beats) over the diastolic pressure (as the heart relaxes between beats). The numbers are written one above or before the other, with the systolic number on top and the diastolic number at the bottom.

blood transfusion: The transfer of blood or blood products from one person (donor) into another person's bloodstream (recipient). Most times, it is done to replace blood cells or blood products lost through severe bleeding. Blood can be given from two sources, your own blood (autologous blood) or from someone else (donor blood).

body mass index (BMI): A measure of body fat based on a person's height and weight.

calorie: A unit of energy-producing potential in food.

cardiovascular disease (CVD): Disease of the heart and blood vessels.

carotid artery: An artery, located on either side of the neck, that supplies the brain with blood.

carotid endarterectomy: Surgery used to remove fatty deposits from the carotid arteries.

cerebrospinal fluid (CSF): Clear fluid that bathes the brain and spinal cord.

cerebrovascular disease: A reduction in the supply of blood to the brain either by narrowing of the arteries through the buildup of plaque on the inside walls of the arteries, called "stenosis," or through blockage of an artery due to a blood clot.

cholesterol: A waxy substance, produced naturally by the liver and also found in foods, that circulates in the blood and helps maintain tissues and cell membranes. Excess cholesterol in the body can contribute to atherosclerosis and high blood pressure.

clipping: Surgical procedure for treatment of brain aneurysms, involving clamping an aneurysm from a blood vessel, surgically removing this ballooned part of the blood vessel, and closing the opening in the artery wall.

computed tomography (CT) scan: A series of cross-sectional x-rays of the brain and head; also called "computerized axial tomography" or "CAT scan."

Coumadin: A commonly used anticoagulant, also known as "warfarin."

dehydration: Excessive loss of body water that the body needs to carry on normal functions at an optimal level. Signs include increasing thirst, dry mouth, weakness or lightheadedness (particularly if worse on standing), and a darkening of the urine or a decrease in urination.

dementia: A group of symptoms caused by disorders that affect the brain. Symptoms may include memory loss, confusion, personality changes, and difficulty with normal activities like eating or dressing. Dementia has many causes, including Alzheimer disease and stroke.

depression: An emotional state involving sadness, lack of energy, and low self-esteem.

dysarthria: Group of speech disorders caused by disturbances in the strength or coordination of the muscles of the speech mechanism as a result of damage to the brain or nerves.

dysphagia: Trouble swallowing.

edema: The swelling of a cell that results from the influx of large amounts of water or fluid into the cell.

embolic stroke: A stroke caused by an embolus.

embolus: A free-roaming clot that usually forms in the heart.

esophagus: Tube that connects the throat with the stomach.

estrogen: A group of female hormones that are responsible for the development of breasts and other secondary sex characteristics in women. Estrogen is produced by the ovaries and other body tissues. Estrogen, along with progesterone, is important in preparing a woman's body for pregnancy.

fat: A source of energy used by the body to make substances it needs. Fat helps your body absorb certain vitamins from food. Some fats are better for your health than others. To help prevent heart disease and stroke, most of the fats you eat should be monounsaturated and polyunsaturated fats.

fatigue: A feeling of lack of energy, weariness or tiredness.

gene: The functional and physical unit of heredity made up of deoxyribonucleic acid (DNA), which has a specific function and is passed from parent to offspring.

global aphasia: Loss of speech caused by a serious injury to the region of the brain that controls speech and language.

heart disease: A number of abnormal conditions affecting the heart and the blood vessels in the heart. The most common type of heart disease is coronary artery disease, which is the gradual buildup of plaque in the coronary arteries—the blood vessels that bring blood to the heart. This disease develops slowly and silently, over decades. It can go virtually unnoticed until it produces a heart attack.

hemiparesis: Weakness on one side of the body.

hemiplegia: Complete paralysis on one side of the body.

hemorrhagic stroke: Sudden bleeding into or around the brain.

heparin: A type of anticoagulant.

high-density lipoprotein (HDL): Also known as the "good cholesterol," a compound consisting of a lipid and a protein that carries a small percentage of the total cholesterol in the blood and deposits it in the liver.

hypertension (high blood pressure): Characterized by persistently high arterial blood pressure defined as a measurement greater than or equal to 140 mm/Hg systolic pressure over 90 mm/Hg diastolic pressure.

intracerebral hemorrhage: Occurs when a vessel within the brain leaks blood into the brain.

ischemic stroke: A blockage of blood vessels supplying blood to the brain, causing a decrease in blood supply.

menopausal hormone therapy (MHT): Replaces the hormones that a woman's ovaries stop making at the time of menopause, easing symptoms like hot flashes and vaginal dryness. MHT is associated with serious risks, including breast cancer, heart disease, and stroke. Women who choose to use MHT should use the lowest dose that helps for the shortest time needed.

neuron: The main functional cell of the brain and nervous system, consisting of a cell body, an axon, and dendrites.

plaque: Fatty cholesterol deposits found along the inside of artery walls that lead to atherosclerosis and stenosis of the arteries.

platelets: Structures found in blood that are known primarily for their role in blood coagulation.

small vessel disease: A cerebrovascular disease defined by stenosis in small arteries of the brain.

speech disorder: Any defect or abnormality that prevents an individual from communicating by means of spoken words. Speech disorders may develop from nerve injury to the brain, muscular paralysis, structural defects, hysteria, or mental retardation.

stenosis: Narrowing of an artery due to the buildup of plaque on the inside wall of the artery.

Stroke Belt: An area of the Southeastern United States with the highest stroke mortality rate in the country.

stroke: Stoppage of blood flow to an area of the brain, causing permanent damage to nerve cells in that region. A stroke can occur either because an artery is clogged by a blood clot (called "ischemic stroke") or an artery tears and bleeds into the brain. A stroke can cause symptoms such as loss of consciousness, problems with movement, and loss of speech.

subarachnoid hemorrhage: Bleeding within the meninges, or outer membranes, of the brain into the clear fluid that surrounds the brain.

transient ischemic attack (TIA): A short-lived stroke that lasts from a few minutes up to 24 hours; often called a "mini-stroke."

traumatic brain injury (TBI): A brain injury that results from a sudden blow to the head. Symptoms may be mild, moderate, or serious, depending on the extent of damage.

ultrasound: A procedure that uses high-energy sound waves to look at tissues and organs inside the body. The sound waves make echoes that form pictures of the tissues and organs on a computer screen (sonogram).

vasospasm: A dangerous side effect of subarachnoid hemorrhage in which the blood vessels in the subarachnoid space constrict erratically, cutting off blood flow.

vitamin: A nutrient that the body needs in small amounts to function and maintain health. Examples are vitamins A, C, and E.

voice: Sound produced by air passing out through the larynx and upper respiratory tract.

Glossary of Terms Related to Stroke

warfarin: A commonly used anticoagulant, also known as "Coumadin."

x-ray: A type of high-energy radiation. In low doses, x-rays are used to diagnose diseases by making pictures of the inside of the body.

yoga: An ancient system of practices used to balance the mind and body through exercise, meditation (focusing thoughts), and control of breathing and emotions.

Chapter 46 | Directory of Organizations That Help Stroke Patients and Their Families

GOVERNMENT AGENCIES THAT PROVIDE INFORMATION ABOUT STROKE

Administration on Aging (AoA)
Administration for Community Living (ACL)
330 C St. S.W.
Washington, DC 20201
Toll-Free: 800-677-1116
Phone: 202-401-4634
Fax: 202-357-3555
Website: acl.gov

Agency for Healthcare Research and Quality (AHRQ)
5600 Fishers Ln.
Seventh Fl.
Rockville, MD 20857
Phone: 301-427-1364
Website: www.ahrq.gov

Centers for Disease Control and Prevention (CDC)
1600 Clifton Rd. N.E.
Atlanta, GA 30333
Toll-Free: 800-CDC-INFO
(800-232-4636)
Toll-Free TTY: 888-232-6348
Website: www.cdc.gov

Centers for Medicare & Medicaid Services (CMS)
7500 Security Blvd.
Baltimore, MD 21244
Toll-Free: 877-267-2323
Phone: 410-786-3000
TTY: 410-786-0727
Toll-Free TTY: 866-226-1819
Website: www.cms.gov

Resources in this chapter were compiled from several sources deemed reliable; all contact information was verified and updated in May 2020.

Eldercare Locator
Toll-Free: 800-677-1116
Website: eldercare.acl.gov
E-mail: eldercarelocator@n4a.org

Eunice Kennedy Shriver National Institute of Child Health and Human Development (NICHD)
Information Resource Center (IRC)
P.O. Box 3006
Rockville, MD 20847
Toll-Free: 800-370-2943
Toll-Free Fax: 866-760-5947
Website: www.nichd.nih.gov
E-mail: NICHDInformation
ResourceCenter@mail.nih.gov

Healthfinder®
U.S. Department of Health and Human Services (HHS)
1101 Wootton Pkwy
Ste. 420
Rockville, MD 20852
Fax: 240-453-8281
Website: health.gov
E-mail: healthfinder@hhs.gov

MedlinePlus
U.S. National Library of Medicine (NLM)
8600 Rockville Pike
Bethesda, MD 20894
Website: medlineplus.gov

National Cancer Institute (NCI)
9609 Medical Center Dr.
Rockville, MD 20892-9760
Toll-Free: 800-4-CANCER
(800-422-6237)
Phone: 240-276-5810
Fax: 240-276-5820
Website: www.cancer.gov
E-mail: NCIGlobalHealth@mail.
nih.gov

National Center for Complementary and Integrative Health (NCCIH)
National Institutes of Health (NIH)
9000 Rockville Pike
Bethesda, MD 20892
Toll-Free: 888-644-6226
Toll-Free TTY: 866-464-3615
Toll-Free Fax: 866-464-3616
Website: www.nccih.nih.gov
E-mail: info@nccih.nih.gov

National Center for Health Statistics (NCHS)
3311 Toledo Rd.
Rm. 2217
Hyattsville, MD 20782-2064
Toll-Free: 800-CDC-INFO
(800-232-4636)
Phone: 301-458-4901
Website: www.cdc.gov/nchs/nhis
E-mail: nhis@cdc.gov

National Heart, Lung, and Blood Institute (NHLBI)

NHLBI Health Information Center
Bldg. 31, 31 Center Dr.
Bethesda, MD 20892
Toll-Free: 877-NHLBI4U
(877-645-2448)
Website: www.nhlbi.nih.gov
E-mail: nhlbiinfo@nhlbi.nih.gov

National Highway Traffic Safety Administration (NHTSA)

1200 New Jersey Ave. S.E.
Washington, DC 20590
Toll-Free: 888-327-4236
Toll-Free TTY: 800-424-9153
Website: www.nhtsa.gov

National Institute of Neurological Disorders and Stroke (NINDS)

NIH Neurological Institute
P.O. Box 5801
Bethesda, MD 20824
Toll-Free: 800-352-9424
Phone: 301-496-5751
Website: www.ninds.nih.gov

National Institute on Aging (NIA)

Bldg 31, 31 Center Dr., MSC 2292
Rm. 5C27
Bethesda, MD 20892
Toll-Free: 800-222-2225
Phone: 301-496-1752
Toll-Free TTY: 800-222-4225
Website: www.nia.nih.gov
E-mail: niaic@nia.nih.gov

National Institute on Alcohol Abuse and Alcoholism (NIAAA)

Toll-Free: 888-MY-NIAAA
(888-69-64222)
Phone: 301-443-3860
Website: www.niaaa.nih.gov
E-mail: niaaaweb-r@exchange.nih.gov

National Institutes of Health (NIH)

9000 Rockville Pike
Bethesda, MD 20892
Phone: 301-496-4000
TTY: 301-402-9612
Website: www.nih.gov
E-mail: NIHinfo@od.nih.gov

National Women's Health Information Center (NWHIC)

Office on Women's Health (OWH)
200 Independence Ave. S.W.
Rm. 712E
Washington, DC 20201
Toll-Free: 800-994-9662
Phone: 202-690-7650
Fax: 202-205-2631
Website: www.womenshealth.gov

Office of Extramural Research (OER)

National Institutes of Health (NIH)
9000 Rockville Pike
Bethesda, MD 20892
Phone: 301-945-7573
Website: grants.nih.gov
E-mail: grantsinfo@od.nih.gov

Office of Minority Health (OMH)
Tower Oaks Bldg., 1101 Wootton Pwky
Ste. 600
Rockville, MD 20852
Toll-Free: 800-444-6472
TDD: 301-251-1432
Fax: 301-251-2160
Website: minorityhealth.hhs.gov
E-mail: info@minorityhealth.hhs.gov

Smokefree.gov
Toll-Free: 800-QUIT-NOW (800-784-8669)
Website: www.smokefree.gov
E-mail: NCISmokefreeTeam@mail.nih.gov

U.S. Department of Health and Human Services (HHS)
200 Independence Ave. S.W.
Washington, DC 20201
Toll-Free: 877-696-6775
Website: www.hhs.gov

U.S. Department of Veterans Affairs (VA)
810 Vermont Ave. N.W.
Washington, DC 20420
Toll-Free: 877-222-VETS (877-222-8387)
Website: www.va.gov

U.S. Equal Employment Opportunity Commission (EEOC)
131 M St. N.E.
Washington, DC 20507
Phone: 202-663-4900
TTY: 202-663-4494
Website: www.eeoc.gov
E-mail: info@eeoc.gov

U.S. Food and Drug Administration (FDA)
10903 New Hampshire Ave.
Silver Spring, MD 20993-0002
Toll-Free: 888-INFO-FDA (888-463-6332)
Website: www.fda.gov

U.S. National Library of Medicine (NLM)
8600 Rockville Pike
Bethesda, MD 20894
Phone: 301-496-4441
Website: www.nlm.nih.gov

U.S. Social Security Administration (SSA)
Office of Earnings & International Operations (OEIO)
P.O. Box 17769
Baltimore, MD 21235-7769
Toll-Free: 800-772-1213
Toll-Free TTY: 800-325-0778
Website: www.ssa.gov

PRIVATE AGENCIES THAT PROVIDE INFORMATION ABOUT STROKE

American Academy of Family Physicians (AAFP)
11400 Tomahawk Creek Pkwy
Leawood, KS 66211-2680
Toll-Free: 800-274-2237
Phone: 913-906-6000
Fax: 913-906-6075
Website: www.aafp.org
E-mail: aafp@aafp.org

American Academy of Neurology (AAN)
201 Chicago Ave.
Minneapolis, MN 55415
Toll-Free: 800-879-1960
Fax: 612-454-2746
Website: www.aan.com
E-mail: memberservices@aan.com

American Academy of Pediatrics (AAP)
National Headquarters
345 Park Blvd.
Itasca, IL 60143
Toll-Free: 800-433-9016
Fax: 847-434-8000
Website: www.aap.org
E-mail: csc@aap.org

American Academy of Physical Medicine and Rehabilitation (AAPM&R)
9700 W. Bryn Mawr Ave.
Ste. 200
Rosemont, IL 60018
Toll-Free: 877-227-6799
Phone: 847-737-6000
Website: www.aapmr.org
E-mail: info@aapmr.org

American Association of Neurological Surgeons (AANS)
5550 Meadowbrook Dr.
Rolling Meadows, IL 60008-3852
Toll-Free: 888-566-AANS
(888-556-2267)
Phone: 847-378-0500
Fax: 847-378-0600
Website: www.aans.org
E-mail: info@aans.org

American Association of Neuroscience Nurses (AANN)
8735 W. Higgins Rd.
Ste. 300
Chicago, IL 60631
Toll-Free: 888-557-2266
Phone: 847-375-4733
Fax: 847-375-6430
Website: aann.org
E-mail: info@aann.org

American College of Obstetricians and Gynecologists (ACOG)
409 12th St. S.W.
Washington, DC 20024-2188
Toll-Free: 800-673-8444
Phone: 202-638-5577
Website: www.acog.org
E-mail: resources@acog.org

American College of Radiology (ACR)
1891 Preston White Dr.
Reston, VA 20191
Toll-Free: 800-227-5463
Phone: 703-648-8900
Website: www.acr.org
E-mail: info@acr.org

American Congress of Rehabilitation Medicine (ACRM)
11654 Plaza America Dr.
Ste. 535
Reston, VA 20190-4700
Phone: 703-435-5335
Toll-Free Fax: 866-692-1619
Website: www.acrm.org
E-mail: info@ACRM.org

American Heart Association (AHA)
National Center
7272 Greenville Ave.
Dallas, TX 75231
Toll-Free: 800-AHA-USA
(800-242-8721)
Website: www.stroke.org

American Medical Association (AMA)
AMA Plaza
330 N. Wabash Ave.
Ste. 39300
Chicago, IL 60611-5885
Phone: 312-464-4782
Website: www.ama-assn.org

American Migraine Foundation (AMF)
19 Mantua Rd.
Mount Royal, NJ 08061
Phone: 856-423-0043
Fax: 856-423-0082
Website: americanmigrainefoundation.org
E-mail: amf@talley.com

American Occupational Therapy Association (AOTA)
6116 Executive Blvd.
Ste. 200
North Bethesda, MD 20852-4929
Toll-Free: 800-SAY-AOTA
(800-729-2682)
Phone: 301-652-6611
Website: www.aota.org
E-mail: customerservice@aota.org

American Physical Therapy Association (APTA)
1111 N. Fairfax St.
Alexandria, VA 22314-1488
Toll-Free: 800-999-APTA
(800-999-2782)
Phone: 703-684-APTA
(703-684-2782)
Fax: 703-684-7343
Website: www.apta.org

American Society of Neurorehabilitation (ASNR)
5841 Cedar Lake Rd.
Ste. 204
Minneapolis, MN 55416
Phone: 952-545-6324
Fax: 952-545-6073
Website: www.asnr.com
E-mail: info@asnr.com

American Speech-Language-Hearing Association (ASHA)
2200 Research Blvd.
Rockville, MD 20850-3289
Toll-Free: 800-638-8255
Phone: 301-296-5700
Fax: 301-296-8580
Website: www.asha.org
E-mail: actioncenter@asha.org

Association of American Medical Colleges
655 K St. N.W.
Ste. 100
Washington, DC 20001-2399
Phone: 202-828-0400
Website: www.aamc.org
E-mail: help@aamc.org

Brain Aneurysm Foundation (BAF)
269 Hanover St.
Hanover, MA 02339
Toll-Free: 888-272-4602
Phone: 781-826-5556
Fax: 781-826-5566
Website: www.bafound.org
E-mail: office@bafound.org

Brain Injury Association of America (BIAA)
1608 Spring Hill Rd.
Ste. 110
Vienna, VA 22182
Toll-Free: 800-444-6443
Phone: 703-761-0750
Fax: 703-761-0755
Website: www.biausa.org
E-mail: info@biausa.org

Brain Injury Recovery Network
840 Central Ave.
Carlisle, OH 45005
Toll-Free: 877-810-2100
Toll-Free Fax: 877-810-2100
Website: www.tbirecovery.org
E-mail: help@tbirecovery.org

Caring.com
2600 S. El Camino Real
Ste. 300
San Mateo, CA 94403
Toll-Free: 800-973-1540
Website: www.caring.com

Children's Hemiplegia and Stroke Association (CHASA)
4101 W. Green Oaks
Ste. 305-149
Arlington, TX 76016
Websites: www.chasa.org

Cleveland Clinic
9500 Euclid Ave.
Cleveland, OH 44195
Toll-Free: 800-223-2273
Phone: 216-444-2200
Website: my.clevelandclinic.org

Family Caregiver Alliance® (FCA)
National Center on Caregiving (NCC)
101 Montgomery St.
Ste. 2150
San Francisco, CA 94104
Toll-Free: 800-445-8106
Phone: 415-434-3388
Website: www.caregiver.org
E-mail: info@caregiver.org

Get Ahead of Stroke
Society of NeuroInterventional Surgery (SNIS)
12587 Fair Lakes Cir.
Ste. 353
Fairfax, VA 22033
Phone: 703-691-2272
Fax: 703-537-0650
Website: getaheadofstroke.org

Hazel K. Goddess Fund for Stroke Research in Women
785 Park Ave.
Ste. 3E
New York, NY 10021
Website: www.thegoddessfund.org

HeartHealthyWomen.org
Cardiovascular Research Foundation (CRF)
111 E. 59th St.
New York, NY 10022-1122
Phone: 212-851-9300
Website: www.hearthealthywomen.org

Internet Stroke Center
Department of Neurology and Neurotherapeutics
5323 Harry Hines Blvd.
Dallas, TX 75390
Phone: 214-648-3111
Website: www.strokecenter.org
E-mail: info@strokecenter.org

Job Accommodation Network (JAN)
P.O. Box 6080
Morgantown, WV 26506-6080
Toll-Free: 800-526-7234
Phone: 304-293-7186
Toll-Free TTY: 877-781-9403
Fax: 304-293-5407
Website: askjan.org
E-mail: jan@askjan.org

National Alliance for Caregiving (NAC)
1730 Rhode Island Ave. N.W.
Ste. 812
Washington, DC 20036
Phone: 202-918-1013
Fax: 202-918-1014
Website: www.caregiving.org
E-mail: info@caregiving.org

National Aphasia Association (NAA)
P.O. Box 87
Scarsdale, NY 10583
Website: www.aphasia.org
E-mail: naa@aphasia.org

National Brain Tumor Society (NBTS)
55 Chapel St.
Ste. 200
Newton, MA 02458
Phone: 617-924-9997
Fax: 617-924-9998
Website: www.braintumor.org
E-mail: development@braintumor.org

National Center for Learning Disabilities (NCLD)
1 Thomas Cir. N.W.
Ste. 700
Washington, DC 20005
Phone: 212-545-7510
Website: www.ncld.org

National Rehabilitation Information Center (NARIC)
8400 Corporate Dr., Ste. 500
Landover, MD 20785
Toll-Free: 800-346-2742
Phone: 301-459-5900
Fax: 301-459-4263
Website: www.naric.com

National Stroke Association (NSA)
9707 E. Easter Ln.
Ste. B
Centennial, CO 80112
Toll-Free: 800-STROKES
(800-787-6537)
Fax: 303-649-1328
Website: www.stroke.org
E-mail: info@stroke.org

Shirley Ryan AbilityLab
(formerly known as Rehabilitation
Institute of Chicago (RIC))
355 E. Erie
Chicago, IL 60611
Toll-Free: 844-355-ABLE
(844-355-2253)
Phone: 312-238-1000
Fax: 312-238-1369
Website: www.sralab.org

Society for Vascular Surgery (SVS)
9400 W. Higgins Rd., Ste. 315
Rosemont, IL 60018-4975
Toll-Free: 800-258-7188
Phone: 312-334-2300
Fax: 312-334-2320
Website: vascular.org
E-mail: vascular@vascularsociety.org

Stroke Awareness Foundation
51 E. Campbell Ave.
Ste. 106-M
Campbell, CA 95008
Phone: 408-370-5282
Website: www.strokeinfo.org
E-mail: info@strokeinfo.org

Stroke Support Association
P.O. Box 8340
Long Beach, CA 90808
Phone: 562-537-0556
Website: strokesupportassoc.org
E-mail: info@strokesupportassoc.
org

Well Spouse Association
63 W. Main St.
Ste. H
Freehold, NJ 07728
Toll-Free: 800-838-0879
Phone: 732-577-8899
Website: www.wellspouse.org
E-mail: info@wellspouse.org

INDEX

INDEX

Page numbers followed by 'n' indicate a footnote. Page numbers in *italics* indicate a table or illustration.